Fundamentals of

Anatomy and Physiology Workbook

Fundamentals of

Anatomy and Physiology Workbook

For Nursing and Healthcare Students

SECOND EDITION

Suzanne Evans, PhD

Professor (Retd), School of Biomedical Sciences & Pharmacy, Faculty of Health and Medicine, University of Newcastle, New South Wales, Australia

Ian Peate, OBE FRCN EN(G) RGN DipN(Lond) RNT BEd(Hons) MA(Lond) LLM Hon DUniv (BNU)

Editor-in-Chief, *British Journal of Nursing*; Consultant Editor, *Journal of Paramedic Practice*; Consultant Editor, *International Journal for Advancing Practice*; Visiting Professor, Northumbria University; Visiting Professor, Buckinghamshire New University; Visiting Senior Clinical Fellow, University of Hertfordshire

WILEY

This edition first published 2027

Edition History
John Wiley & Sons Ltd (1e, 2017)

Registered Office(s)
John Wiley & Sons, Inc., 111 River Street, Hoboken, NJ 07030, USA
John Wiley & Sons Ltd, New Era House, 8 Oldlands Way, Bognor Regis, West Sussex, PO22 9NQ, UK

For details of our global editorial offices, customer services, and more information about Wiley products visit us at www.wiley.com.

The manufacturer's authorized representative according to the EU General Product Safety Regulation is Wiley-VCH GmbH, Boschstr. 12, 69469 Weinheim, Germany, e-mail: Product_Safety@wiley.com.

Wiley also publishes its books in a variety of electronic formats and by print-on-demand. Some content that appears in standard print versions of this book may not be available in other formats.

Library of Congress Cataloging-in-Publication Data
Names: Evans, Suzanne author | Peate, Ian author
Title: Fundamentals of anatomy and physiology workbook : for nursing and healthcare students / Suzanne Evans, PhD, Ian Peate, OBE FRCN EN(G) RGN DipN(Lond) RNT BEd(Hons) MA(Lond) LLM Hon DUniv (BNU).
Description: Second edition. | Hoboken, NJ : Wiley, 2027. | Includes bibliographical references.
Identifiers: LCCN 2026006131 (print) | LCCN 2026006132 (ebook) | ISBN 9781394324248 paperback | ISBN 9781394324361 adobe pdf | ISBN 9781394324309 epub
Subjects: LCSH: Human physiology | Human anatomy | LCGFT: Study guides
Classification: LCC QP34.5 .Q8614 2027 Suppl. (print) | LCC QP34.5 (ebook)
LC record available at https://lccn.loc.gov/2026006131
LC ebook record available at https://lccn.loc.gov/2026006132

Cover Design: Wiley
Cover Images: PIXOLOGICSTUDIO/Getty Images, Vorobyeva/Shutterstock

Set in 9.5/12.5pt Source Sans Pro by Straive, Pondicherry, India
Printed and bound by CPI Group (UK) Ltd, Croydon, CR0 4YY

C9781394324248_080826

Contents

Preface

We are delighted to present this new edition of the workbook *Fundamentals of Anatomy and Physiology Workbook: For Nursing and Healthcare Students.* The book is designed to accompany the best-selling *Fundamentals of Anatomy and Physiology for Nursing and Healthcare Students,* now in its fourth edition. Since the publication of the first edition, the workbook has been widely adopted by students and educators alike as a supportive resource for mastering the foundational concepts of human anatomy and physiology. Its interactive, learner-centred approach continues to resonate with those beginning their journey into healthcare education.

This new edition builds on the strengths of the original while responding to feedback from students, lecturers and clinical educators. Learning the names, locations and functions of the many structures and systems of the human body can be a challenging and, at times, overwhelming experience. For many students, particularly those new to higher education or returning to study after a break, anatomy and physiology represent one of the more complex and content-heavy areas of the curriculum. Our aim remains to make this learning process not only manageable but also enjoyable.

As in the previous edition, this workbook offers a wide range of anatomically accurate line drawings for students to label and colour. These exercises are not simply artistic tasks; they are grounded in pedagogical research that demonstrates the benefits of active, multi-sensory learning. Colouring and labelling body structures supports both visual and kinaesthetic learning styles, helping students to encode and retrieve key information more effectively.

Chapters follow a systems-based structure aligned with the parent textbook, allowing for integrated learning. Students can study one body system at a time, such as the musculoskeletal, cardiovascular or nervous systems, reinforcing their understanding through repetition, practice and application. This approach also helps learners make connections between structure and function and between anatomy and clinical relevance.

Self-assessment activities, clear illustrations and detailed terminology are used to reflect current best practice in clinical language. The self-tests are designed to encourage active recall and support students in applying anatomical and physiological knowledge to real-world care scenarios. Whether preparing for examinations, placements or professional practice, students will find these exercises invaluable in consolidating learning and building confidence.

Importantly, *Fundamentals of Anatomy and Physiology Workbook: For Nursing and Healthcare Students* is intended as a companion resource, not a replacement, for core texts. It works best when used alongside *Fundamentals of Anatomy and Physiology for Nursing and Healthcare Students*, reinforcing and revising key concepts introduced in the main textbook.

We hope this new edition continues to support students in becoming safe, competent and compassionate healthcare professionals. We remain grateful to the many students and educators whose feedback has shaped this edition, and we welcome ongoing input to ensure future editions remain relevant and useful in an ever-evolving healthcare education landscape.

Suzanne Evans
Newcastle
New South Wales

Ian Peate
London

Acknowledgements

Suzanne wishes to thank her family for their patience and support; Ian wishes to thank his partner Jussi Lahtinen for his ongoing support.

Prefixes, suffixes

Prefix: a prefix is positioned at the beginning of a word to modify or change its meaning. 'Pre' means 'before'. Prefixes may also indicate a location, number or time.

Suffix: the ending part of a word that changes the meaning of the word.

Prefix or suffix	Meaning	Example(s)
a-, an-	not, without	analgesic, apathy
ab-	from; away from	abduction
abdomin(o)-	of or relating to the abdomen	abdomen
acous(io)-	of or relating to hearing	acoumeter, acoustician
acr(o)-	extremity, topmost	acrocrany, acromegaly, acro-osteolysis, acroposthia
ad-	at, increase, on, toward	adduction
aden(o)-, aden(i)-	of or relating to a gland	adenocarcinoma, adenology, adenotome, adenotyphus
adip(o)-	of or relating to fat or fatty tissue	adipocyte
adren(o)-	of or relating to adrenal glands	adrenal artery
-aemia	blood condition	anaemia
aer(o)-	air, gas	aerosinusitis
-aesthesio-	sensation	anaesthesia
alb-	denoting a white or pale colour	albino
-alge(si)-	pain	analgesic
-algia, alg(i)o-	pain	myalgia
all(o-)	denoting something as different, or as an addition	alloantigen, allopathy
ambi-	denoting something as positioned on both sides; describing both of two	ambidextrous
amni-	pertaining to the membranous fetal sac (amnion)	amniocentesis
an-	not, without	analgesia
ana-	back, again, up	anaplasia
andr(o)-	pertaining to a man	android, andrology
angi(o)-	blood vessel	angiogram
ankyl(o)-, ancyl(o)-	denoting something as crooked or bent	ankylosis

Prefix or suffix	Meaning	Example(s)
ante-	describing something as positioned in front of another thing	antepartum
anti-	describing something as 'against' or 'opposed to' another	antibody, antipsychotic
arteri(o)-	of or pertaining to an artery	arteriole, artery
arthr(o)-	of or pertaining to the joints, limbs	arthritis
articul(o)-	joint	articulation
-ase	enzyme	lactase
-asthenia	weakness	myasthenia gravis
ather(o)-	fatty deposit, soft gruel-like deposit	atherosclerosis
atri(o)-	an atrium (especially heart atrium)	atrioventricular
aur(i)-	of or pertaining to the ear	aural
aut(o)-	self	autoimmune
axill-	of or pertaining to the armpit (uncommon as a prefix)	axilla
bi-	twice, double	binary
bio-	life	biology
blephar(o)-	of or pertaining to the eyelid	blepharoplast
brachi(o)-	of or relating to the arm	brachium of inferior colliculus
brady-	'slow'	bradycardia
bronch(i)-	bronchus	bronchiolitis obliterans
bucc(o)-	of or pertaining to the cheek	buccolabial
burs(o)-	bursa (fluid sac between the bones)	bursitis
carcin(o)-	cancer	carcinoma
cardi(o)-	of or pertaining to the heart	cardiology
carp(o)-	of or pertaining to the wrist	carpopedal
-cele	pouching, hernia	hydrocele, varicocele
-centesis	surgical puncture for aspiration	amniocentesis
cephal(o)-	of or pertaining to the head (as a whole)	cephalalgy
cerebell(o)-	of or pertaining to the cerebellum	cerebellum
cerebr(o)-	of or pertaining to the brain	cerebrology
chem(o)-	chemistry, drug	chemotherapy
chol(e)-	of or pertaining to bile	cholecystitis
cholecyst(o)-	of or pertaining to the gall bladder	cholecystectomy
chondr(i)o-	cartilage, gristle, granule, granular	chondrocalcinosis
-chrom(ato)-	colour	haemochromatosis

Prefix or suffix	Meaning	Example(s)
-cidal, -cide	killing, destroying	bacteriocidal
cili-	of or pertaining to the cilia, the eyelashes; eyelids	ciliary
circum-	denoting something as 'around' another	circumcision
col-, colo-, colono-	colon	colonoscopy
colp(o)-	of or pertaining to the vagina	colposcopy
contra-	against	contraindicate
coron(o)-	crown	coronary
cost(o)-	of or pertaining to the ribs	costochondral
crani(o)-	belonging or relating to the cranium	craniology
-crine, -crin(o)-	to secrete	endocrine
cry(o)-	cold	cryoablation
-cutane-	skin	subcutaneous
cyan(o)-	denotes a blue color	cyanopsia
cycl-	circle, cycle	cyclical
cyst(o)-, cyst(i)-	of or pertaining to the urinary bladder	cystotomy
cyt(o)-	cell	cytokine
-cyte	cell	leucocyte
-dactyl(o)-	of or pertaining to a finger, toe	dactylology, polydactyly
dent-	of or pertaining to teeth	dentist
dermat(o)-, derm(o)-	of or pertaining to the skin	dermatology
-desis	binding	arthrodesis
dextr(o)-	right, on the right side	dextrocardia
di-	two	diplopia
dia-	through, during, across	dialysis
digit-	of or pertaining to the finger *[rare as a root]*	digit
-dipsia	suffix meaning '(condition of) thirst'	polydipsia, hydroadipsia, oligodipsia
dors(o)-, dors(i)-	of or pertaining to the back	dorsal, dorsocephalad
duodeno-	duodenum	duodenal atresia
dynam(o)-	force, energy, power	hand-strength dynamometer
-dynia	pain	vulvodynia
dys-	bad, difficult, defective, abnormal	dysphagia, dysphasia
ec-	out, away	ectopia, ectopic pregnancy
ect(o)-	outer, outside	ectoblast, ectoderm
-ectasia, -ectasis	expansion, dilation	bronchiectasis, telangiectasia

Prefix or suffix	Meaning	Example(s)
-ectomy	denotes a surgical operation or removal of a body part; resection, excision	mastectomy
-emesis	vomiting condition	haematemesis
encephal(o)-	of or pertaining to the brain; also see **cerebr(o)-**	encephalogram
endo-	denotes something as 'inside' or 'within'	endocrinology, endospore
eosin(o)-	red	eosinophil granulocyte
enter(o)-	of or pertaining to the intestine	gastroenterology
epi-	on, upon	epicardium, epidermis, epidural, episclera, epistaxis
erythr(o)-	denotes a red colour	erythrocyte
-oesophageal, -oesophago-	gullet	oesophagus
ex-	out of, away from	excision, exophthalmos
exo-	denotes something as 'outside' another	exoskeleton
extra-	outside	extradural haematoma
faci(o)-	of or pertaining to the face	facioplegic
fibr(o)	fibre	fibroblast
fossa	a hollow or depressed area; trench or channel	fossa ovalis
front-	of or pertaining to the forehead	frontonasal
galact(o)-	milk	galactorrhoea
gastr(o)-	of or pertaining to the stomach	gastric bypass
-genic	formative, pertaining to producing	cardiogenic shock
gingiv-	of or pertaining to the gums	gingivitis
glauc(o)-	denoting a grey or bluish-grey colour	glaucoma
gloss(o)-, glott(o)-	of or pertaining to the tongue	glossology
gluco-	sweet	glucocorticoid
glyc(o)-	sugar	glycolysis
-gnosis	knowledge	diagnosis, prognosis
gon(o)-	seed, semen; also, reproductive	gonorrhoea
-gram, **-gramme**	record or picture	angiogram
-graph	instrument used to record data or picture	electrocardiograph
-graphy	process of recording	angiography
gyn(aec)o-	woman	gynaecomastia
halluc-	to wander in mind	hallucinosis
haemat-, haemato- (haem-,)	of or pertaining to blood	haematology
haemangi-, haemangio-	blood vessels	haemangioma

Prefix or suffix	Meaning	Example(s)
hemi-	one-half	cerebral hemisphere
hepat- (hepatic-)	of or pertaining to the liver	hepatology
heter(o)-	denotes something as 'the other' (of two), as an addition, or different	heterogeneous
hist(o)-, histio-	tissue	histology
home(o)-	similar	homeopathy
hom(o)-	denotes something as 'the same' as another or common	homosexuality
hydr(o)-	water	hydrophobe
hyper-	denotes something as 'extreme' or 'beyond normal'	hypertension
hyp(o)-	denotes something as 'below normal'	hypovolaemia
hyster(o)-	of or pertaining to the womb, the uterus	hysterectomy, hysteria
iatr(o)-	of or pertaining to medicine, or a physician	iatrogenic
-iatry	denotes a field in medicine of a certain body component	podiatry, psychiatry
-ics	organised knowledge, treatment	obstetrics
ileo-	ileum	ileocaecal valve
infra-	below	infrahyoid muscles
inter-	between, among	interarticular ligament
intra-	within	intramural
ipsi-	same	ipsilateral hemiparesis
ischio-	of or pertaining to the ischium, the hip joint	ischioanal fossa
-ism	condition, disease	dwarfism
-ismus	spasm, contraction	hemiballismus
iso-	denoting something as being 'equal'	isotonic
-ist	one who specialises in	pathologist
-itis	inflammation	tonsillitis
-ium	structure, tissue	pericardium
juxta- (iuxta-)	near to, alongside or next to	juxtaglomerular apparatus
karyo-	nucleus	eukaryote
kerat(o)-	cornea (eye or skin)	keratoscope
kin(e)-, kin(o)-, kinesi(o)-	movement	kinaesthesia
kyph(o)-	humped	kyphoscoliosis
labi(o)-	of or pertaining to the lip	labiodental
lacrim(o)-	tear	lacrimal canaliculi
lact(i)-, lact(o)-	milk	lactation
lapar(o)-	of or pertaining to the abdomen wall, flank	laparotomy

Prefix or suffix	Meaning	Example(s)
laryng(o)-	of or pertaining to the larynx, the lower throat cavity where the voice box is	larynx
latero-	lateral	lateral pectoral nerve
-lepsis, -lepsy	attack, seizure	epilepsy, narcolepsy
lept(o)-	light, slender	leptomeningeal
leuc(o)-, leuk(o)-	denoting a white colour	leucocyte
lingu(a)-, lingu(o)-	of or pertaining to the tongue	linguistics
lip(o)-	fat	liposuction
lith(o)-	stone, calculus	lithotripsy
-logist	denotes someone who studies a certain field	oncologist, pathologist
-logy	denotes the academic study or practice of a certain field	haematology, urology
lymph(o)-	lymph	lymphoedema
lys(o)-, -lytic	dissolution	lysosome
-lysis	destruction, separation	paralysis
macr(o)-	large, long	macrophage
-malacia	softening	osteomalacia
mamm(o)-	of or pertaining to the breast	mammogram
mammill(o)-	of or pertaining to the nipple	mammoplasty, mammillitis
manu-	of or pertaining to the hand	manufacture
mast(o)-	of or pertaining to the breast	mastectomy
meg(a)-, megal(o)-, -megaly	enlargement, million	splenomegaly, megametre
melan(o)-	black colour	melanin
mening(o)-	membrane	meningitis
meta-	after, behind	metacarpus
-meter	instrument used to measure or count	sphygmomanometer
-metry	process of measuring	optometry
metr(o)-	pertaining to conditions or instruments of the uterus	metrorrhagia
micro-	denoting something as small, or relating to smallness, millionth	microscope
milli-	thousandth	millilitre
mon(o)-	single	infectious mononucleosis
morph(o)-	form, shape	morphology
muscul(o)-	muscle	musculoskeletal system
my(o)-	of or relating to muscle	myoblast
-myc(o)-	fungus	onychomycosis

Prefix or suffix	Meaning	Example(s)
myel(o)-	of or relating to bone marrow or spinal cord	myeloblast
myri-	ten thousand	myriad
myring(o)-	eardrum	myringotomy
narc(o)-	numb, sleep	narcolepsy
nas(o)-	of or pertaining to the nose	nasal
necr(o)-	death	necrosis, necrotising fasciitis
neo-	new	neoplasm
nephr(o)-	of or pertaining to the kidney	nephrology
neur(i)-, neur(o)-	of or pertaining to nerves and the nervous system	neurofibromatosis
normo-	normal	normocapnia
ocul(o)-	of or pertaining to the eye	oculist
-odont(o)-	of or pertaining to teeth	orthodontist
odyn(o)-	pain	stomatodynia
-oesophageal, oesophago-	gullet	gastro-oesophageal reflux
-oid	resemblance to	sarcoidosis
-ole	small or little	arteriole
olig(o)-	denoting something as 'having little, having few'	oliguria
-oma (singular), **-omata** (plural)	tumour, mass, collection	sarcoma, teratoma
onco-	tumour, bulk, volume	oncology
onych(o)-	of or pertaining to the nail (of a finger or toe)	onychophagy
oo-	of or pertaining to the egg, a woman's egg, the ovum	oogenesis
oophor(o)-	of or pertaining to the woman's ovary	oophorectomy
ophthalm(o)-	of or pertaining to the eye	ophthalmology
optic(o)-	of or relating to chemical properties of the eye	opticochemical
orchi(o)-, orchid(o)-, orch(o)-	testis	orchiectomy, orchidectomy
-osis	a condition, disease or increase	harlequin type ichthyosis, psychosis, osteoporosis
osseo-	bony	osseous
ossi-	bone	peripheral ossifying fibroma
ost(e)-, oste(o)-	bone	osteoporosis
ot(o)-	of or pertaining to the ear	otology
ovo-, ovi-, ov-	of or pertaining to the eggs, the ovum	ovogenesis
pachy-	thick	pachyderma

Prefix or suffix	Meaning	Example(s)
paed-, paedo-	of or pertaining to the child	paediatrics. paedophilia
palpebr-	of or pertaining to the eyelid *[uncommon as a root]*	palpebra
pan-, pant(o)-	denoting something as 'complete' or containing 'everything'	panophobia, panopticon
papill-	of or pertaining to the nipple (of the chest/breast)	papillitis
papul(o)-	indicates papulosity, a small elevation or swelling in the skin, a pimple, swelling	papulation
para-	alongside of, abnormal	paracyesis
-paresis	slight paralysis	hemiparesis
parvo-	small	parvovirus
path(o)-	disease	pathology
-pathy	denotes (with a negative sense) a disease, or disorder	sociopathy, neuropathy
pector-	breast	pectoralgia, pectoriloquy, pectorophony
ped-, -ped-, -pes	of or pertaining to the foot; -footed	pedoscope
pelv(i)-, pelv(o)-	hip bone	pelvis
-penia	deficiency	osteopenia
-pepsia	denotes something relating to digestion, or the digestive tract	dyspepsia
peri-	denoting something with a position 'surrounding' or 'around' another	periodontal
-pexy	fixation	nephropexy
phaco-	lens, lens-shaped	phacolysis, phacometer, phacoscotoma
-phage, -phagia	forms terms denoting conditions relating to eating or ingestion	sarcophagia
-phago-	eating, devouring	phagocyte
-phagy	forms nouns that denote 'feeding on' the first element or part of the word	haematophagy
pharmaco-	drug, medication	pharmacology
pharyng(o)-	of or pertaining to the pharynx, the upper throat cavity	pharyngitis, pharyngoscopy
phleb(o)-	of or pertaining to the (blood) veins, a vein	phlebography, phlebotomy
-phobia	exaggerated fear, sensitivity	arachnophobia
phon(o)-	sound	phonograph, symphony
phot(o)-	of or pertaining to light	photopathy
phren(i)-, phren(o)-, phrenico	the mind	phrenic nerve, schizophrenia
-plasia	formation, development	achondroplasia
-plasty	surgical repair, reconstruction	rhinoplasty
-plegia	paralysis	paraplegia

Prefix or suffix	Meaning	Example(s)
pleio-	more, excessive, multiple	pleiomorphism
pleur(o)-, pleur(a)	of or pertaining to the ribs	pleurogenous
-plexy	stroke or seizure	cataplexy
pneum(o)-	of or pertaining to the lungs	pneumonocyte, pneumonia
pneumat(o)-	air, lung	pneumatocele
-poiesis	production	haematopoiesis
poly-	denotes a 'plurality' of something	polymyositis
post-	denotes something as 'after' or 'behind' another	postoperation, postmortem
pre-	denotes something as 'before' another (in [physical] position or time)	premature birth
presby(o)-	old age	presbyopia
prim-	denotes something as 'first' or 'most important'	primary
proct(o)-	anus, rectum	proctology
prot(o)-	denotes something as 'first' or 'most important'	protoneurone
pseud(o)-	denotes something false or fake	pseudoephedrine
psych(e)-, psych(o)-	of or pertaining to the mind	psychology, psychiatry
psor-	itching	psoriasis
-ptosis	falling, drooping, downward placement, prolapse	apoptosis, nephroptosis
-ptysis	(a spitting), spitting	haemoptysis
pulmon-, pulmo-	of or relating to the lungs	pulmonary
pyel(o)-	pelvis	pyelonephritis
py(o)-	pus	pyometra
pyr(o)-	fever	antipyretic
quadr(i)-	four	quadriceps
radio-	radiation	radiowave
ren(o)-	of or pertaining to the kidney	renal
retro-	backwards, behind	retroversion, retroverted
rhin(o)-	of or pertaining to the nose	rhinoplasty
rhod(o)-	denoting a rose-red colour	rhodophyte
-rrhage	burst forth	haemorrhage
-rrhagia	rapid flow of blood	menorrhagia
-rrhaphy	surgical suturing	gastrorrhaphy
-rrhexis	rupture	karyorrhexis
-rrhoea	flowing, discharge	diarrhoea
-rupt	break or burst	erupt, interrupt

Prefix or suffix	Meaning	Example(s)
salping(o)-	of or pertaining to tubes, e.g. fallopian tubes	salpingectomy, salpingopharyngeus muscle
sangui-, sanguine-	of or pertaining to blood	sanguine
sarco-	muscular, flesh-like	sarcoma
scler(o)-	hard	scleroderma
-sclerosis	hardening	atherosclerosis, multiple sclerosis
scoli(o)-	twisted	scoliosis
-scope	instrument for viewing	endoscope
-scopy	use of instrument for viewing	endoscopy
semi-	one-half, partly	semiconscious
sial(o)-	saliva, salivary gland	sialagogue
sigmoid(o)-	sigmoid, s-shaped curvature	sigmoid colon
sinistr(o)-	left, left side	sinistrocardia
sinus-	of or pertaining to the sinus	sinusitis
somat(o)-, somatico-	body, bodily	somatic
-spadias	slit, fissure	hypospadias, epispadias
spasmo-	spasm	spasmodic dysphonia
sperma-, spermo-, spermato-	semen, spermatozoa	spermatogenesis
splen(o)-	spleen	splenectomy
spondyl(o)-	of or pertaining to the spine, the vertebra	spondylitis
squamos(o)-	denoting something as ‘full of scales’ or ‘scaly’	squamous cell
-stalsis	contraction	peristalsis
-stasis	stopping, standing	cytostasis, homeostasis
-staxis	dripping, trickling	epistaxis
-stenosis	abnormal narrowing in a blood vessel or other tubular organ or structure	restenosis, stenosis
stomat(o)-	of or pertaining to the mouth	stomatogastric, stomatognathic system
-stomy	creation of an opening	colostomy
sub-	beneath	subcutaneous tissue
super-	in excess, above, superior	superior vena cava
supra-	above, excessive	supraorbital vein
tachy-	denoting something as fast, irregularly fast	tachycardia
-tension, -tensive	pressure	hypertension
tetan-	rigid, tense	tetanus

Prefix or suffix	Meaning	Example(s)
thec-	case, sheath	intrathecal
therap-	treatment	hydrotherapy, therapeutic
therm(o)-	heat	thermoregulation
thorac(i)-, thorac(o)-, thoracico-	of or pertaining to the upper chest, chest; the area above the breast and under the neck	thorax
thromb(o)-	of or relating to a blood clot, clotting of blood	thrombus, thrombocytopenia
thyr(o)-	thyroid	thyroxine
thym-	emotions	dysthymia
-tome	cutting instrument	osteotome
-tomy	act of cutting; incising, incision	gastrostomy
tono-	tone, tension, pressure	tonometer
-tony	tension	neurotony
top(o)-	place, topical	topical anaesthetic
tort(i)-	twisted	torticollis
tox(i)-, tox(o)-, toxic(o)-	toxin, poison	toxoplasmosis
trache(a)-	trachea	tracheotomy
trachel(o)-	of or pertaining to the neck	tracheloplasty
trans-	denoting something as moving or situated 'across' or 'through'	transfusion
tri-	three	triangle
trich(i)-, trichia, trich(o)-	of or pertaining to hair, hair-like structure	trichocyst
-tripsy	crushing	lithotripsy
-trophy	nourishment, development	pseudohypertrophy
tympan(o)-	eardrum	tympanocentesis
-ula, -ule	small	nodule
ultra-	beyond, excessive	ultraviolet
un(i)-	one	unilateral hearing loss
ur(o)-	of or pertaining to urine, the urinary system; (specifically) pertaining to the physiological chemistry of urine	urology
uter(o)-	of or pertaining to the uterus or womb	uterus
vagin-	of or pertaining to the vagina	vagina
varic(o)-	swollen or twisted vein	varicose
vas(o)-	duct, blood vessel	vasoconstriction
vasculo-	blood vessel	vascular
ven-	of or pertaining to the (blood) veins, a vein	vein, venospasm

Prefix or suffix	Meaning	Example(s)
ventr(o)-	of or pertaining to the belly; the stomach cavities	ventrodorsal
ventricul(o)-	of or pertaining to the ventricles; any hollow region inside an organ	cardiac ventriculography
-version	turning	anteversion, retroversion
vesic(o)-	of or pertaining to the bladder	vesical arteries
viscer(o)-	of or pertaining to the internal organs, the viscera	viscera
xanth(o)-	denoting a yellow colour	xanthopathy
xen(o)-	foreign, different	xenograft
xer(o)-	dry, desert-like	xerostomia
zo(o)-	animal, animal life	zoology
-zym(o)-	fermentation	enzyme, lysozyme

How to use your textbook

It is entirely up to you how you use this book for each of us knows best how we learn. You can dip in and out of the chapters as you wish. The first four chapters set the scene, and it may be advisable to consider these chapters first prior to moving into the various systems.

Following are the icons used in the book:

Colouring. You are asked to colour in the elements of the diagram. The more colours that you have available to you, the more effective and enjoyable your artistic work will be. You should have at least a range of 10 colours. Using felt-tipped pens is not recommended as this may cause the colours to 'bleed' through the page. If lighter colours are used, they are less likely to cover up detail.

Generally, you should use whatever colours please you. There are universally agreed colours that are used in anatomy texts. For example,

- red for arteries
- blue for veins
- purple for capillaries
- yellow for nerves
- green for lymph vessels and lymph nodes.

Identifying. Invites you to identify the various components/structures in the diagram; label the diagram.

Pairing. Here you are required to match the pairs. You are provided with a range of sentences that should be paired up to make meaningful paragraphs.

SCRAMBLE

Scrambled words. Time yourself to unscramble the words.

Wordplay. A number of activities to test your knowledge of terminology and concepts are included, such as **crosswords** and **word searches**.

About the companion website

This book is accompanied by a companion website.

www.wiley.com/go/anatomyworkbook

To access the website materials, click on the link under Related Resources on the book's page on wiley.com. You can also find this by searching www.wiley.com for the ISBN 9781394324248.

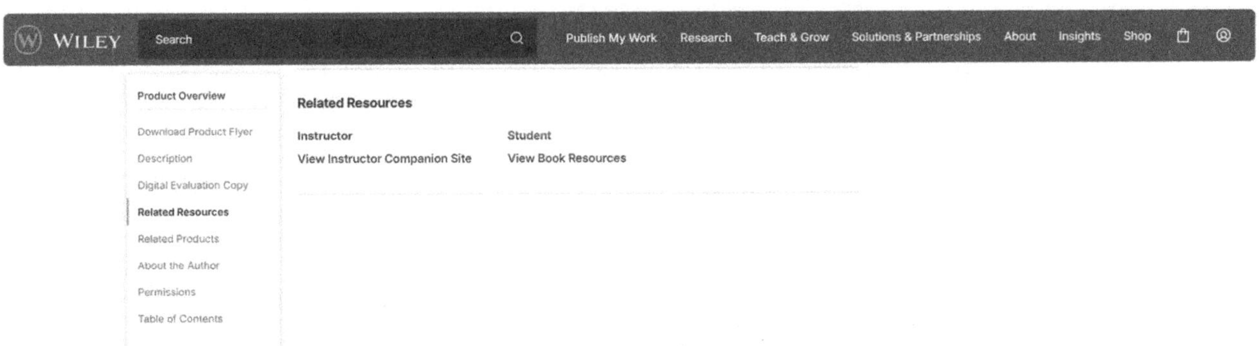

This website includes:
Answers to the questions in this workbook.

CHAPTER 1

Language and terminology

1 Anatomical directions

Using the anatomical position as a reference, complete the following statements:

(a) The hand is ______________ to the elbow.

(b) The elbow is ______________ to the hand.

(c) The ears are ______________ to the nose.

(d) The kneecap is on the ______________ surface of the body.

(e) The cervical vertebrae are ______________ to the lumbar vertebrae.

(f) The sternum is ______________ to the armpit.

(g) The buttocks are on the ______________ surface of the body.

(h) The bones are ______________ to the muscles.

(i) The epidermis is ______________ to the dermis.

2 Planes

(a) Label the three planes on the following diagram:

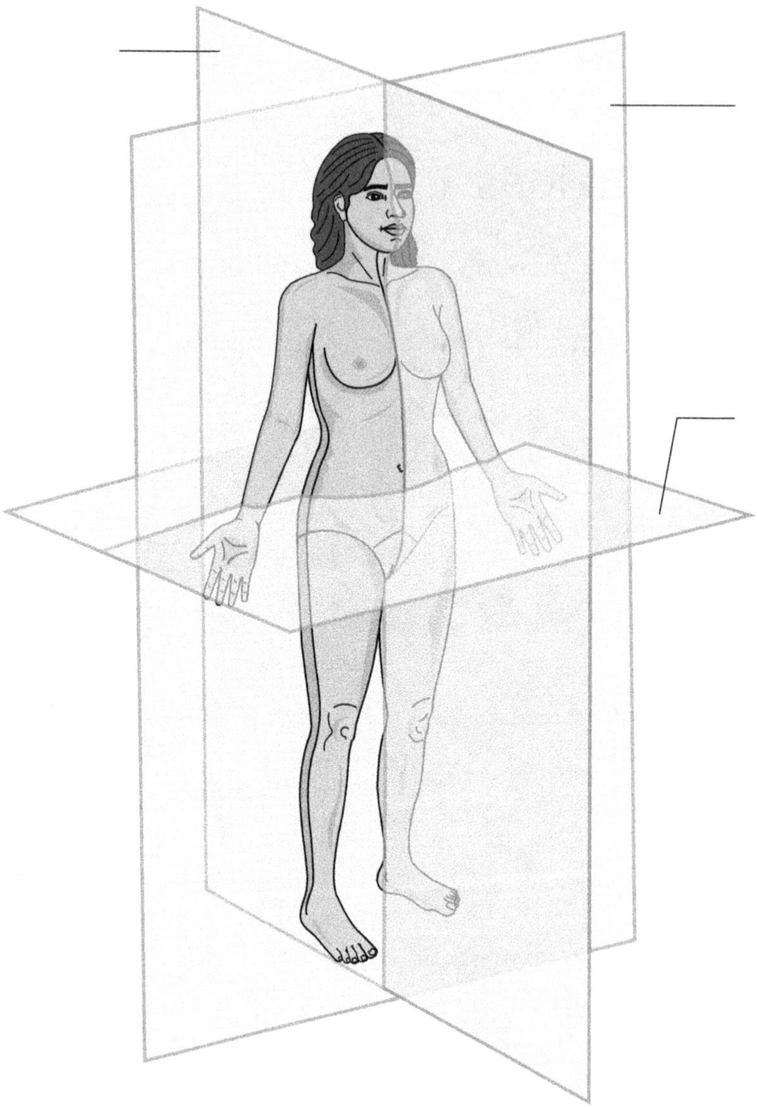

Source: Peate and Nair (2021) / Reproduced with permission of John Wiley & Sons.

(b) Identify the planes through which the following structures have been cut to produce the sections shown.

I. Eye, ______________________________ section.

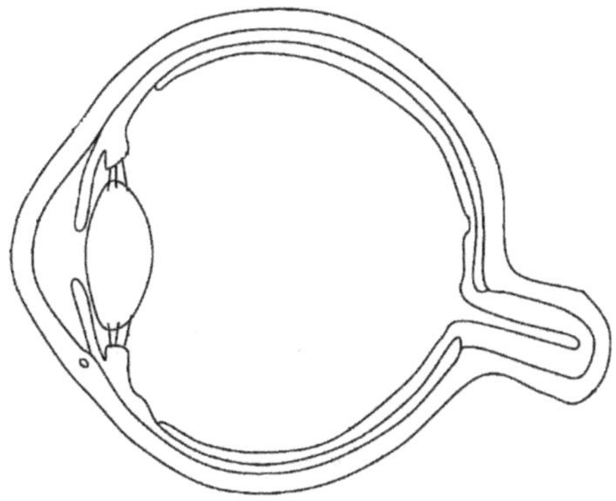

II. Spinal cord, ______________________ section.

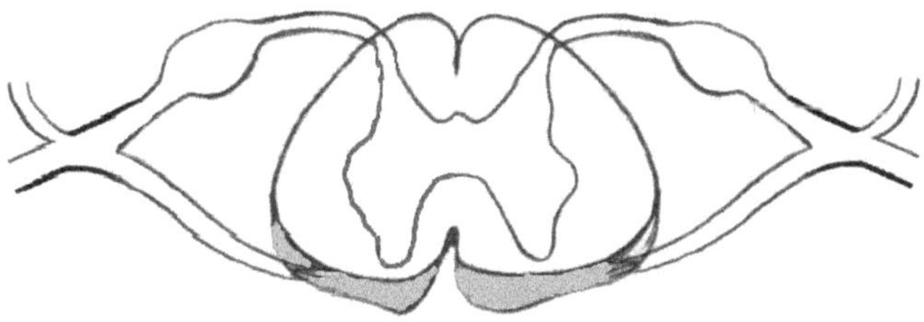

III. Knee joint, ______________________ section.

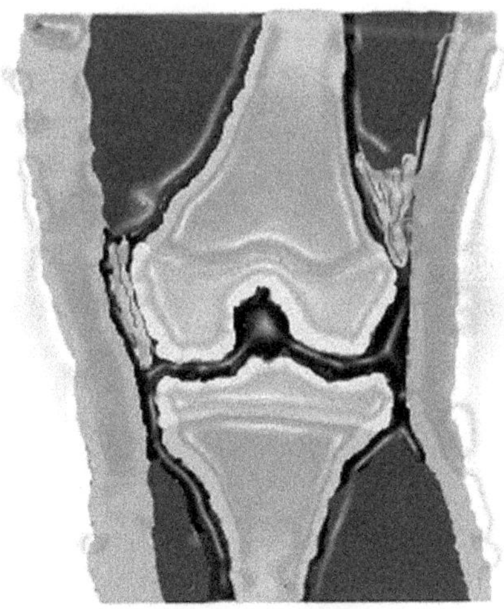

IV. Heart, ____________________ section

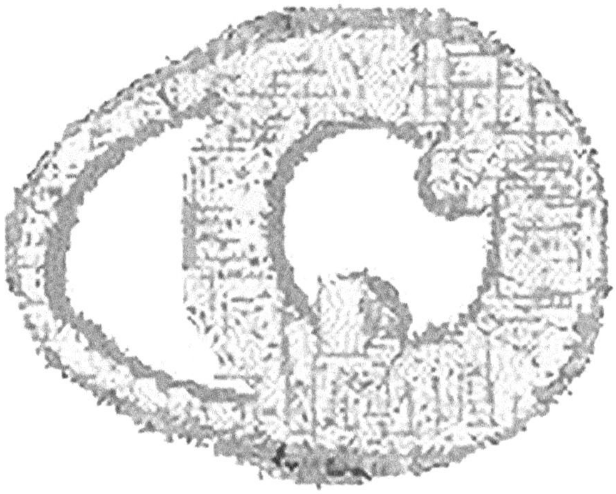

3 Anatomical regions and areas

Complete the following table with the corresponding anatomical term or the region or area the term describes:

Region or area	Anatomical term
Head	
	Occipital
Eyes	
	Popliteal
Spinal column/backbone	
	Perineal
Fingers	
	Brachial
Neck	
	Carpal
Feet	
	Pectoral
Mouth	
	Inguinal
Nose	
	Cubital
Navel	
	Gluteal
Ribs	
	Plantar
Kneecap	
	Femoral
Pubis	
	Mammary
Armpit	

4 Body cavities

Colour and label the body cavities on the following diagram:

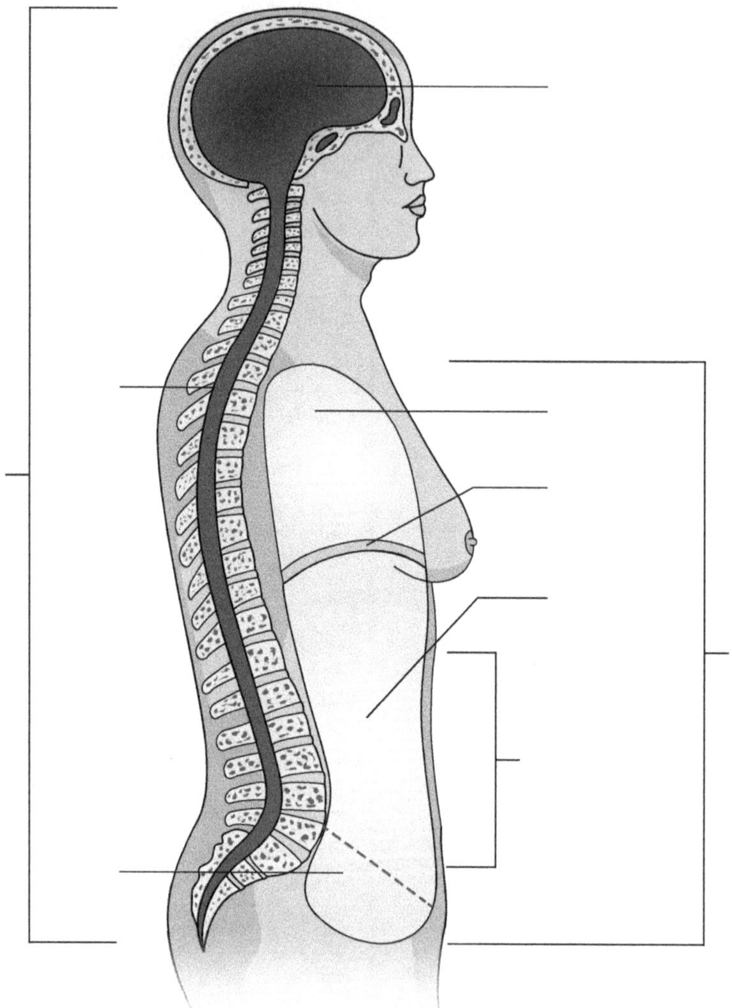

Source: Peate and Nair (2021) / Reproduced with permission of John Wiley & Sons.

5 Combining terms

Select the appropriate root and prefix from the boxes below to create terms with the meanings given in the table. Each root and prefix can only be used once.

(a) Lower than normal blood pressure	
(b) A slowed heart rate	
(c) Inside the spinal canal	
(d) An increased rate of breathing	
(e) Lack of oxygen	
(f) Small cells	
(g) Drinking a lot	
(h) A sense of unease, anxiety or unhappiness	
(i) Abnormally high rate and depth of breathing	
(j) Between cells	

Prefixes	**Roots**
Hyper-	cardia
Hypo-	cytic
Poly-	oxia
Tachy-	dipsia
Brady-	phoria
Intra-	ventilation
Inter-	pnoea
An-	thecal
Dys-	cellular
Micro-	tension

6 Word scramble

Time yourself to unscramble these words.

Scrambled	Answer
GEPASTHONEIS	
ADIPITICHO	
RECTEAOBANIX	
IONACLOSMO	
POSONSIRG	
SEAQLUEE	

7 Definitions

For the following terms, underline the root and then give the meaning of the term:

Term	Meaning
Haemostasis	
Hyperalgesia	
Acidosis	
Vasospasm	
Endometriosis	
Cystitis	
Atherosclerosis	
Pericarditis	
Cytotoxic	
Thrombocytopenia	

8 Procedures

Match the procedures with their suffixes, then complete each suffix with a root word to create an example of a specific procedure.

Making an opening to the outside from a structure or organ	-otomy
Viewing the inside of a structure or organ	-ectomy
Cutting into a structure or organ	-oscopy
Removing a structure or organ	-ostomy

9 Abbreviations

Write the following instructions out in full, without abbreviations:

(a) Tx Bactrim DS tabs po bid, pc. 1st dose stat.

____

(b) Hx recurrent UTI, pain on PU, BMI 32.

____

(c) Hx Hyperemesis gravidarum (Primigrav). Tx Ondansetron 6 mg po tid.

____

(d) BP 160/90, HR 131, RR 19.

____

(e) NSAID PRN

____

10 Concise language

In the brackets, write the correct terms for the conditions described in the highlighted text.

(a) The patient had an elevated heart rate ( ), but abnormally low blood pressure ( ). The skin was pale, suggesting narrowing of the blood vessels ( ) and urine output over the previous 12 hours had been extremely low ( ).

(b) Before starting any treatment for excessive mucus discharge from the nose ( ), it is important to check for inflammation of the mucous membranes of the nose ( ), or of the skin around the nose ( ), to help determine whether the problem is due to a microscopic invader spread from another person ( ), or a hypersensitive immune response to something in the environment ( ).

(c) Cancer chemotherapy usually involves the use of drugs that are poisonous to living cells ( ). Many kill the cells while they are undergoing division involving duplicating all their genetic material and splitting in two, giving a complete copy of the genetic material to each new cell ( ). Because these drugs act while the cell is dividing, they tend to have the most damaging effect on the specialised collections of cells ( ) of the body that divide rapidly, such as skin, hair follicles and gut linings, and less effect on those that divide more slowly, such as cells of the nervous system ( ).

11 Prefixes and suffixes

Use the clues and their prefixes/suffixes to complete the terms.

(a) Irrational feeling of mistrust and persecution:	para___
(b) Endocrine gland:	para___
(c) Healthcare professional skilled in emergency care:	para___
(d) Paralysis of the legs and lower body:	para___
(e) Organism living in or on another organism:	para___
(f) Pain on urination:	___uria
(g) Blood in the urine:	___uria
(h) Production of a large volume of urine:	___uria
(i) Abnormally high level of calcium in the urine:	___uria

(j) Presence in the urine of the oxygen-carrying protein normally found in muscle:	___uria
(k) Medical specialisation dealing with the heart:	cardio___
(l) Return of a heart in arrhythmia to normal rhythm:	cardio___
(m) Record of electrical activity of the heart from the body surface:	___cardio___
(n) Disease of the heart muscle:	cardio___
(o) Increased heart rate:	___cardia
(p) Increased levels of ketone bodies in blood:	___osis
(q) Blood pH below the normal range:	___osis
(r) Death of cells:	___osis
(s) Blue colouration of skin or mucous membranes:	___osis
(t) Too much iron in the body:	___osis

12 Common suffix

Complete the following puzzle using the same suffix in each term:

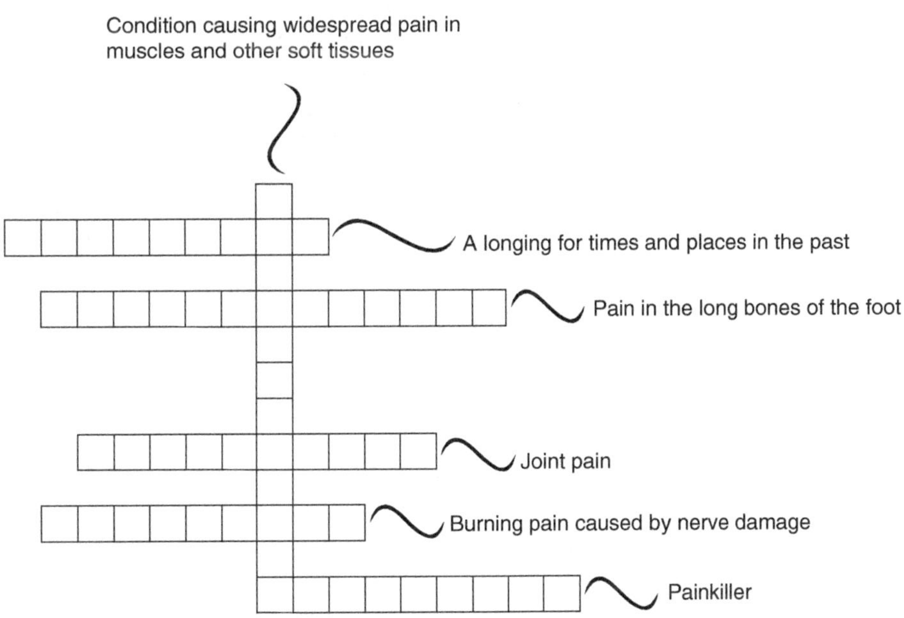

13 Crossword

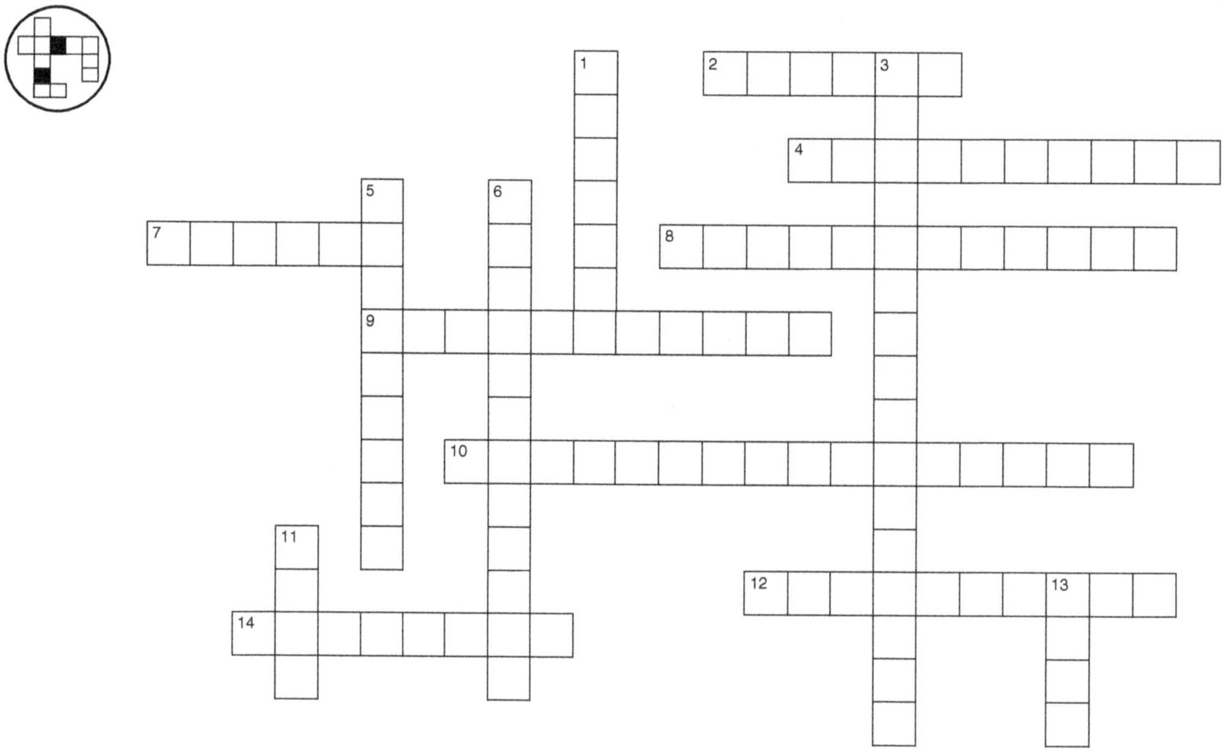

Across

2. Directional term meaning 'towards the middle'
4. Disease caused by medical intervention
7. Lying face up
8. Worsening of an illness
9. Between ribs
10. Physiological control of body temperature
12. Disease acquired at a hospital
14. Concerning the head

Down

1. Condition that continues over an extended period
3. Hardening of the arteries
5. The cause of a disease
6. Higher-than-normal body temperature
11. An ophthalmic preparation should be put in the ____
13. Suffix meaning inflammation

14 Find the errors

The following passage contains several errors for you to find and correct:

The patient was admitted with significant abdominal pain, and a prognosis of appendicitis was made. Surgery was performed to remove the inflamed appendix (an appendostomy). Recovering in the ward, the patient was given algesic medication to control any postoperative pain, administered by means of a patient-controlled delivery system. The nurse noted on the chart that pain control was to be administered STAT, meaning as and when needed by the patient.

Multiple-choice questions

15. The anatomical position:
- A. is the position patients are placed in for examination
- B. has arms extended to the side with palms facing forwards
- C. has head turned to one side
- D. depends on the position of the patient

16. When referring to structure a on the body trunk, which is higher up and closer to the midline of the body than structure b, the correct terminology would be:
- A. Structure a is posteromedial to structure b
- B. Structure a is anterior to structure b
- C. Structure a is superomedial to structure b
- D. Structure a is inferomedial to structure b

17. A patient has sustained a fracture of the tibia close to the ankle. This would be described as:
- A. the distal end of the tibia
- B. the proximal ankle
- C. the deep tibia
- D. the origin of the tibia

18. A frontal plane divides the body into:
- A. equal right and left halves
- B. upper and lower halves
- C. front and back halves
- D. None of the above

19. The urinary bladder is located in the:
- A. dorsal cavity
- B. thoracic cavity
- C. abdominal cavity
- D. pelvic cavity

20. The term bacteraemia means:

A. abnormal composition of blood

B. a type of bacteria

C. bacteria in the blood

D. None of the above

21. A person is having the interior wall of the urinary bladder visualised using an instrument placed inside the bladder. This procedure would be called a:

A. cystotomy

B. cytology

C. cystoscopy

D. cystectomy

22. A patient is brought into hospital suffering from agonising abdominal pain that started about an hour before arrival. This pain would be described as:

A. severe and acute

B. chronic and acute

C. intense and chronic

D. acute on chronic

23. A young patient is diagnosed with a condition known as juvenile idiopathic arthritis. This means that the condition involves:

A. inflammation of soft tissues, occurs in childhood and is caused by medical treatment

B. inflammation of the joints and immature behaviour and has no identifiable cause

C. inflammation of the arteries and reduced intelligence and occurs in childhood

D. inflammation of the joints, occurs in childhood and has no identifiable cause

24. When communicating with patients and colleagues, acronyms and abbreviations should be used:

A. as often as possible, to save time

B. only when you know it will be understood by the listener/reader

C. to show you are a qualified healthcare professional

D. to maintain secrecy when talking about patients

CHAPTER 2

Basic scientific principles of physiology

1 Levels of organisation

Identify the levels of body organisation represented by the following examples:

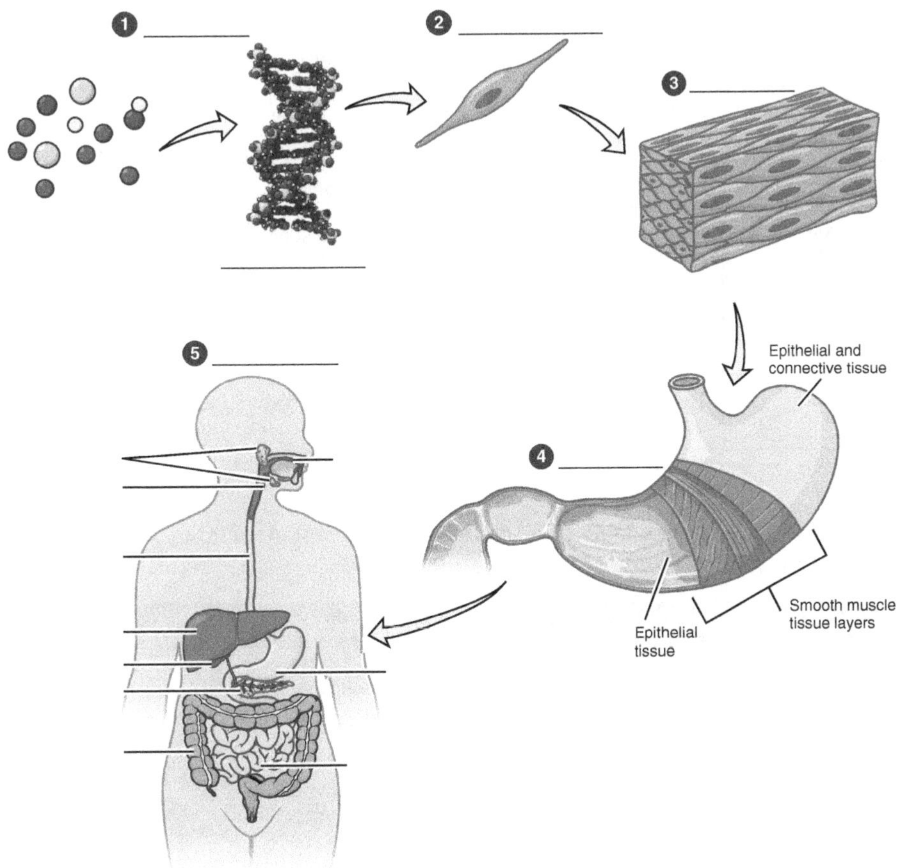

Source: Tortora (2009) / Reproduced with permission of John Wiley & Sons.

2 Elements

(a) Colour in the metals, metalloids and non-metals on the periodic table below:

	1	2	3	4	5	6	7	8	9	10	11	12	13	14	15	16	17	18
1	1 H																1 H	2 He
2	3 Li	4 Be											5 B	6 C	7 N	8 O	9 F	10 Ne
3	11 Na	12 Mg											13 Al	14 Si	15 P	16 S	17 Cl	18 Ar
4	19 K	20 Ca	21 Sc	22 Ti	23 V	24 Cr	25 Mn	26 Fe	27 Co	28 Ni	29 Cu	30 Zn	31 Ga	32 Ge	33 As	34 Se	35 Br	36 Kr
5	37 Rb	38 Sr	39 Y	40 Zr	41 Nb	42 Mo	43 Tc	44 Ru	45 Rh	46 Pd	47 Ag	48 Cd	49 In	50 Sn	51 Sb	52 Te	53 I	54 Xe
6	55 Cs	56 Ba	71 Lu	72 Hf	73 Ta	74 W	75 Re	76 Os	77 Ir	78 Pt	79 Au	80 Hg	81 Tl	82 Pb	83 Bi	84 Po	85 At	86 Rn

☐ Metals ☐ Metalloids ☐ Non-metals

(b) Match the statements on the right of the table to the appropriate elements.

Oxygen	Its atoms bond to each other to form long chains which form the basis of all organic compounds.
Hydrogen	An alkaline earth metal. Its ions are biologically very important.
Nitrogen	The ionised form of this element is the most abundant cation in the body.
Carbon	The lightest of all the elements. Two atoms bind together to form an explosive gas.
Calcium	Two atoms of this element bind together to form a highly reactive gas which constitutes 21% of air by volume.
Sodium	Two atoms of this element bind together to form a gas which constitutes 78% of air by volume.

(c) Complete the following table by filling in the chemical symbol for each element and identifying the metals and non-metals:

Element	Chemical symbol	Metal or non-metal
Iron		
Hydrogen		
Carbon		
Nitrogen		

Oxygen		
Calcium		
Potassium		
Sodium		
Chlorine		
Sulphur		
Phosphorus		

3 Atoms

(a) In the atom shown below, coloured circles represent protons, neutrons and electrons. Fill in the key to identify which is which and show the charge of each.

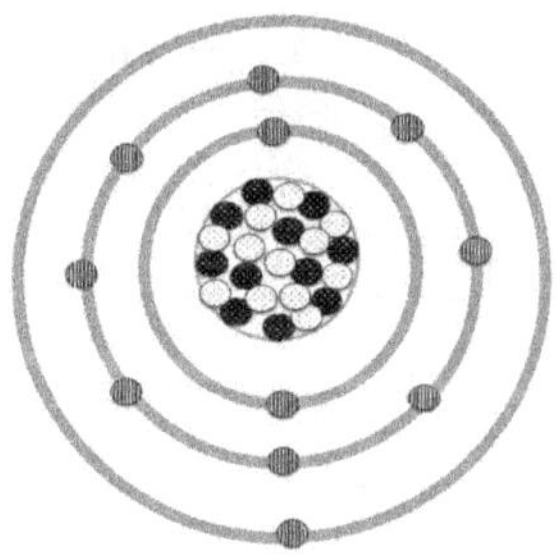

i. ● =	ii. ○ =	iii. ◍ =

(b) Identify the atoms shown below, giving their names and chemical symbols.

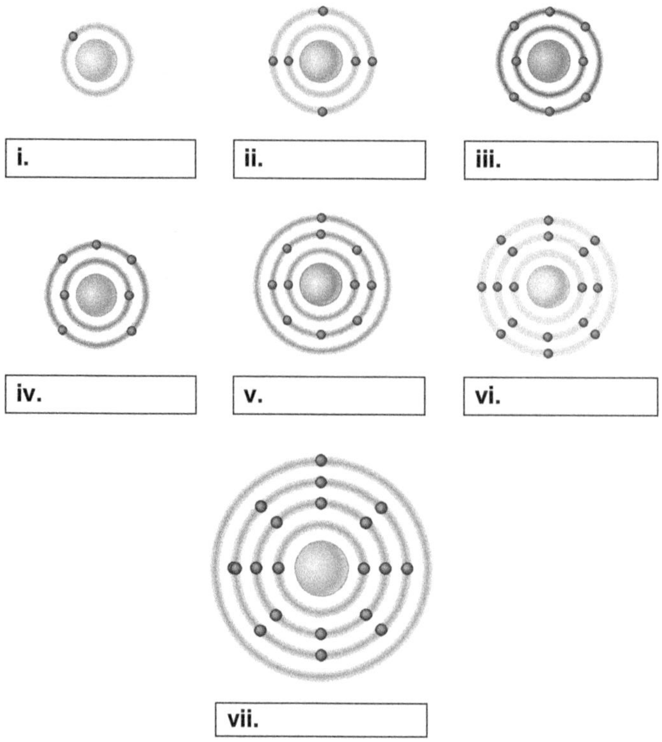

Source: Suzanne Evans (2025).

(c) Fill in the atomic numbers and mass numbers of the elements listed in the following table:

	Atomic number	**Mass number**
Hydrogen		
Carbon		
Nitrogen		
Oxygen		
Sodium		
Magnesium		
Chlorine		
Potassium		
Calcium		
Iron		
Copper		
Zinc		

4 Chemical bonding

(a) For each of these atoms, circle on the statements the number of electrons exchanged and the chemical symbol each would have on becoming an ion.

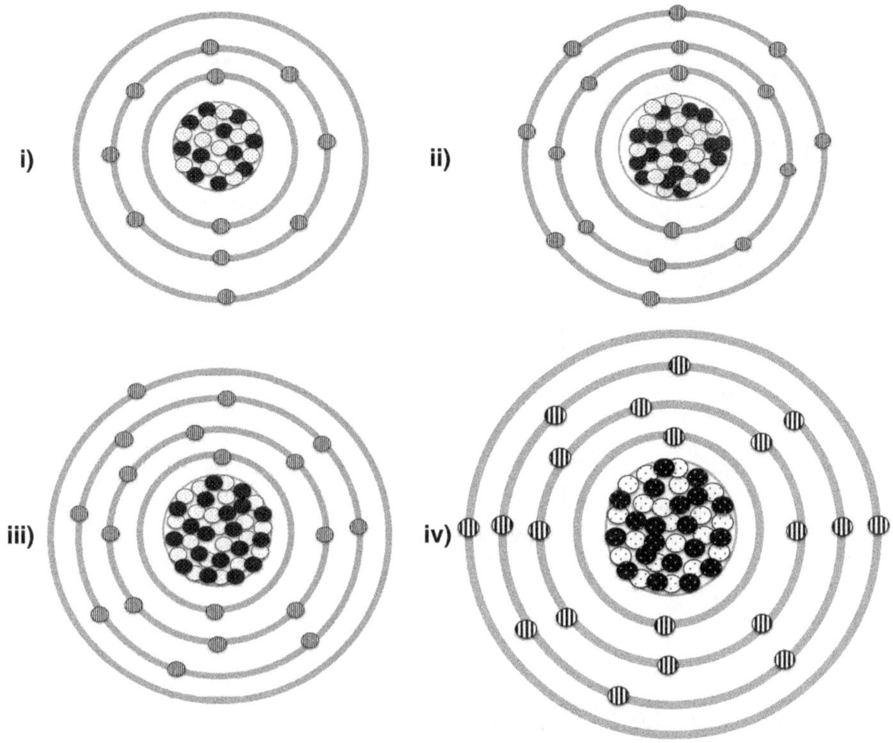

Source: Suzanne Evans (2025).

Atom i would lose/gain 1/2/3/4 electrons to become ______________

Atom ii would lose/gain 1/2/3/4 electrons to become______________

Atom iii would lose/gain 1/2/3/4 electrons to become______________

Atom iv would lose/gain 1/2/3/4 electrons to become______________

(b) Identify the following as either ionic or covalent compounds:

	Ionic or Covalent?
Sodium chloride	
Water	
Potassium chloride	
Calcium phosphate	
Oxygen (O_2)	
Organic compounds	

5 Molecular characteristics

Place a tick in the boxes below to indicate which of the molecules shown has the characteristics listed.

	Covalent molecule	Polar molecule	Contains a double bond	Contains a triple bond
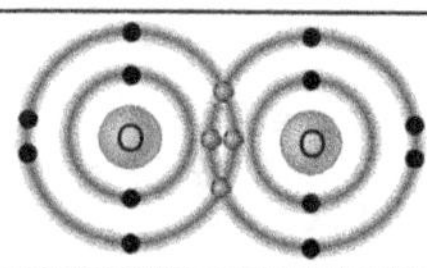				
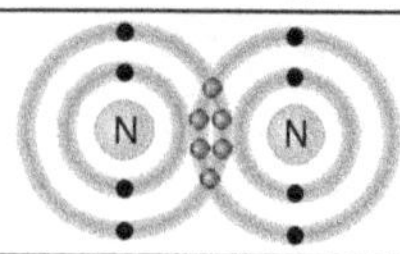				
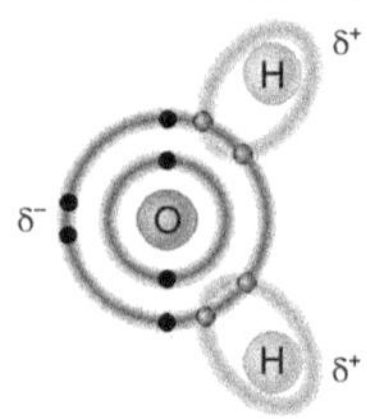				

6 Chemical characteristics

Match the pairs.

A pure substance made up of two or more elements chemically bonded together	Non-metals
They donate electrons to other atoms when reacting	Metalloids
They accept electrons from atoms when reacting	Metals
They are neither metals nor non-metals – they are sometimes referred to as semi-metals	A compound such as H_2O (water), NaCl (salt), CO_2 (carbon dioxide)

7 Chemical formulae

Fill in the names of the substances represented by the chemical formulae shown below.

Chemical formula	Name
KCl	
MgO	
NaCl	
$NaHCO_3$	
HCO_3^-	
$CaCO_3$	
CH_4	
CO	
CO_2	

8 Chemical groups

Match the compounds with their chemical groups:

Oleic acid	Disaccharide
Glucose	Polysaccharide
Acetic acid	Fatty acid
Lactose	Organic acid
Starch	Inorganic acid
Hydrochloric acid	Monosaccharide

9 Crossword

Across

1. An atom will become a/an ____________after accepting electrons
2. An atom will become a/an__________ after donating electrons
4. The majority of elements in the periodic table are _________
5. Electrons _________ the nucleus of an atom
8. A metal reacting with a non-metal will bond this way
10. Ionic compounds dissolved in water become _________ solutions
12. A reading of less than 7 on the pH scale indicates a/an ____________
13. The concentration of these ions in a solution will determine its alkalinity
14. The chemical symbol of the element iron
15. Sub-atomic particle with weight but no charge
18. When this atom donates an electron, only a proton remains

Down

1. The number of protons in the nucleus provides this
3. Atoms react chemically to increase their _________
6. Element required for healthy bones and teeth
7. Sub-atomic particle with no weight and a negative charge
9. A non-metal reacting with another non-metal will bond in this way
11. Maximum number of electrons held by 2nd and 3rd atomic shells
16. Polar covalent molecule essential for life
17. Element that forms the basis of organic compounds

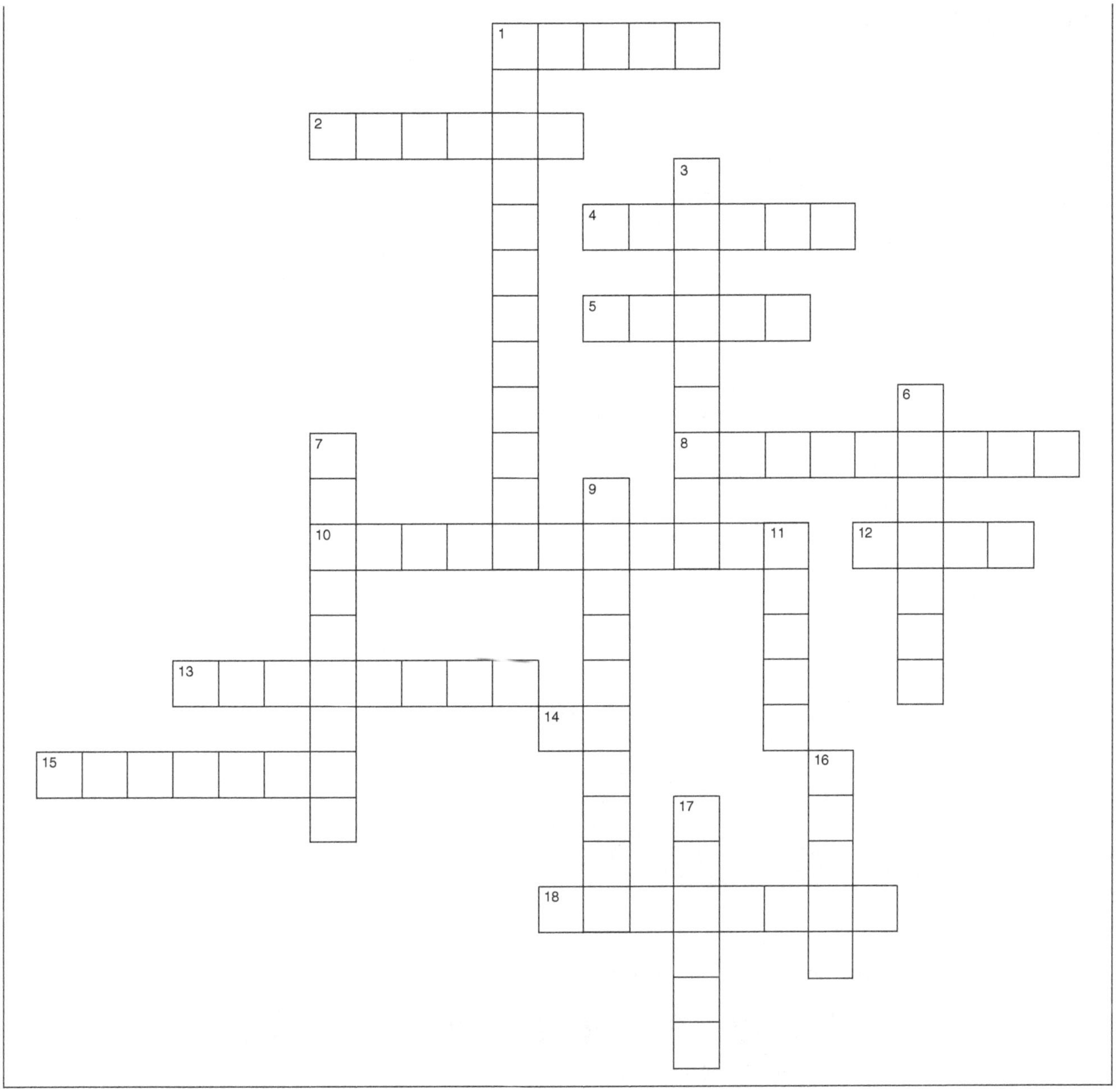
1
2
3
4
5
6
7
8
9
10
11
12
13
14
15
16
17
18

10 Electrolytes

(a) Write a "T" or "F" in each box to indicate whether the statement is true or false.

☐	An electrolyte solution conducts electricity by the movement of ions within the solution.
☐	An electrolyte solution contains free electrons which conduct the current within the solution.
☐	Electrolytes help physiological function, but are not necessary for normal function.
☐	The levels of electrolytes within the body are carefully regulated.
☐	All electrolytes are charged.

(b) Match the pairs.

The major anion outside cells	Potassium
The major cation inside cells	Bicarbonate
Vital for maintaining acid–base balance	Sodium
The most abundant cation in the body, vital for fluid balance	Chloride

(c) In the following table, show how electrolytes differ in their ability to conduct electrical current.

Type of electrolyte	Conduction of electrical current
Strong electrolytes	
Weak electrolytes	
Non-electrolytes	

11 Acids and bases

(a) Complete the following table, showing whether the substances listed are acidic, alkaline or neutral.

Substance	pH (acidic, alkaline or neutral)
Milk	
Water	
Vinegar	
Orange juice	
Coconut water	
Salt	
Ammonia	
Tea	
Oven cleaner	
Stomach contents	
Blood	

(b) Complete the boxes on the pH scale below to indicate neutral, acidic, alkaline, very acidic and very alkaline.

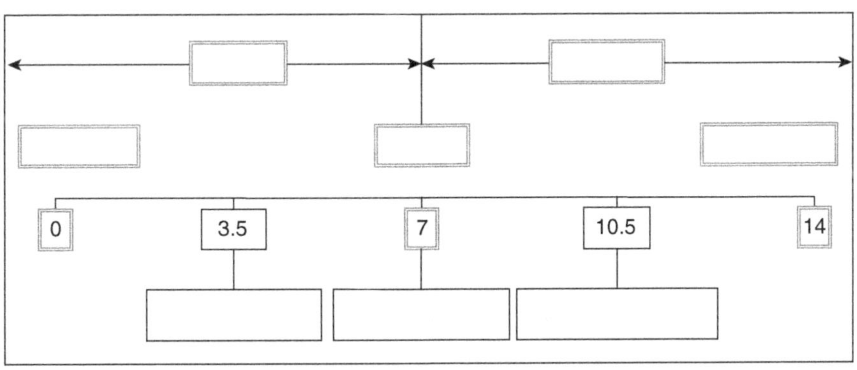

Source: Peate and Nair (2011) / Reproduced with permission of John Wiley & Sons.

(c) Match the pairs.

A strong acid means	only some of the acid molecules form ions in solution
A weak acid means	ten times the concentration of H^+ ions
A pH change of 7 to 6 means	a higher pH
More OH^- ions present in a solution mean	a lower pH
More H^+ ions present in a solution mean	nearly all the acid molecules form ions in solution

12 Crossword

Across

1. The most abundant substance in the human body
3. Anatomy is the study of ________
5. A substance that cannot be broken down by chemical means
9. The maintenance of a stable internal environment
10. A molecule with a total number of electrons greater than the total number of protons

Down

2. Releases hydroxyl ions in solution
3. Physiology is the study of ________
4. Makes up 20% of air
6. An element that conducts both heat and electricity
7. Releases hydrogen ions in solution
8. Humans are ________-based life forms

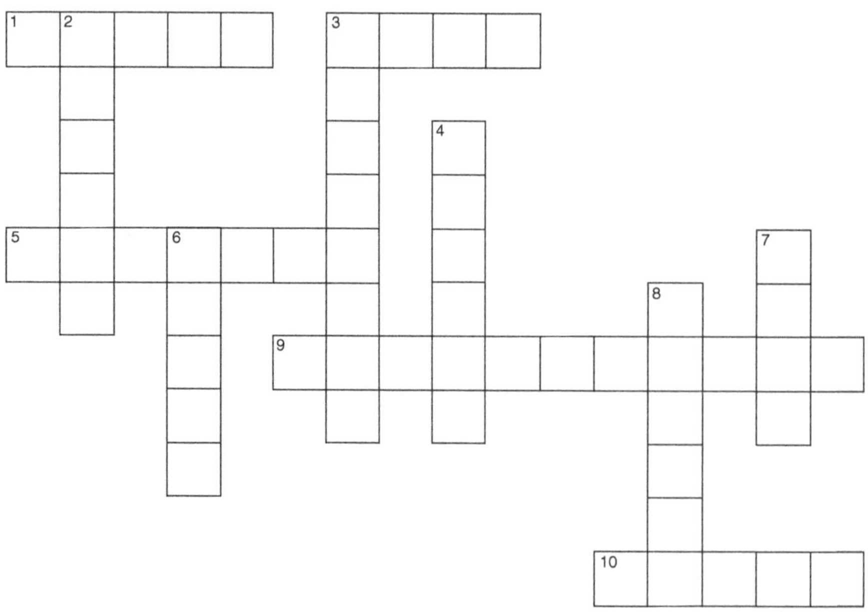

13 Homeostasis

(a) Identify the key elements of a homeostatic feedback loop in the following figure:

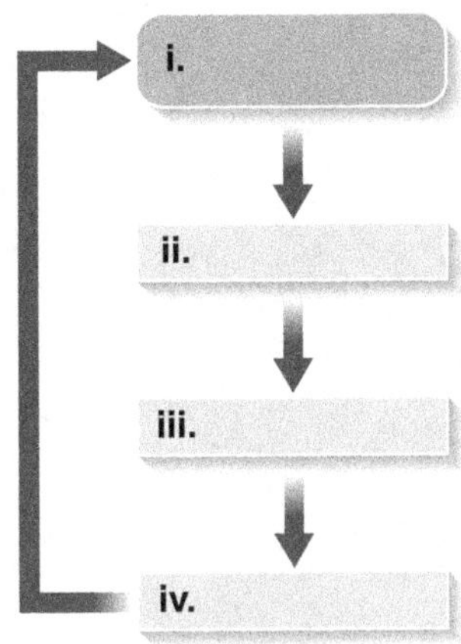

Source: Peate and Nair (2015) / Reproduced with permission of John Wiley & Sons.

(b) Using a rise in body temperature as the stimulus, complete the following diagram to show how temperature regulation is brought about:

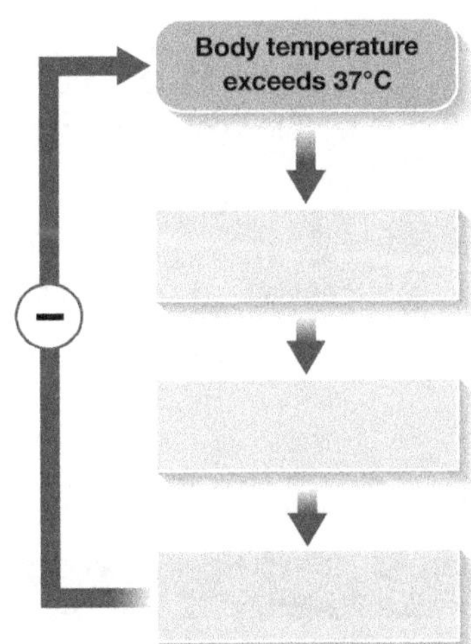

Source: Peate and Nair (2015) / Reproduced with permission of John Wiley & Sons.

(c) Fill in the key components of the following response loop:

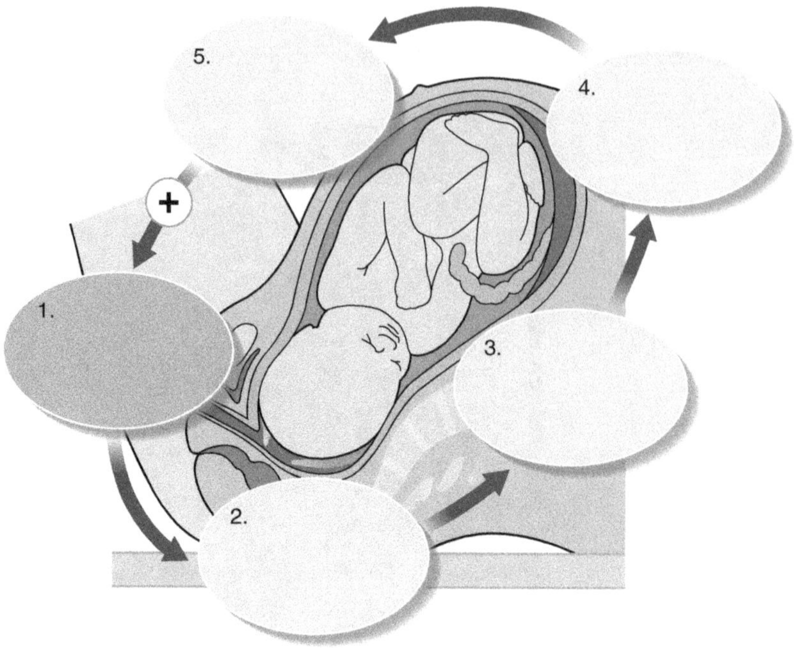

Source: Peate and Nair (2015) / Reproduced with permission of John Wiley & Sons.

(d) Match the pairs.

The control centre is	a tissue or organ that alters its activity to produce the response required
An effector is	a change in physiological state that can elicit or evoke a response in a cell, tissue or organism
Homeostasis is	the brain
A stimulus is	a reaction to a specific stimulus
A response is	maintenance of physiological variables within a certain range

(e) Time yourself to unscramble these words.

Scrambled	Answer
LAXETERN	
MEQUILIRIBU	
MASSIHOOTES	
TROFFECES	

14 Units of measurement

Complete the following tables:

Quantity	Name	Symbol
Length	metre	
Mass	kilogram	
Time	second	
Current	ampere	
Temperate	kelvin	
Amount of substance	mole	
Luminous intensity	candela	

Prefix	Symbol	Meaning	Scientific notation
tera	T		10^{12}
giga	G		10^{9}
mega	M		10^{6}
kilo	k		10^{3}
hecto	h		10^{2}
deca	da		10^{1}
deci	d		10^{-1}
centi	c		10^{-2}
milli	m		10^{-3}

1 kilogram = ________ grams
1 gram = ________ milligrams
1 milligram = ________ grams
1 microgram = ________ grams

1 litre = ________ millilitres
100 millilitre = ________ decilitres
1 millilitre = ________ microlitres

15 Crossword

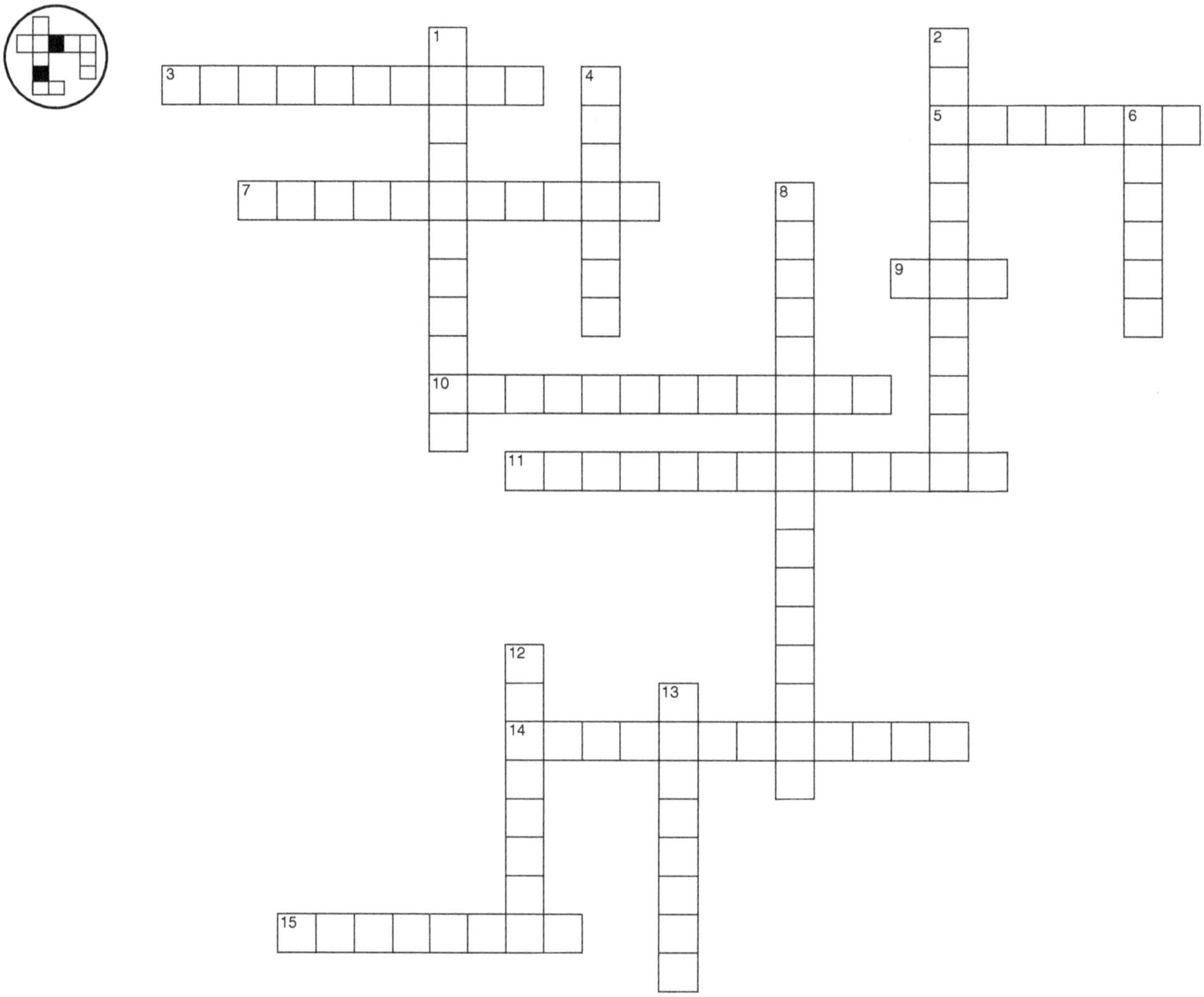

Across

3. Form long chains to make proteins
5. Milk sugar
7. A solution that passes electrical current
9. Good cholesterol
10. Three fatty acids attached to glycerol, used by cells for energy
11. Receptors that detect changes in blood pressure
14. H_2CO_3
15. A polysaccharide stored in liver and muscle cells

Down

1. Blood pH is rapidly buffered by a reaction between hydrogen ions and ______ ions
2. An acid reacts with a base to produce _____
4. Enzymes are this type of molecule
6. The most abundant electrolyte in the body
8. The secretion of insulin to reduce blood glucose is an example of________________
12. An increase in free hydrogen ions in a solution would cause the pH to ______
13. These feedback loops are inherently unstable, producing rapid, dramatic changes

16 Snap shot

Body temperature represents heat production and heat loss. If heat generated equals heat lost, the core body temperature will be stable and there will be a state of homeostasis.

(a) What are the various sites and methods used to take temperature?

(b) What are the clinical indications for temperature taking?

(c) What are the intrinsic factors that may influence temperature?

(d) Define hypothermia.

(e) Define fever.

(f) Define hyperthermia.

Multiple-choice questions

17. The ionisation of NaCl

A. is an enzymatic reaction
B. has no impact on pH
C. produces a cation (Na^+) and an anion (Cl^-)
D. causes acidosis

18. What is true of iodine and radioactive iodine?

A. They have the same atomic numbers
B. Neither has an atomic mass
C. Neither has electrons
D. Both create a biohazard

19. Which of the following is not true of sodium?

A. It is highly reactive
B. Its atoms contain more protons than electrons
C. Its ions are the main determinants of body fluid volume
D. It is an alkali metal

20. Water is:

A. a molecule
B. an aqueous solvent
C. a compound
D. All of the above

21. ATP is:

A. a buffer, adding K^+ to a solution
B. an energy-transfer molecule
C. an enzyme
D. measured by light

22. Which of the following has donated an electron?

A. ATP
B. Cl^-
C. Na^+
D. HCO_3^-

23. The building blocks of life are known as:

A. enzymes
B. proteins
C. atoms
D. All of the above

24. Which of the following carries a positive electrical charge?

A. Enzymes
B. Proteins
C. Atoms
D. Protons

25. Which of the following carries a negative electrical charge?

A. Electrons

B. Proteins

C. Atoms

D. Protons

26. What is the chemical notation for potassium chloride?

A. KCl

B. PCl

C. NaCl

D. Ca

CHAPTER 3

Cells

1 Cell types

(a) The following figure shows examples of some cells of the human body. Identify the five cell types and draw a circle around the nucleus of each cell.

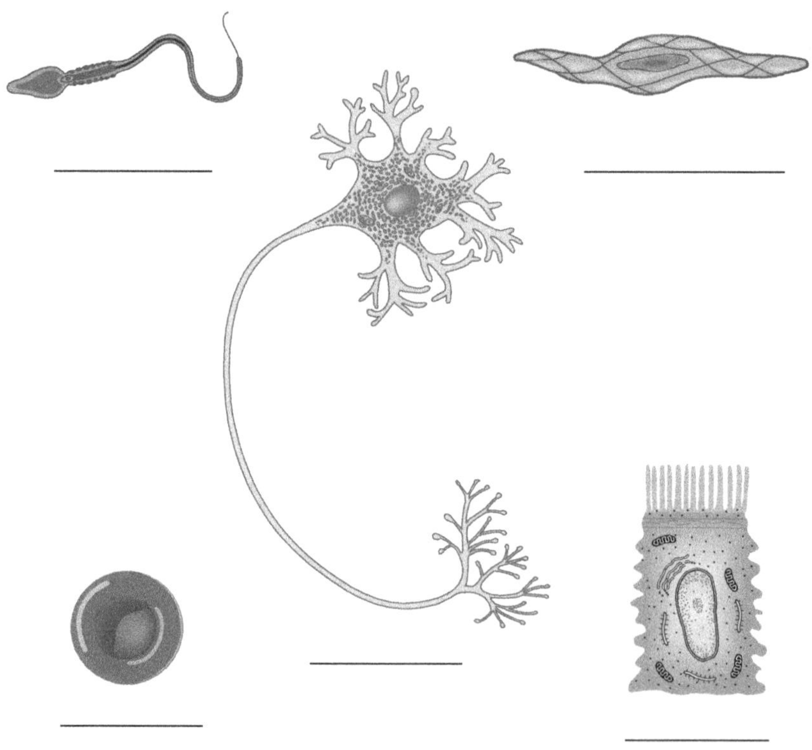

Source: Tortora and Derrickson (2005) / Reproduced with permission of John Wiley & Sons.

(b) One of the cells illustrated does not possess a nucleus. Name the cell, describe why the nucleus is missing in this case and what the consequences are for the cell.

____

____

____

____

2 Cell organelles

(a) Add the labels listed to the following figure:

- Microfilament
- Mitochondrion
- Golgi complex
- Plasma membrane
- Ribosome
- Lysosome
- Smooth endoplasmic reticulum
- Rough endoplasmic reticulum
- Flagellum
- Nucleus
- Cytoplasm

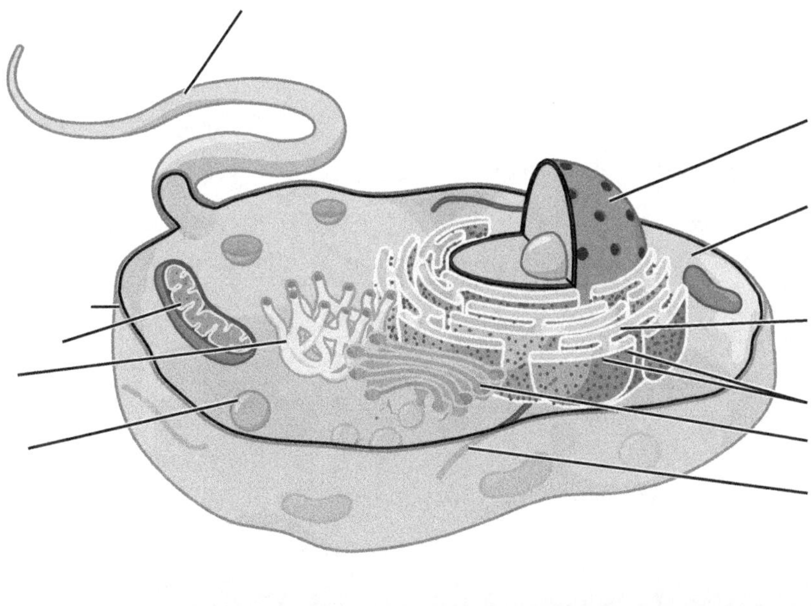

(b) Complete the following table with the cell organelles that perform each of the functions listed.

Component	Function
	Moves fluid over the cell surface
	Fluid bathing organelles
	Brace and support the cell structure
	Carry out protein transport, modification of drugs and synthesis of lipids and steroids
	Package proteins for secretion
	Digest harmful substances and faulty proteins
	Provide structural support and cell movement
	Increase cell surface area
	Holds the DNA
	Regulates movement of substances in and out of the cell
	Synthesise proteins
	Power the cell

SCRAMBLE

(c) Time yourself to unscramble these words.

Scrambled	Answer
BREMMANE	
BROOMEISS	
GIGOL YDOB	
LESSOOMY	
RONTIDOMHIONC	
CENSULU	

(d) Match the pairs.

Humans are	unicellular
Some organisms such as bacteria are	the cell
Fluid and electrolytes are constantly moved between	flagellum
The basic structural, functional and biological unit of all known living organisms is	the nucleus
To survive and reproduce, cells need	multicellular
To move around, cells use a	the intracellular and extracellular compartments

3 Cell membrane

(a) In the following figure, colour the hydrophobic and hydrophilic regions of the cell membrane phospholipids and identify:

- cytosol
- glycolipids
- glycoproteins
- lipid bilayer

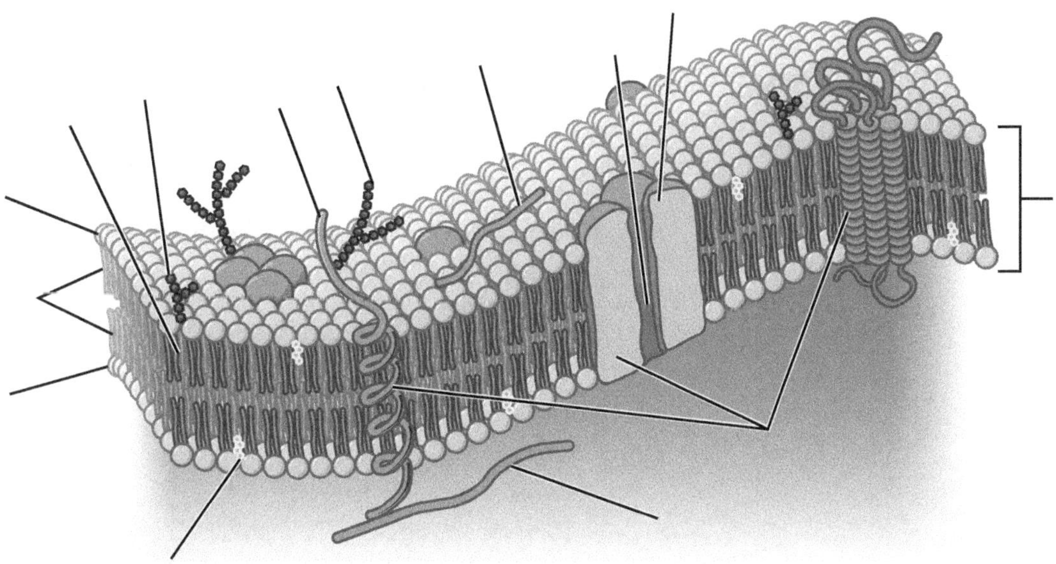

Source: Peate and Nair (2015) / Reproduced with permission of John Wiley & Sons.

(b) Match the pairs.

Cell membrane	water-loving
Cell membranes are made of	separates and protects a cell from its surrounding environment
Cell membrane thickness	self-sealing
Hydrophilic means	a double layer of lipids
Hydrophobic means	varies from 7.5 to 10 nm
The lipid bilayer is	water-hating

(c) Match the pairs.

Cytoplasm without structures is	the cytoskeleton
The cytoplasm is more than	the fatty membrane
Cell organelles are held together by	integral or peripheral proteins
The cell membrane anchors to	cytosol
Membrane proteins are categorised as	carry out metabolic reactions near the inner surface
Some protein molecules in the cell membrane	80% water

4 Energy production in the cell

(a) Identify the various parts of the mitochondrion and use colours to differentiate between them in the following figure:

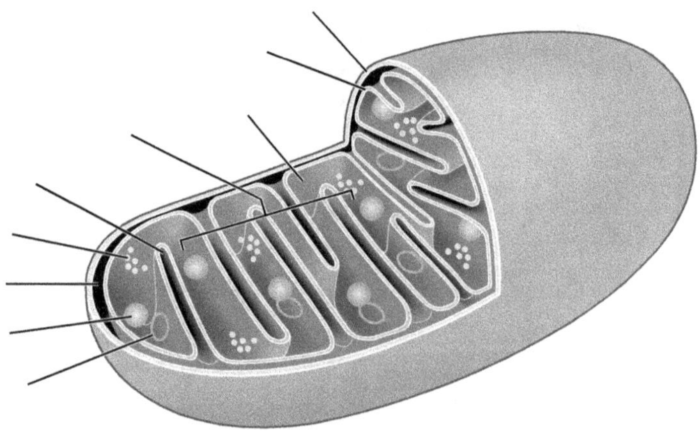

Source: Peate and Nair (2015) / Reproduced with permission of John Wiley & Sons.

(b) Match the pairs.

The cell's power producers	in the mitochondrion
The mitochondria are located	adenosine triphosphate
Cellular respiration occurs	in the cytoplasm
The mitochondria	are the mitochondria
The energy made by the mitochondria is in the form of	generate fuel for cell activity

5 Production of lipids and proteins in the cell

(a) In the following figure, identify the smooth endoplasmic reticulum, the rough endoplasmic reticulum and the ribosomes. Colour the smooth and rough endoplasmic reticulum to differentiate between them.

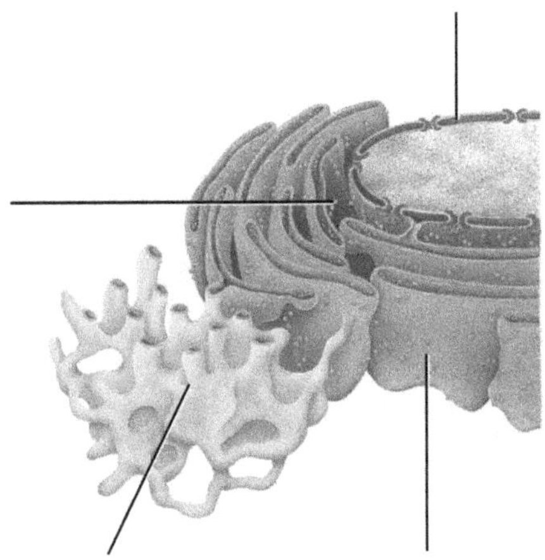

Source: Jenkins and Tortora (2013) / Reproduced with permission of John Wiley & Sons.

(b) Match the pairs.

The endoplasmic reticulum	abundant in mammalian liver and gonad cells
The endoplasmic reticulum	is a network without any ribosomes
Cells with a lot of endoplasmic reticulum	is an organelle of the cell
Rough endoplasmic reticulum	are found in the pancreas and liver
Smooth endoplasmic reticulum	has ribosomes attached to its surface
Smooth endoplasmic reticulum is	works closely with the Golgi apparatus

6 The command centre of the cell

(a) In the following figure, identify the components of the nucleus and colour in the chromatin, the nuclear pores, the nuclear envelope and the nucleolus.

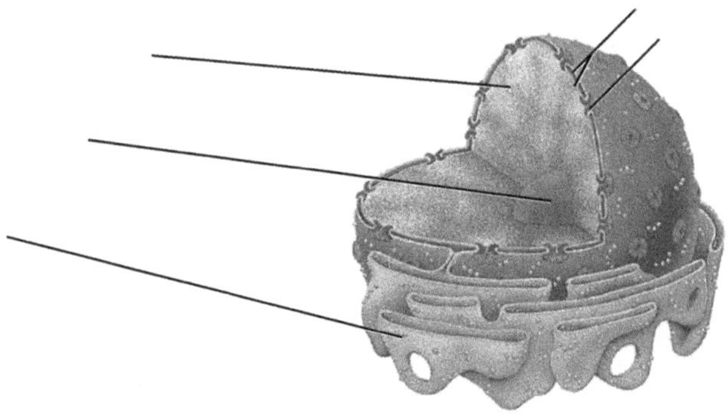

Source: Jenkins and Tortora (2013) / Reproduced with permission of John Wiley & Sons.

(b) Match the pairs.

The genetic information of cells is packaged in the form of	deoxyribonucleic acid (DNA) replication
The nucleus is a characteristic feature of	nucleolus
One of the key functions of the cell nucleus is	ribosomal subunits from proteins and ribosomal RNA (rRNA)
Inside the nucleus is the	most eukaryotic cells
There is no membrane surrounding the	nucleolus
The nucleolus makes	chromatin

7 Terminology

Look up the meanings of the prefixes and suffixes in the following terms, write them into the table and then give the meaning of the complete terms.

(a)

Hydrophilic	
Hydro- =	-philic =
Meaning:	

(b)

Lysosome	
Lyso- =	-some =
Meaning:	

(c)

Ribosome	
Ribo- =	-some =
Meaning:	

(d)

Cytoplasm	
Cyto- =	-plasm =
Meaning:	

(e)

Phagocyte	
Phago- =	-cyte =
Meaning:	

(f)

Exocytosis		
Exo- =	-cyto =	-osis =
Meaning:		

(g)

Erythrocyte	
Erythro- =	-cyte =
Meaning:	

(h)

Intracellular	
Intra- =	-cellular =
Meaning:	

8 Concentration gradients

Fill in the chemical symbols for each ion both inside and outside the cell, indicating by the size of the symbol and an arrow the concentration gradient for each. The first is completed as an example.

(a) Bicarbonate

(b) Protein

(c) Sodium

(d) Chlorine

(e) Potassium

(f) Calcium

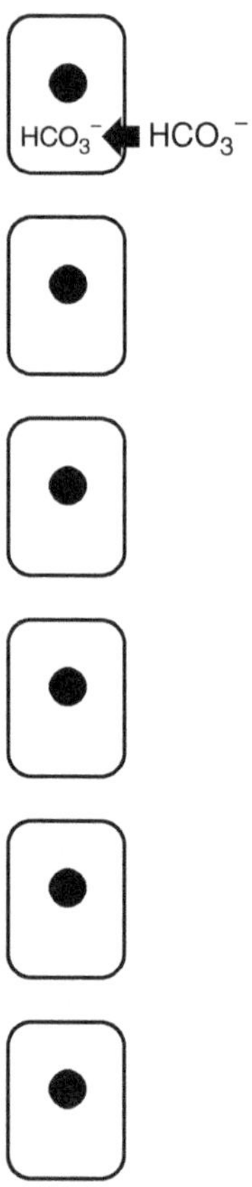

9 Regulation of electrolytes and water

Fill in the following crosswords with the names of the hormones responsible for controlling the levels of the substances listed below.

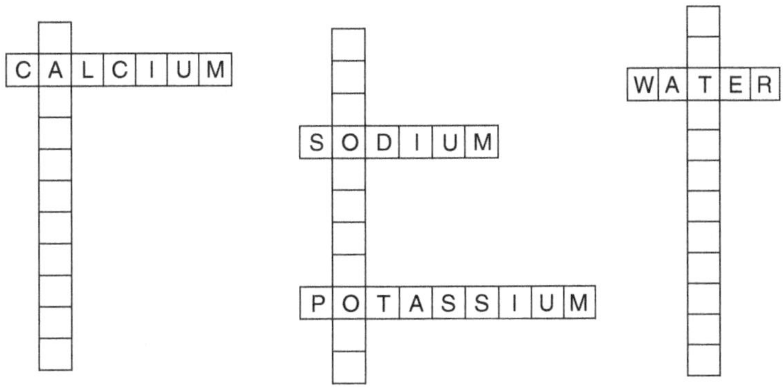

10 Snap shot

Intravenous electrolyte administration

Hypokalaemia and hyperkalaemia can be life threatening, as can other electrolyte disturbances. Some patients require electrolyte replacement, and this can be administered in a number of ways. Discuss some of the issues related to intravenous electrolyte administration.

11 Crossword

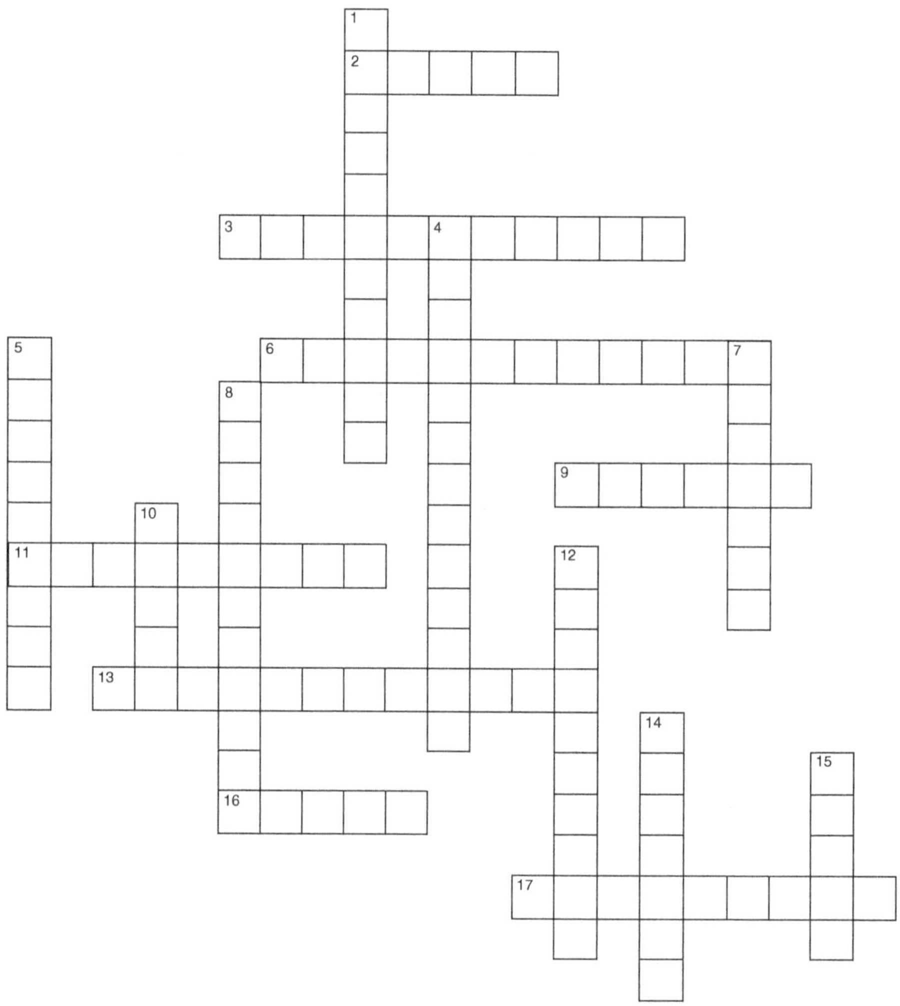

Across

2. Endoplasmic reticulum studded with ribosomes
3. Water-loving
6. Made of microtubules, it stiffens and supports the cell
9. Cells that shorten to produce movement
11. Engulf and destroy worn-out organelles or foreign particles in the cell
13. Energy-producing sites of the cell
16. On the outer surface of the cell, where they move to 'waft' substances around
17. Responsible for making proteins in a cell

Down

1. Microorganisms lacking a membrane-bound nucleus
4. Fatty molecules forming the cell membrane
5. Structure that allows a sperm cell to swim
7. Location of the cell's genetic material
8. Water-hating
10. Packages proteins for secretion
12. Organisms made of cells with a membrane-bound nucleus
14. Cells specialised to communicate using electrical signals
15. The main constituent of cytoplasm

12 Spot the errors

Find and correct the errors in the following passage:

All living things are made up of many cells, which means they are multicellular. Cells are of many different types, specialised for certain functions and containing different organelles, depending on their particular function. Some genetic material, in the form of DNA, is carried by all cells, but only sperm and egg cells carry a complete set of a person's DNA, as they are involved in reproducing a new individual. Other cells just contain the DNA they require to do their particular function. This is why only certain cells can be cloned.

Multiple-choice questions

13. What is the spherical organelle that contains the genetic material?
- A. Ribosomes
- B. Mitochondria
- C. Nucleus
- D. Enzyme

14. What is protoplasm found inside the nucleus known as?
- A. Riboflavin
- B. Cytoplasm
- C. Mitochondria
- D. Nucleoplasm

15. Which of the following is a passive process?
- A. The movement of sodium ions out of the cell against their concentration gradient
- B. The movement of potassium ions into the cell by Na^+/K^+ ATP-ase
- C. The movement of potassium out of the cell down its concentration gradient
- D. None of the above

16. For osmosis to occur, a membrane must be:
- A. fully permeable to all molecules
- B. non-expandable
- C. composed of a double layer of lipid molecules
- D. permeable to some molecules but not others

17. When administering a fluid intravenously, to ensure no damage to cells, the fluid must be:
- A. hypotonic
- B. isotopic
- C. hyperosmolar
- D. isotonic

18. Some red blood cells are placed in a solution of solutes to which the membrane is impermeable. The concentration of these solutes is higher than the intracellular solute concentration. Which of the following will occur as a result?

A. There would be no movement of water between the inside and outside of the cells
B. There would be movement of water out of the cell, causing cell shrinkage
C. There would be movement into the cell, causing swelling
D. None of the above would occur

19. What would be the effect on cells of a substance that stops the Na^+/K^+ pump?

A. Na^+ concentration inside the cell would increase, while K^+ concentration inside the cell would decrease
B. Na^+ concentration inside the cell would decrease, while K^+ concentration inside the cell would increase
C. Na^+ concentration inside the cell would remain the same, while K^+ concentration inside the cell would increase
D. None of the above would occur

20. Centrioles:

A. have no role to play in human survival
B. are only present in certain circumstances
C. are only associated with cellular destruction
D. are associated with cellular reproduction

21. Microfilaments:

A. only provide structural support
B. only provide for cell movement
C. provide structural support and cell movement
D. provide cellular nutrition

22. Hydrophilic means:

A. water-loving
B. water-hating
C. water-loving and water-hating
D. self-healing

23. Which of the following is an isotonic solution?

A. 0.9% NaCl solution
B. 9% NaCl solution
C. 200 mM $MgCl_2$ solution
D. 400 mM NaCl solution

24. Which of the following is a passive form of transport, requiring no input of energy?

A. Osmosis
B. Exocytosis
C. Phagocytosis
D. All of the above

25. A cell without a nucleus would be unable to:

A. create ATP
B. respire
C. synthesise proteins
D. move

CHAPTER 4

Genetics

1 Deoxyribonucleic acid (DNA)

(a) Label the chemical components of the DNA double helix on the following figure:

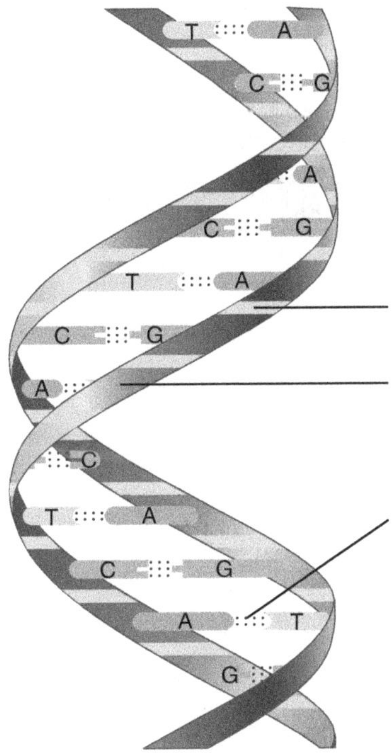

Source: Tortora and Derrickson (2014) / Reproduced with permission of John Wiley & Sons.

(b) Fill in the bases that will pair with each of the bases on the DNA base sequence shown below.

A	G	C	A	G	G	A	T	T
↓	↓	↓	↓	↓	↓	↓	↓	↓

(c) Match the pairs.

Genes	Thymine
The base that binds with adenine	The sides of the DNA ‘ladder’
Chain of alternating deoxyribose and phosphate groups	Hydrogen
The base that binds with guanine	Nucleotide
The type of bond that holds the bases together	Sections of DNA
A molecule of deoxyribose, phosphate and a base bonded together	Cytosine

(d) Time yourself to unscramble these words.

Scrambled	Unscrambled
SEENITGC	
DENISECLOUT	
ELIXH	
HYMINTE	
NINAGUE	

2 Chromosomes

(a) On the following diagram, colour in and label the following:

- DNA double helix
- Histones
- Nucleosome
- Chromatids
- Centromere

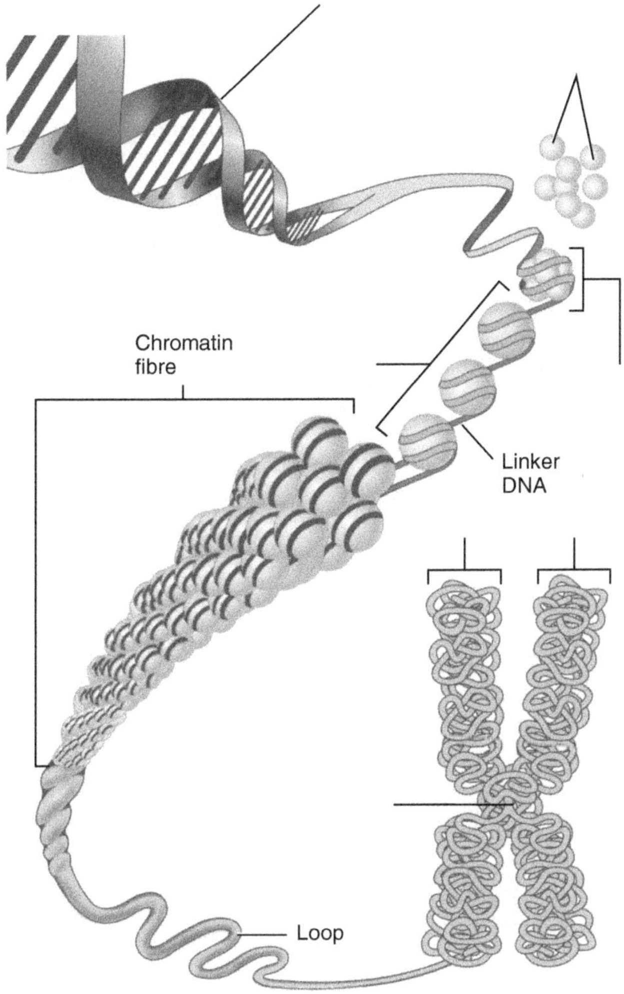

Source: Tortora and Derrickson (2009) / Reproduced with permission of John Wiley & Sons.

(b) Spot the errors.

Find and correct the errors in the following paragraph:

Chromosomes are long strings of DNA wrapped around special proteins known as nucleotides and wound up tightly enough to make them compact. Not only is this important as it protects the DNA, but it also allows the chromosomes to fit into the cytoplasm of the cells. Every one of your cells, with the exception of white blood cells, contains a complete set of your chromosomes. The chromosomes are visible with a light microscope at all times and are usually lined up along the equator of the cell.

(c) Match the pairs.

Chromosomes are thread-like structures of DNA	requires the process of meiosis
Each chromosome is made of	and unwind (decondense), losing their chromosome shape once it is completed
Normal growth and function	a double helix of DNA wrapped around some globular proteins and tightly coiled
Chromosomes are condensed for cell division	the centromere
Those with Down syndrome have	found inside the nucleus of a cell
Sexual reproduction	requires mitosis
The narrow region where two chromatids come together is	three copies of chromosome 21

(d) Complete the following puzzle using the same suffix in each term:

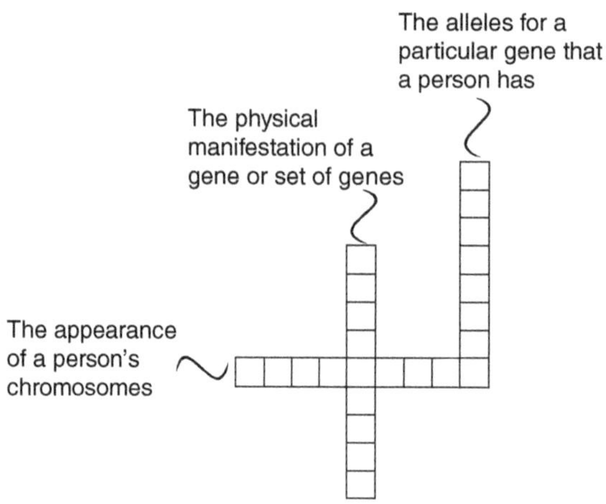

3 Ribonucleic acid (RNA)

(a) Colour in and name the bases on the figure below.

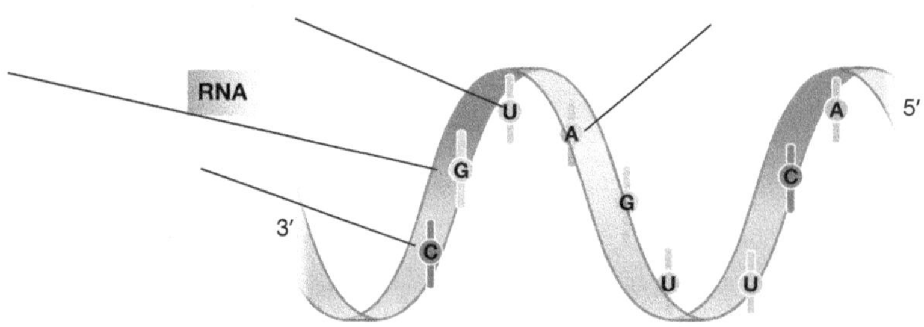

Source: Peate and Nair (2011) / Reproduced with permission of John Wiley & Sons.

(b) List the three types of RNA and their functions.

____

____

____

____

____

____

(c) Label the following diagram showing the synthesis of proteins within the ribosome.

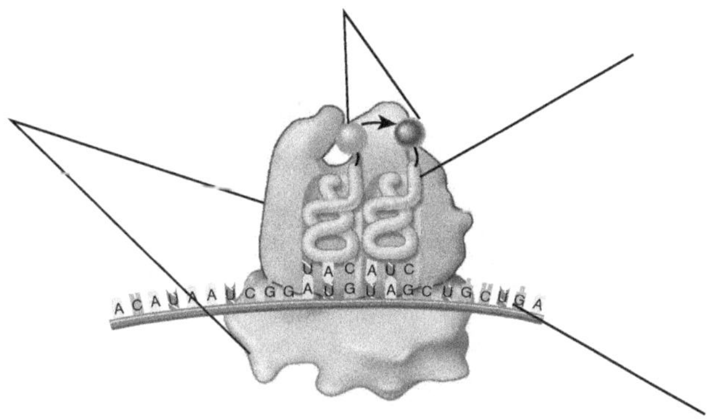

Source: Tortora and Derrickson (2009) / Reproduced with permission of John Wiley & Sons.

(d) Match the pairs.

RNA	Takes the transcripted gene code out of the nucleus into the cytoplasm
Transfer RNA (tRNA)	Makes up part of both ribosomal subunits
Messenger RNA (mRNA)	Consists of a single strand of nucleotides
Ribosomal RNA (rRNA)	Carries a base triplet and the amino acid for which it encodes

4 Transcription

(a) Fill in the bases on mRNA that will pair with each of the bases on the DNA base sequence shown here:

A	G	C	A	G	G	A	T	T	DNA
↓	↓	↓	↓	↓	↓	↓	↓	↓	
									mRNA

5 DNA replication

(a) On the following diagram, colour in the two old DNA strands and then the two new strands, then label the hydrogen bond, a phosphate group and a deoxyribose sugar and fill in the missing bases on the new strands:

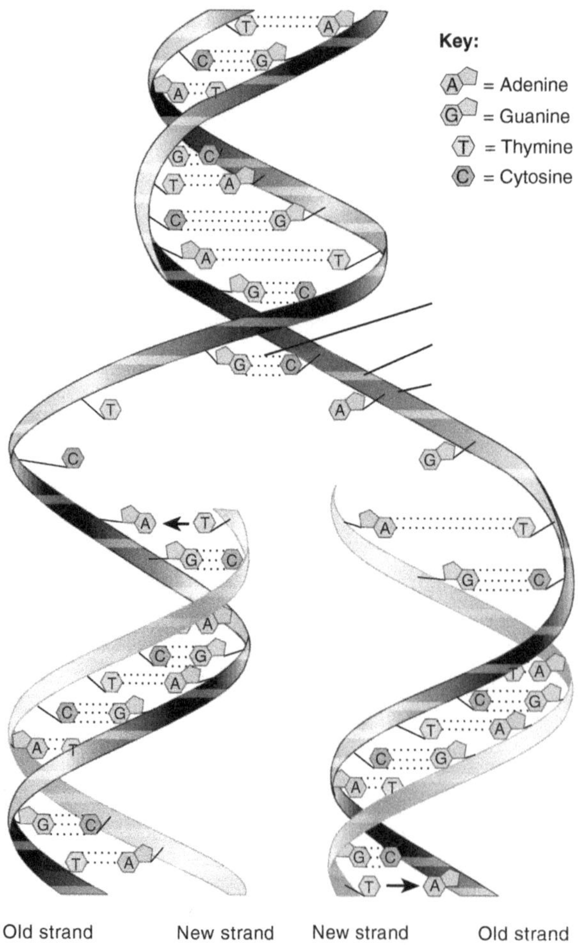

Source: Tortora and Derrickson (2009) / Reproduced with permission of John Wiley & Sons.

(b) Circle the correct options in the following sentence:

DNA replication results in 1 / 2 DNA molecule / molecules, each molecule containing 0 / 1 / 2 original strand / strands and 0 / 1 / 2 new strand / strands.

6 Protein synthesis

(a) Match the pairs.

In order to synthesise a protein	the RNA attaches to a ribosome where the information is converted into a corresponding sequence of amino acids, forming a new protein molecule
The gene is then copied	onto mRNA
Messenger RNA	connects the sequence of bases (in triplets) to specific amino acids
In the ribosome	the strands of DNA on the chromosome containing the gene separate at the point where the gene is located, exposing the base sequence
During translation	carries the copied gene sequence to the ribosome
Transfer RNA	the genetic information encoded on mRNA is translated to produce a new protein

(b) Select one term from the boxes shown below to fill each of the gaps in the text.

Nucleus | Ribose | Translation | Ribosome

Replication | Transcription | Codon | Deoxyribose

The site of translation is the ____________________.

The sugar found in the backbone of mRNA is ____________________.

The first step in cell division is ____________________.

The first step in protein synthesis is ____________________.

The sugar found in the backbone of DNA is ____________________.

The site of transcription is the ____________________.

tRNA brings amino acids to the ribosome during ____________________.

The sequence of three nucleotides specifying an amino acid is the ____________________.

7 Mitosis and Meiosis

Place a tick in the columns to show which characteristics belong to each process.

	Mitosis	Meiosis
The process begins with the duplication of the chromosomes		
Chromosomes line up individually across the middle of the cell		
Corresponding pairs of chromosomes align together across the middle of the cell		
Chromosome pairs separate and migrate to opposite ends of the cell		
Chromatids pull apart and migrate to opposite ends of the cell		
The cell divides to produce two diploid daughter cells		
The cell divides to produce two haploid daughter cells		
The new cells divide again to produce four haploid daughter cells		

8 Meiosis

(a) Identify the two main stages of meiosis.

Stage of meiosis	Name
1.	
2.	

(b) Identify the four subdivided stages associated with meiosis I.

Stage of meiosis I	Name
1.	
2.	
3.	
4.	

(c) Identify the four stages associated with meiosis II.

Stage of meiosis II	Name
1.	
2.	
3.	
4.	

(d) On the following diagram, colour in the DNA of each chromosome to show the process of crossing over:

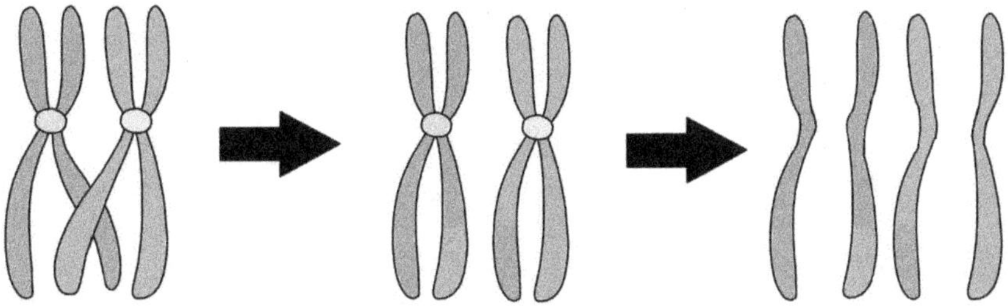

(e) The process and stages of mitosis are identical to which major stage of meiosis?

____

(f) Match the pairs.

During metaphase in meiosis I	further divide again
During metaphase in mitosis	In the sex cells (ova and sperm)
Meiosis occurs	Chromosome pairs line up along the cell equator
In meiosis II both of the cells produced in meiosis I	DNA replication occurs in the diploid cells
During the interphase that precedes meiosis I	Chromosomes line up individually along the cell equator

9 Snap shot – Cystic fibrosis

This is a well-known disease that is inherited as an autosomal recessive disorder and affects 1 in 2500 children born in the United Kingdom. A faulty gene causes the condition. The gene is transmitted as an autosomal recessive disorder whereby both parents carry the faulty gene and there is a 1 in 4 chance of each pregnancy leading to a child with cystic fibrosis.

On the following diagram, label the body systems predominantly affected by cystic fibrosis.

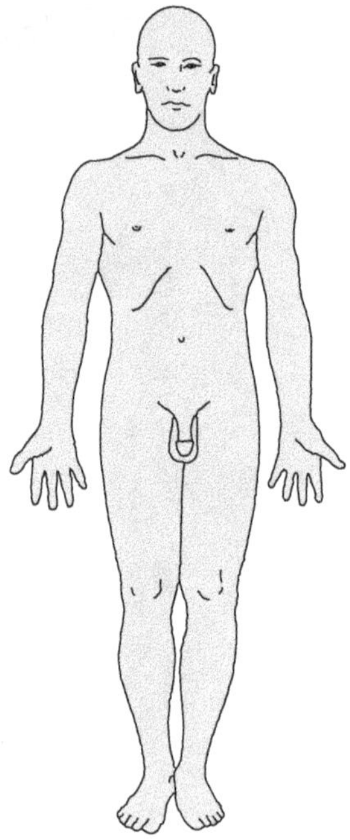

10 Inheritance

Mary has an inherited form of kidney disease. The allele that causes the disease is autosomal recessive (a).

(a) What does autosomal mean? ____________________

(b) What does recessive mean? ____________________

(c) Mary's partner has two normal alleles (A). Fill in the Punnett square shown here and write in the probability that any children of Mary and her partner will also have the disease:
Probability of children inheriting the disease =

	a	a
A		
A		

(d) What would the risk of children inheriting the disease be if Mary's partner was a carrier of the abnormal allele (a)? Use the following Punnett square.
Probability of children inheriting the disease =

11 Genetic conditions

(a) Match the pairs.

Three copies of chromosome 21	results in Turner syndrome
An abnormal X-linked recessive gene	results in Down syndrome
A missing or partial X chromosome in females	results in Klinefelter syndrome
An additional X chromosome in males	is expressed in males since there is no paired chromosome to override them

(b) Make notes about the characteristics of Down, Turner and Klinefelter syndromes.

12 Crossword

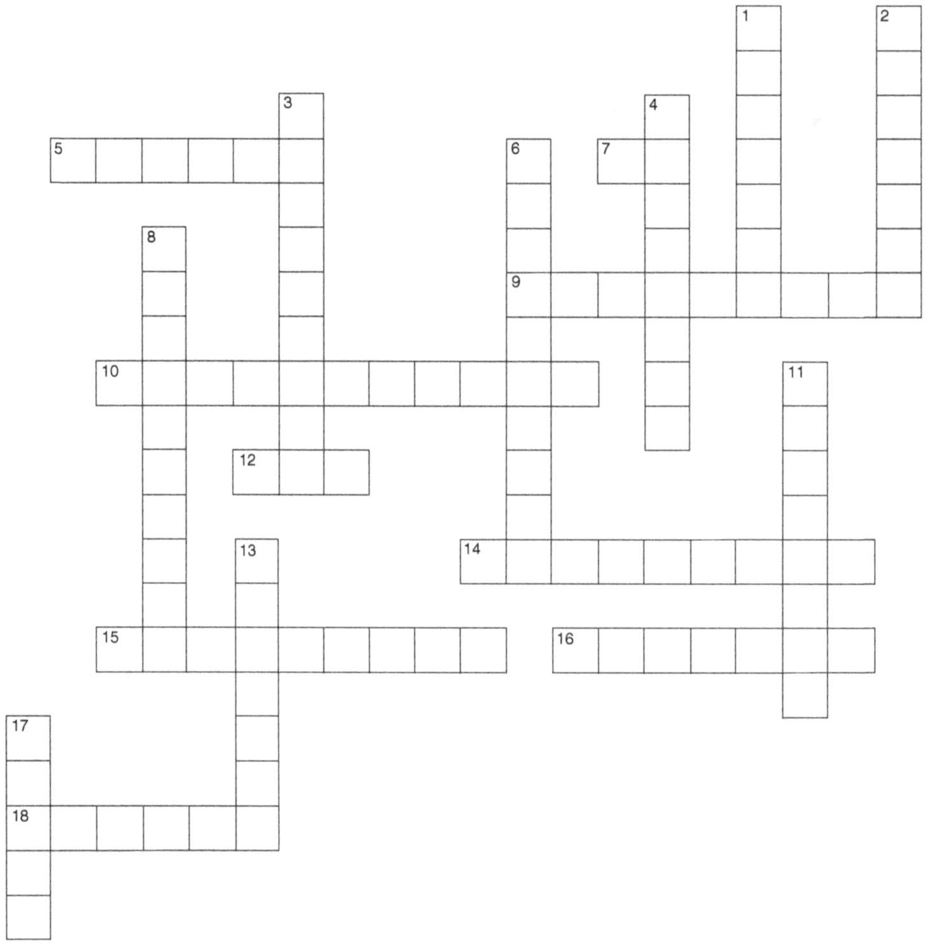

Across

5. An organism's complete set of genetic material

7. Sex chromosomes in males

9. Short, repeating DNA sequences at the ends of chromosomes that protect them during the process of replication

10. The process by which a copy of the cell's DNA is made prior to cell division

12. Number of strands in an RNA molecule

14. Phase of mitosis when chromosomes line up along the equator of the cell

15. A person needs two of these alleles for the gene to be expressed

16. An inherited disorder that is recessive and usually carried by females and expressed by males

18. The sugar in RNA

Down

1. Spool-like protein structure that DNA is tightly wrapped around

2. Process by which the nucleus of a cell divides to create two new nuclei, each containing an identical copy of DNA

3. Type of inheritance in which alleles can be recessive or dominant

4. The bases are joined by this type of bonding

6. The constricted region of linear chromosomes

8. The resting period of a cell

11. Type of RNA that carries an amino acid to the ribosomes and matches it with a specific codon

13. Thymine always pairs with this

17. There are __________ different types of RNA in a cell

Multiple-choice questions

13. Approximately how many genes does each cell in the human body contain?
- A. 2000–3000 genes
- B. 200–300 genes
- C. 250 000–350 000 genes
- D. 25 000–35 000 genes

14. What is a gene?
- A. A section of deoxyribonucleic acid coding for a particular protein
- B. A chromatid, one half of a chromosome
- C. A section of ribonucleic acid with a triplet of bases
- D. None of the above

15. What does guanine always pair with?
- A. Adenine
- B. Cytosine
- C. Uracil
- D. Thymine

16. What is a nucleotide?
- A. A molecule consisting of a base and a phosphate group
- B. A molecule consisting of a base (either adenine, thymine, guanine or cytosine)
- C. A molecule consisting of deoxyribose, phosphate and base groups
- D. A molecule consisting of deoxyribose and phosphate groups

17. In DNA, which base pairs with adenine?
- A. Cytosine
- B. Guanine
- C. Thymine
- D. Uracil

18. How many chromosomes do human body cells have?
- A. 4 chromosomes
- B. 6 chromosomes
- C. 46 chromosomes
- D. 460 chromosomes

19. A person's outward appearance is their:
- A. genotype
- B. chromosomal complement
- C. allele type
- D. phenotype

20. What do ribosomes consist of?
- A. Two parts, a large subunit and a small subunit
- B. Three parts, a large subunit and a small subunit
- C. Two parts, two large subunit and a small subunit
- D. Two parts, a large subunit and three small subunits

21. A recessive allele:

A. is always expressed

B. is only expressed when a person has two copies

C. is only expressed in males

D. is only carried by females

22. A person has a disease-causing dominant allele. The person's partner does not have the disease. What is the chance that the disease will be passed on to any children they have?

A. 25%

B. 50%

C. 75%

D. 100%

CHAPTER 5

Tissues

1 Major tissue types

Fill in the major tissue types against the following descriptions:

(a) ________________ tissue consists of specialised cells in an extracellular matrix.

(b) __________________ consists of sheets of cells, either single or multilayered.

(c) __________________ and ________________ tissue consists of electrically excitable cells.

2 Epithelial tissue

(a) Identify the simple, stratified and pseudostratified epithelia in the following diagram and colour and identify the squamous, cuboidal and columnar cells.

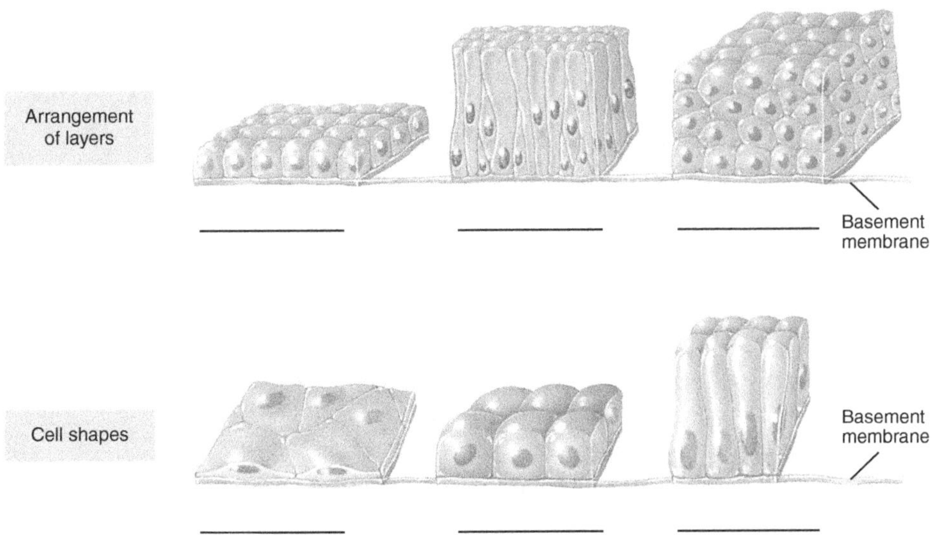

Source: Tortora and Derrickson (2009) / Reproduced with permission of John Wiley & Sons.

(b) Match the pairs.

The overall function of the epithelium is	the cells are closely packed
Epithelial tissue is classified by	coverings of external and internal surfaces, hollow organs, tubes and vessels
In epithelia there is usually	a basement membrane on which the cells lie
The intracellular substance in epithelia is minimal and	to provide protective coverings, linings and glands
Epithelial tissue may be	shape and depth
Epithelial tissue is located in	simple, stratified or glandular

3 Time yourself to unscramble these words

Scrambled	Unscrambled
DSLANG	
SUESIT	
NAMEBERM	
GROANS	
FAIRTSTIED	
CURATEINLLILAR	
VEINCONECT	
KEELSLAT	

4 Connective tissue

(a) Briefly describe the roles of the connective tissue cells listed in the following table:

Cell	Role
Adipocytes	
Primary blast cells	
Macrophages	
Plasma cells	
Mast cells	
Leukocytes	

(b) Label the following figure and colour in the nerve and blood vessel, and use colour to differentiate between the connective tissue and the epithelium.

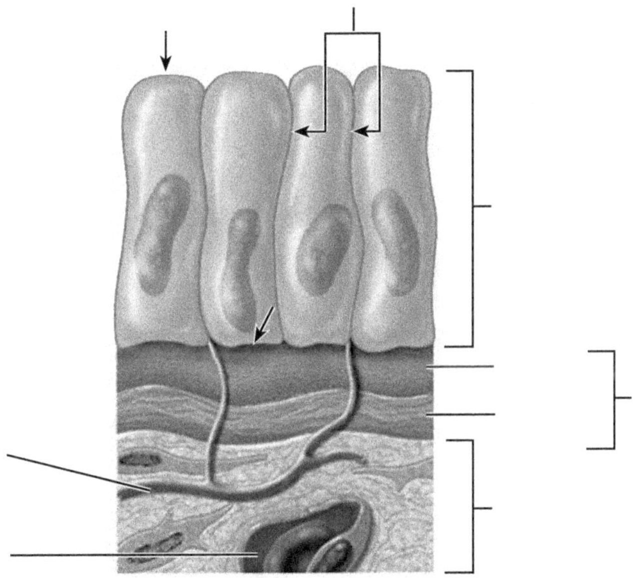

Source: Tortora and Derrickson (2009) / Reproduced with permission of John Wiley & Sons.

(c) Match the pairs.

Connective tissue	secrete substances that form the extracellular matrix
Connective tissues that stretch and recoil contain	support, binding, protection, insulation
Connective tissues with strength and resilience contain	elastin fibres
The cells of connective tissue	is not present on body surfaces
Atypical connective tissues are	collagen fibres
Connective tissue provides	lymph and blood

5 Membranes

Name the type of membrane found in each of the pictured locations.

(a) ________________ membrane

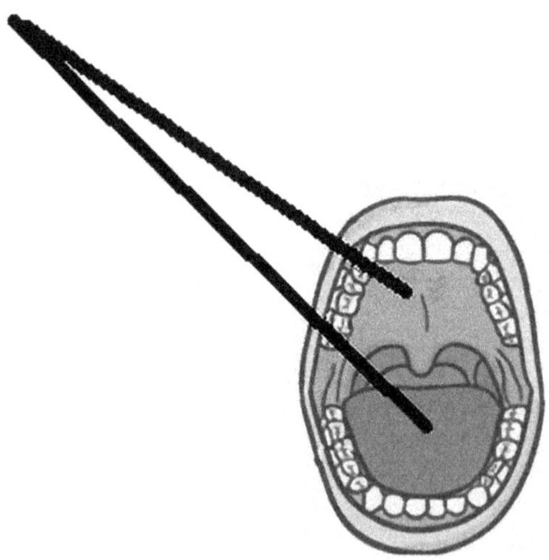

(b) ________________ membrane

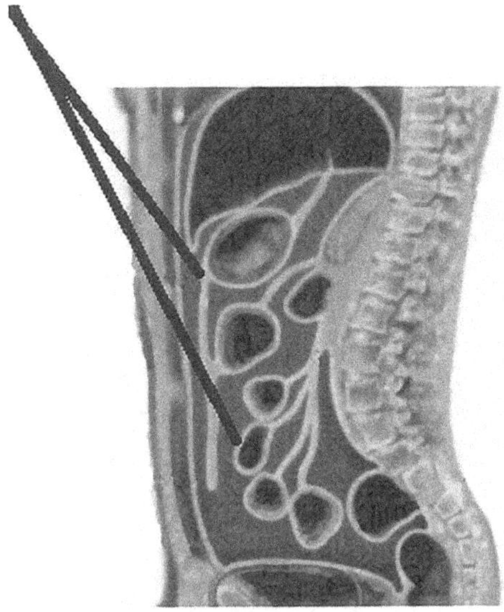

(c) ________________ membrane

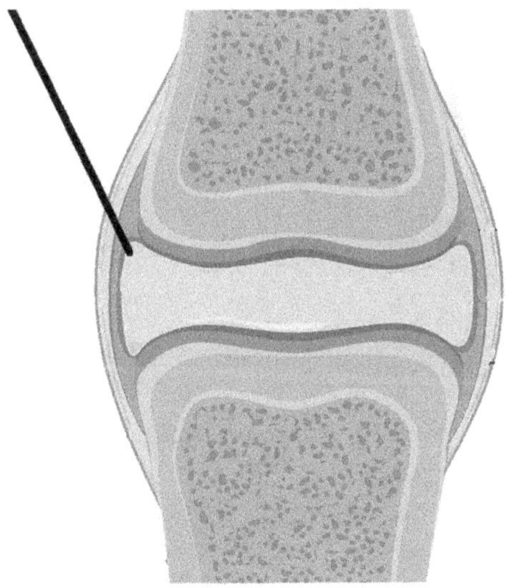

(d) ________________ membrane

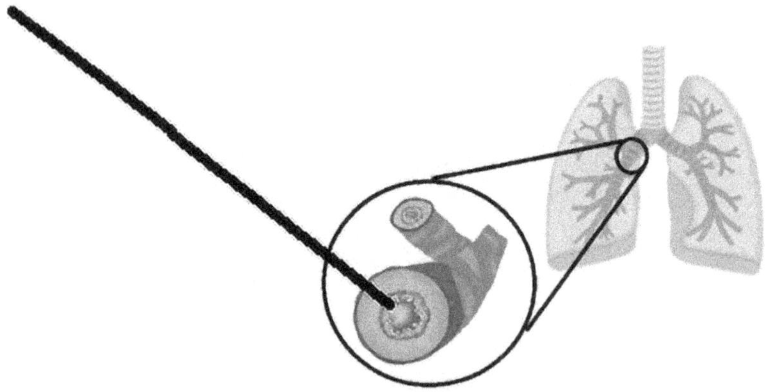

6 Nervous tissue

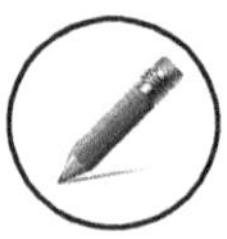

(a) Label the following figure:

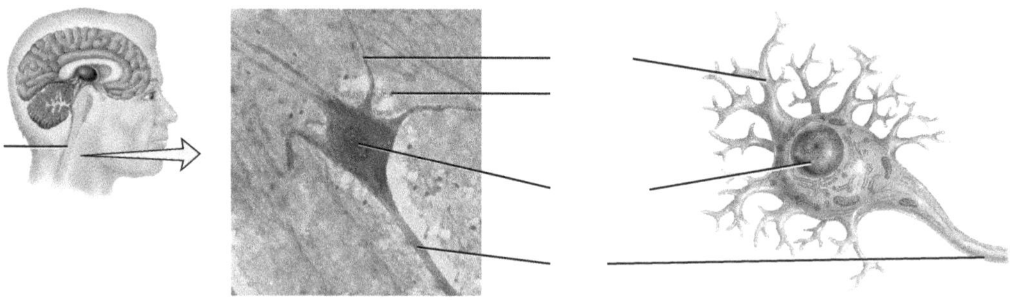

Source: Tortora and Derrickson (2009) / Reproduced with permission of John Wiley & Sons.

(b) Match the pairs.

The function of the nervous tissue is	at a synapse
Nervous tissue is composed of	neurones and glial cells
The neuroglial cells	initiate, receive, conduct and transmit information
The neurones	to receive and transmit neural impulses
Axons frequently terminate	support the neurones

7 Muscle

(a) Label the following diagram:

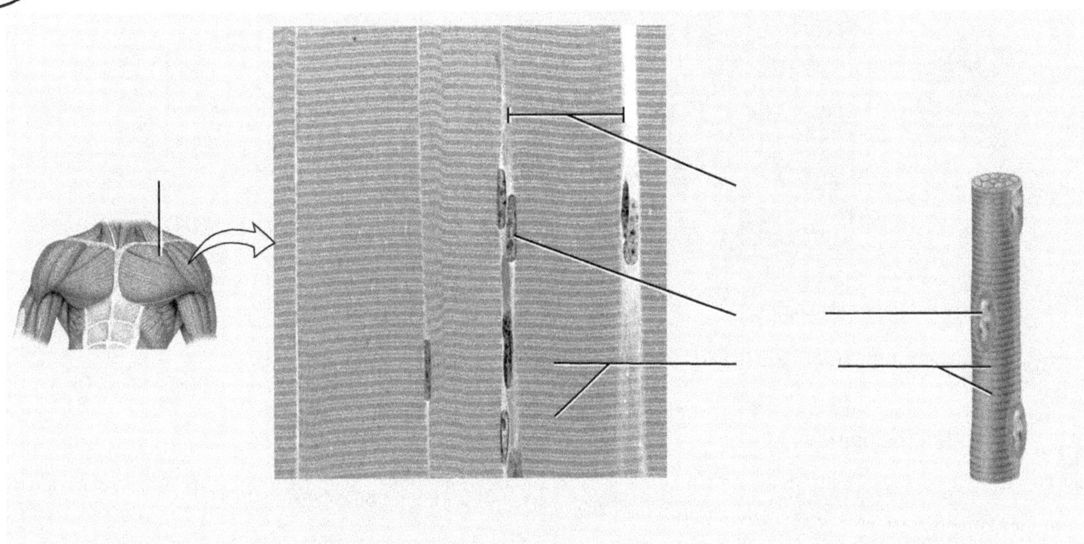

Source: Tortora and Derrickson (2009) / Reproduced with permission of John Wiley & Sons.

(b) Match the pairs.

Skeletal muscle is found	by tendons
Skeletal muscle is also known as	actively contract to generate movement
Muscle is composed of cells that	long muscle fibres
Muscle tissue contains	protective functions
Skeletal muscle also has	striated muscle
Skeletal muscle is attached to bone	adjacent to the skeleton

(c) Label the following diagram:

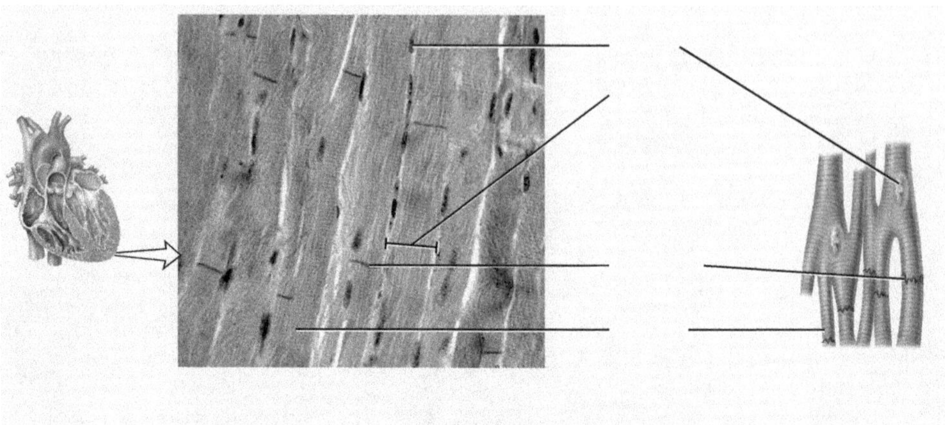

Source: Tortora and Derrickson (2009) / Reproduced with permission of John Wiley & Sons.

(d) Match the pairs.

Cardiac muscle fibres are	under voluntary control
Both cardiac and skeletal muscles are	multinucleate
Cardiac muscle is not	run the full length of the muscle
Skeletal muscle fibres are	striated
Skeletal muscle fibres	Connected end to end and branched

(e) Label the following diagram:

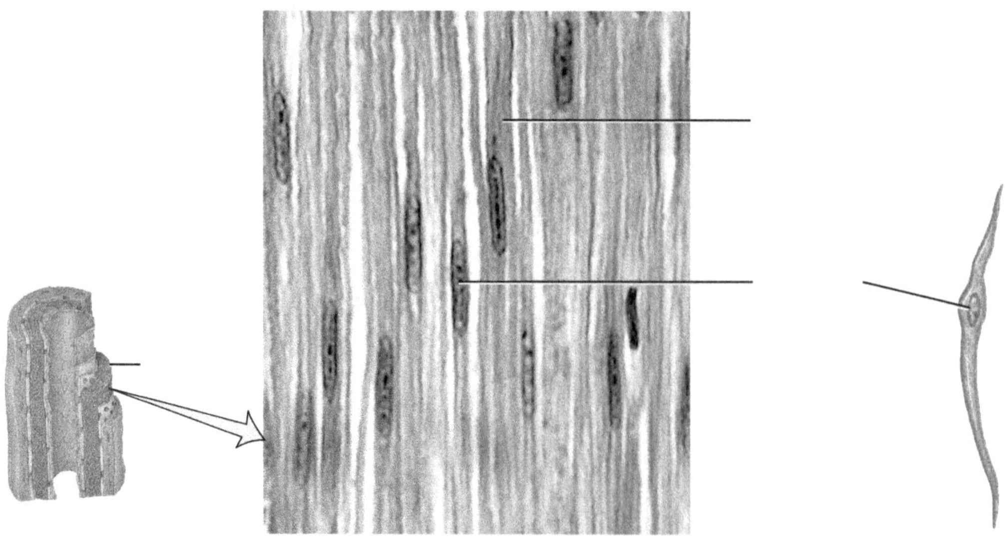

Source: Tortora and Derrickson (2009) / Reproduced with permission of John Wiley & Sons.

(f) Match the pairs.

Smooth muscle is	stimulated by involuntary neurogenic impulses and has slow, rhythmical contractions
Smooth muscle is involuntary	non-striated
Smooth muscle is held together by	in the walls of hollow internal structures and vessels
Smooth muscle is found	connective tissue with bands of elastic protein wrapped around them
Smooth muscle tends to	myosin and actin filaments over each other
Contraction of smooth muscle is caused by the sliding of	have greater elasticity than striated muscle

8 Tissue identification

Match the descriptions with the tissue and microscopic appearance.

Sheets of cells of various sizes, form linings in hollow structures which need to stretch	Compact bone	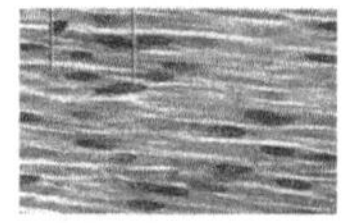
Collagen fibres are densely and regularly packed with fibroblasts scattered throughout. A very strong tissue found in tendons and ligaments	Adipose tissue	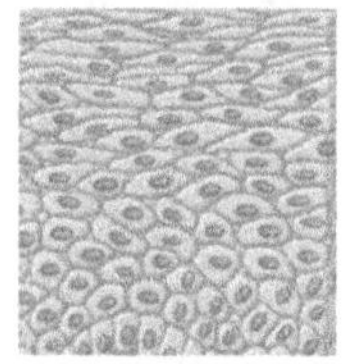
Thin, roughly hexagonal cells existing in multiple layers. The top layers are easily sloughed off and replaced	Dense connective tissue	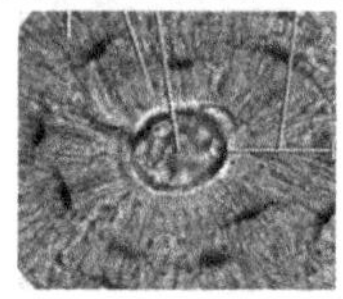
Fibres consist of regular contractile units which form striations	Transitional epithelium	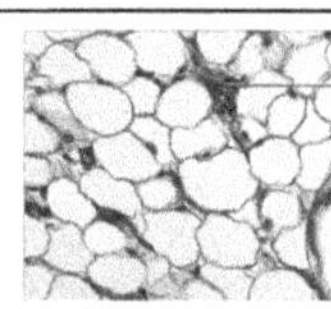
Loose tissue composed mainly of fat containing cells with extracellular matrix	Columnar epithelium	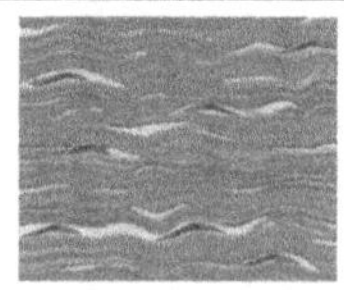
Collagen matrix covered in hardened inorganic salts arranged in dense, concentric rings	Smooth muscle	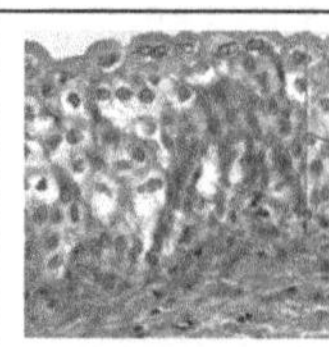
Consists of a row of roughly rectangular cells with both secretory and absorptive functions. May also have cilia to move extracellular substances around	Skeletal muscle	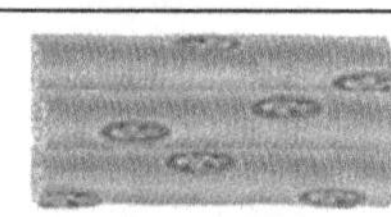
Consists of short contractile cells with no striations. Function together as a unit, but cells are distinct	Squamous epithelium	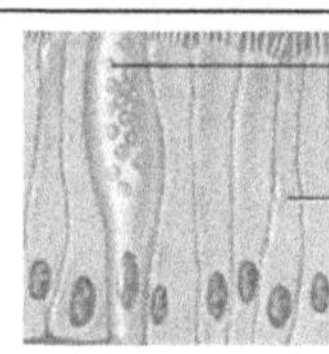

Source: Tortora and Derrickson (2017) / Reproduced with permission of John Wiley & Sons.

9 Terminology

Look up the meanings of the prefixes and suffixes in the following terms, write them into the table and then give the meaning of the complete terms.

Histology	
Hist- =	-ology =
Meaning:	

Fibroblast	
Fibro- =	-blast =
Meaning:	

Chondrocyte	
Chondro- =	-cyte =
Meaning:	

Osteoblast	
Osteo- =	-blast =
Meaning:	

Osteoclast	
Osteo- =	-clast =
Meaning:	

Avascular	
A- =	-vascular =
Meaning:	

Macrophage	
Macro- =	-phage =
Meaning:	

10 Spot the errors

Correct the errors in the following paragraph:

When tissue is damaged, it can be repaired either by regeneration of new, functional tissue or by a repair that leaves a fibrous scar, consisting of non-functional tissue. Which of these occurs depends on the tissue – tissues which readily undergo mitosis, such as nervous and muscle tissues, are able to regenerate by producing new cells by cell division. The number of stem cells in a tissue gives a clue to how readily it will regenerate – a large number of stem cells suggests that the damage will be repaired with fibrous tissue, whereas complete regeneration is likely in tissue with low stem cell numbers. Repaired tissue is usually repaired with connective tissue, produced by fibroblasts, but regenerated tissue involves the replacement of the tissue's own cells.

11 Snap shot

Pressure sores are an injury to the skin and underlying tissue. They can range from mild reddening of the skin to severe tissue damage and sometimes infection that can extend into muscle and bone.
Describe the four stages of development of pressure sores.

12 Crossword

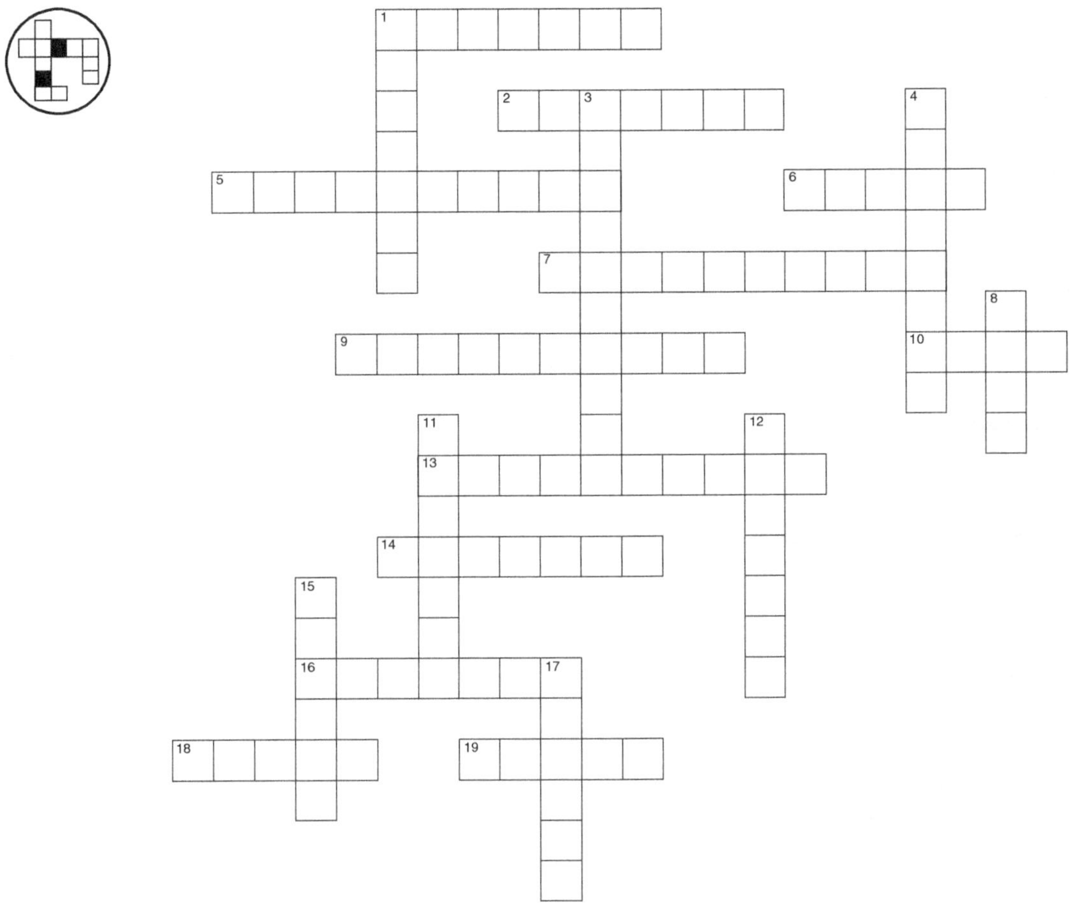

Across

1. Strongly staining structure in tissue sample sections
2. A prefix meaning cartilage
5. Connective tissue cell that makes collagen; important in tissue repair
6. A prefix meaning bone
7. Tissues that can be extremely strong
9. Makes sheets, linings and glands
10. Nerve impulses travel some distance down this
13. Muscles and nerves use this type of activation to function
14. Connective tissue containing fat cells
16. Groups of cells with similar structure and function
18. Microscopic hairs on a cell that beat to move extracellular substances around
19. Fluid connective tissue vital for transport of substances

Down

1. Glial cells support these
3. Cell that resorbs bone tissue
4. The diaphragm is made of this muscle
8. The number of main tissue types in the human body
11. Attach skeletal muscle to bone
12. Muscle type found in the heart
15. The extracellular substance found in connective tissue
17. The muscle type responsible for movements of the digestive tract

Multiple-choice questions

13. Which of the following is not typical of epithelial tissue?
- A. Cells arranged like paving
- B. Squamous, cuboidal or columnar
- C. Large amount of mineral-containing intercellular matrix
- D. Gives rise to endocrine and exocrine glands

14. Adipose tissue is:
- A. a type of connective tissue storing fat
- B. described as pulsatile and voluntary
- C. highly metabolically active
- D. None of the above

15. Osseous tissue:
- A. contains hard mineral-containing intercellular matrix
- B. contains osteocytes
- C. is a kind of connective tissue
- D. All of the above

16. Which of the following is not true of the pleural membranes?
- A. There is a visceral and parietal pleura.
- B. They consist entirely of connective tissue.
- C. They are classified as serous membranes.
- D. They are located in the thorax.

17. The pleura and peritoneum:
- A. are serous membranes
- B. are mucous membranes
- C. are connective tissue membranes
- D. None of the above

18. Epithelial tissue is avascular, meaning that it:
- A. contains adipose tissue
- B. contains no blood vessels
- C. is made of blood vessels
- D. cannot repair itself

19. Epithelial tissue is classified by:
- A. shape, colour and depth
- B. shape, vascularity and depth
- C. shape, weight and depth
- D. shape and depth

20. Connective tissue:
- A. is made up of tightly packed rows of cells
- B. is a highly disorganised tissue
- C. always contains a lot of extracellular matrix
- D. forms sheets covering body surfaces

21. The basic functional unit of the nervous system is:
- A. the glial cell
- B. the synapse
- C. the axon
- D. the neurone

22. Which of the following is under voluntary control?

A. Skeletal muscle
B. Smooth muscle
C. Glands
D. All of the above

23. Cardiac muscle is:

A. composed of non-striated muscle cells
B. under voluntary control
C. composed of branching fibres
D. able to regenerate

24. Connective tissue is able to resist stretching forces due to:

A. a tough, inelastic membrane that wraps around the tissue
B. elastin fibres in the cells
C. collagen fibres in the extracellular matrix
D. the interlocking pattern of the cells

25. Areas of the body that are subject to rubbing and abrasion are usually lined with:

A. dense connective tissue
B. smooth muscle
C. stratified squamous epithelium
D. pseudostratified epithelium

26. Hollow organs are able to contract by virtue of:

A. fibrous connective tissue
B. elastin fibres
C. collagen fibres
D. smooth muscle

CHAPTER 6

Embryology

1 Eggs and sperm

Match the pairs – Oocyte maturation.

Increase in gonadotropins FSH and LH	Causes a surge in FSH and LH
Several oocytes are recruited each month	During ovulation
Oocyte completes meiosis I and starts meiosis II	Stimulates follicle maturation and ovulation
Peaking oestrogen level	Only the dominant follicle is released

Match the pairs – Sperm maturation.

Sperm capacitation	Is the final maturation stage
The acrosome reaction	Is characterised by whipping movements
Hyperactivation	Sperm acquire ability to swim forward
Transiting through the epididymis	Occurs after ejaculation

2 Fertilisation

(a) Label the structures on the diagram below.

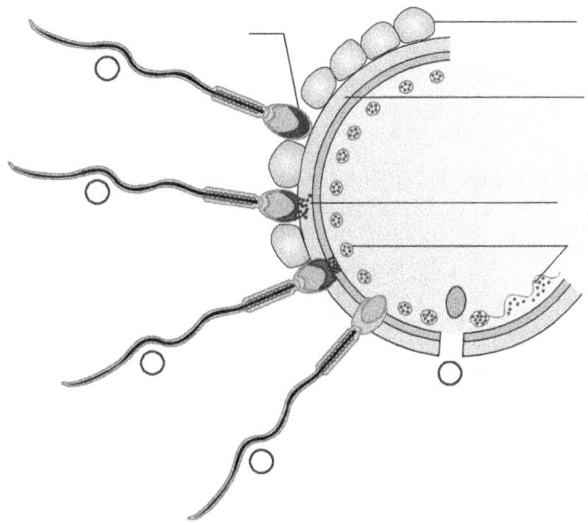

Source: Webster et al. 2018. Reproduced with permission of John Wiley & Sons.

3 Pre-implantation

Name each of the following structures and give the approximate day after fertilisation they would be present.

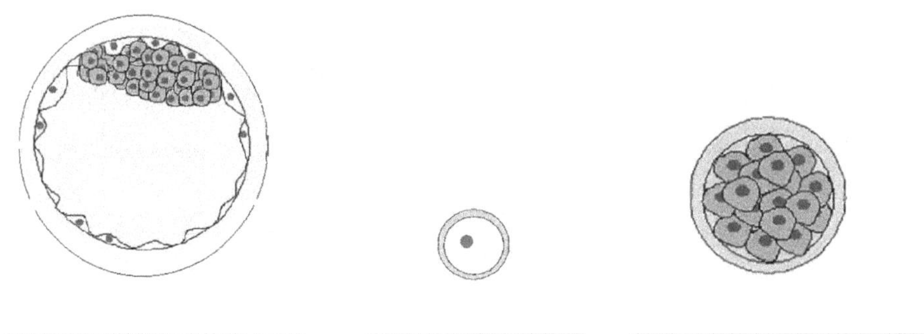

Source: Suzanne Evans 2025.

4 Implantation

Write a 'T' or 'F' in each box to indicate whether the statement is true or false.

(a) Implantation occurs on day 6.	☐
(b) Implantation occurs at the blastocyst stage.	☐
(c) Endometrial cells divide and grow around the blastocyst to embed it.	☐
(d) The trophoblast cells are shed just prior to implantation.	☐
(e) The implantation failure rate is 50% or above.	☐

5 Development

(a) On the timeline below, fill in the boxes to identify gestational age, embryonic age and the trimesters.

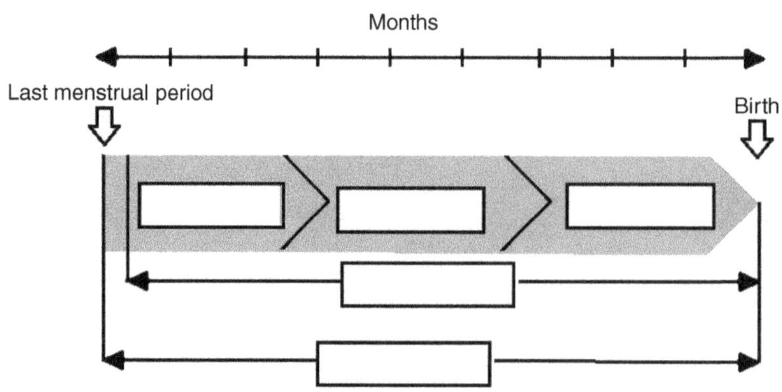

(b) List the embryonic stages shown in the following diagram in the correct order and give the age (in weeks) of the embryo in each case.

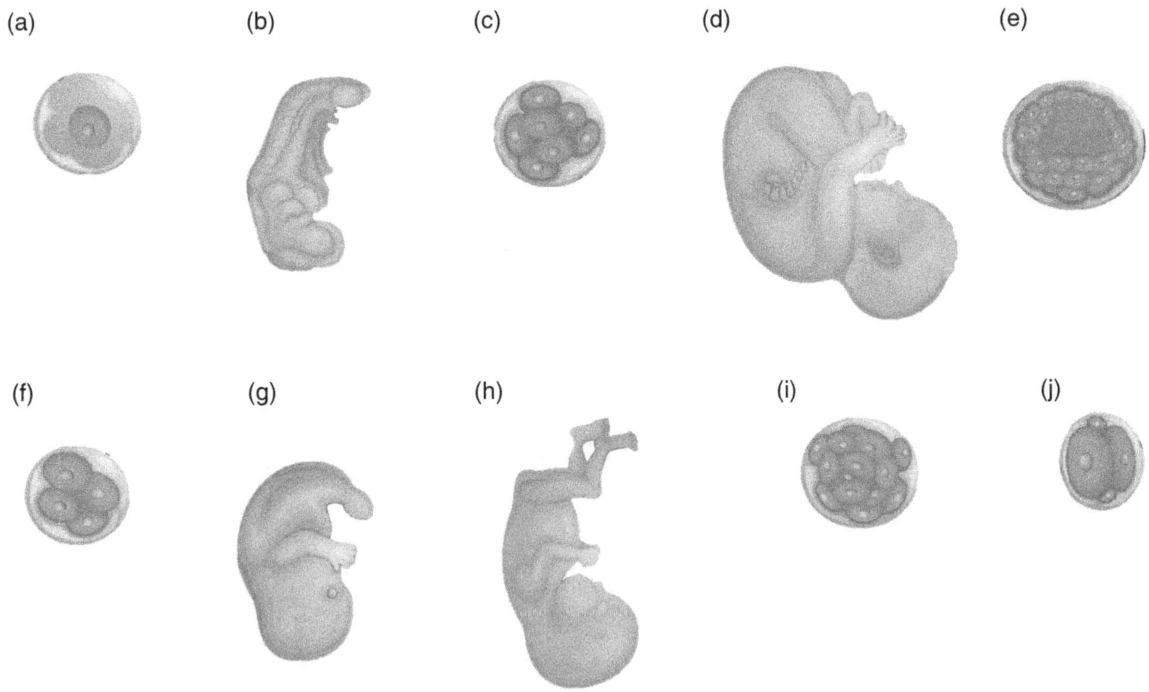

Correct sequence: __________ __________ __________ __________ __________

__________ __________ __________ __________ __________

6 Gastrulation

Label and colour the yolk sac, amniotic cavity and the three germ layers on the diagram below.

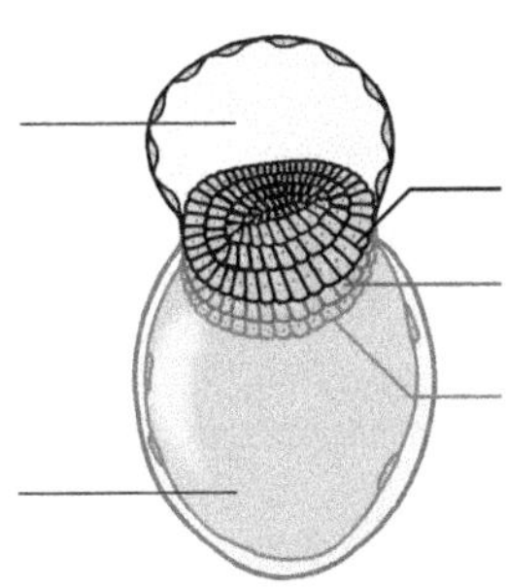

Source: Webster and de Wreede (2016) / Reproduced with permission of John Wiley & Sons.

7 Neurulation

Colour the ectoderm, mesoderm, endoderm and notochord on the diagrams below.

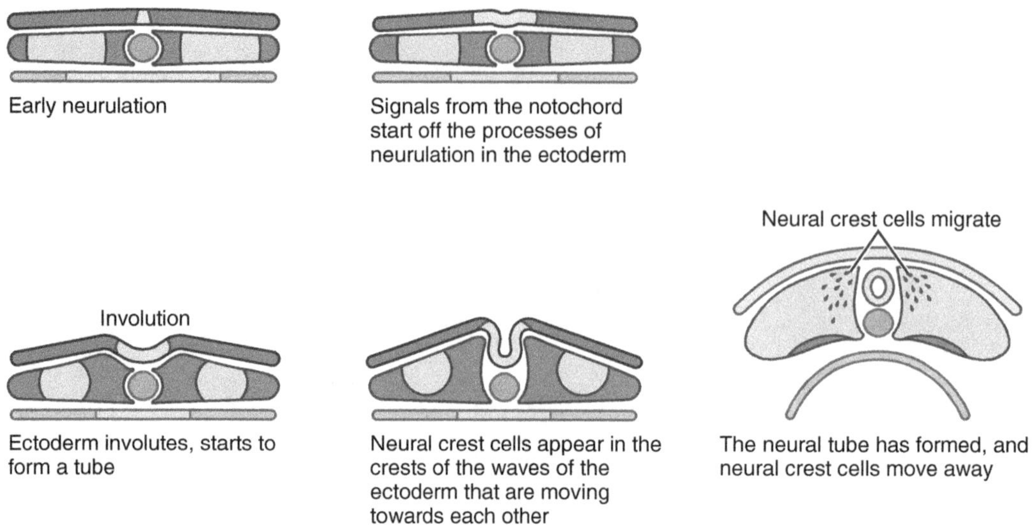

Source: Webster and de Wreede (2016) / Reproduced with permission of John Wiley & Sons.

8 Differentiation of germ layers

Place the following tissues in the correct columns in the table to show which germ cell layer each develops from:
Neurones; Glands; Blood vessels; Cartilage; Epidermis; Bladder; Gastrointestinal tract; Bone; Lungs; Muscles; Heart.

Develops from ectodermal layer	**Develops from mesodermal layer**	**Develops from endodermal layer**

9 Disorders

Match the pairs in the following table:

Trisomy 21	Result of alcohol consumption during pregnancy
Fetal alcohol spectrum disorder (FASD)	Stillbirth
Nuchal transparency high	Pregnancy
Urine human chorionic gonadotropin (hCG) high	Miscarriage
Loss of pregnancy after 20 weeks' gestation	Down syndrome
Loss of pregnancy prior to 20 weeks' gestation	Likely chromosomal abnormality

10 Formation of the placenta

Identify and colour the maternal and fetal tissues in the following diagrams:

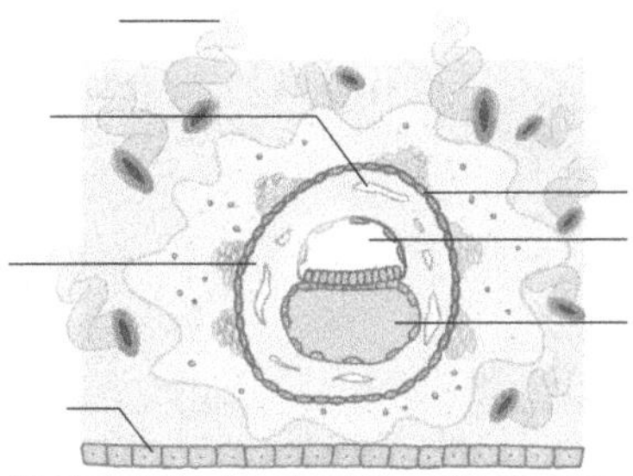

The blastocyst has implanted into the endometrium and the cells of the trophoblast invade the maternal tissue. (End of week 2)

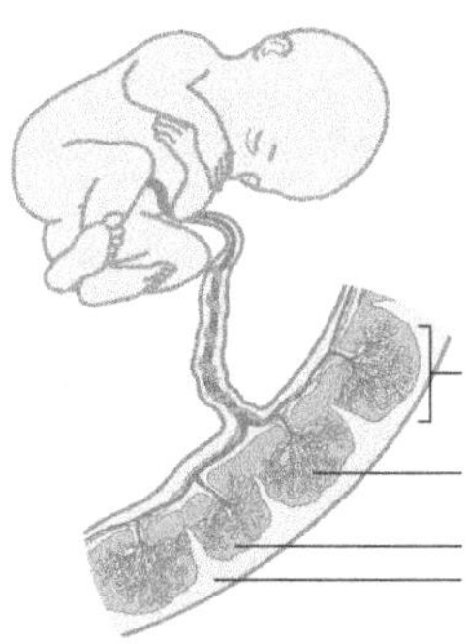

The structure of the placenta

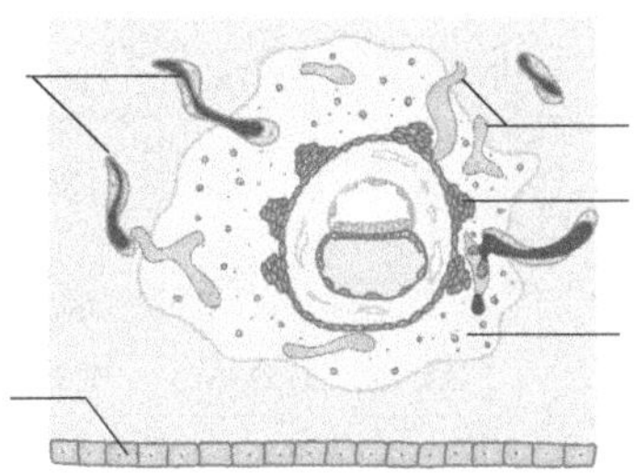

The syncytiotrophoblast meets and erodes the maternal endometrial blood vessels, and lacunae within the syncytiotrophoblast form pools of blood that will become interconnected. The cells of the cytotrophoblast start to form chorionic

Source: Webster and de Wreede (2016) / Reproduced with permission of John Wiley & Sons.

11 Word scramble

Time yourself to unscramble these words.

Scrambled	Unscrambled
BREMOY	
EGOINOSES	
THLABORSTOP	
AMUROL	
RERITEMTS	
CEFILLOL	

12 Definitions

For the following terms, underline the root and then give the meaning of the term:

Term	Meaning
Polyspermy	
Ovulation	
Macrosomia	
Microsomia	
Antenatal	
Prenatal	
Embryology	

13 Abbreviations

Write the following information out in a form that could be understood by a patient, without abbreviations.

(a) Primigrav. ♀, GA 38 wks, BP 142/89 mm Hg, Proteinuria ++, HELLP. Diag Pre-E.

(b) Female G3 P1, p/w VB at 7 wks GA.

(c) BB, NSVD, AFP low, ? DS

14 Prefixes and suffixes

Look up the meanings of the prefixes and suffixes in the following terms, write them into the table and then give the meaning of the complete terms.

Trophoblast	
Tropho- =	-blast =
Meaning:	

Blastocyst	
Blasto- =	-cyst =
Meaning:	

Gonadotropin	
Gonado- =	-tropin =
Meaning:	

Oocyte	
Oo- =	-cyte =
Meaning:	

Syncytiotrophoblast			
Syn- =	cyt- =	tropho- =	-blast =
Meaning:			

Progesterone		
Pro- =	gest- =	-sterone =
Meaning:		

Oestrogen	
Oestro- =	-gen =
Meaning:	

15 Crossword

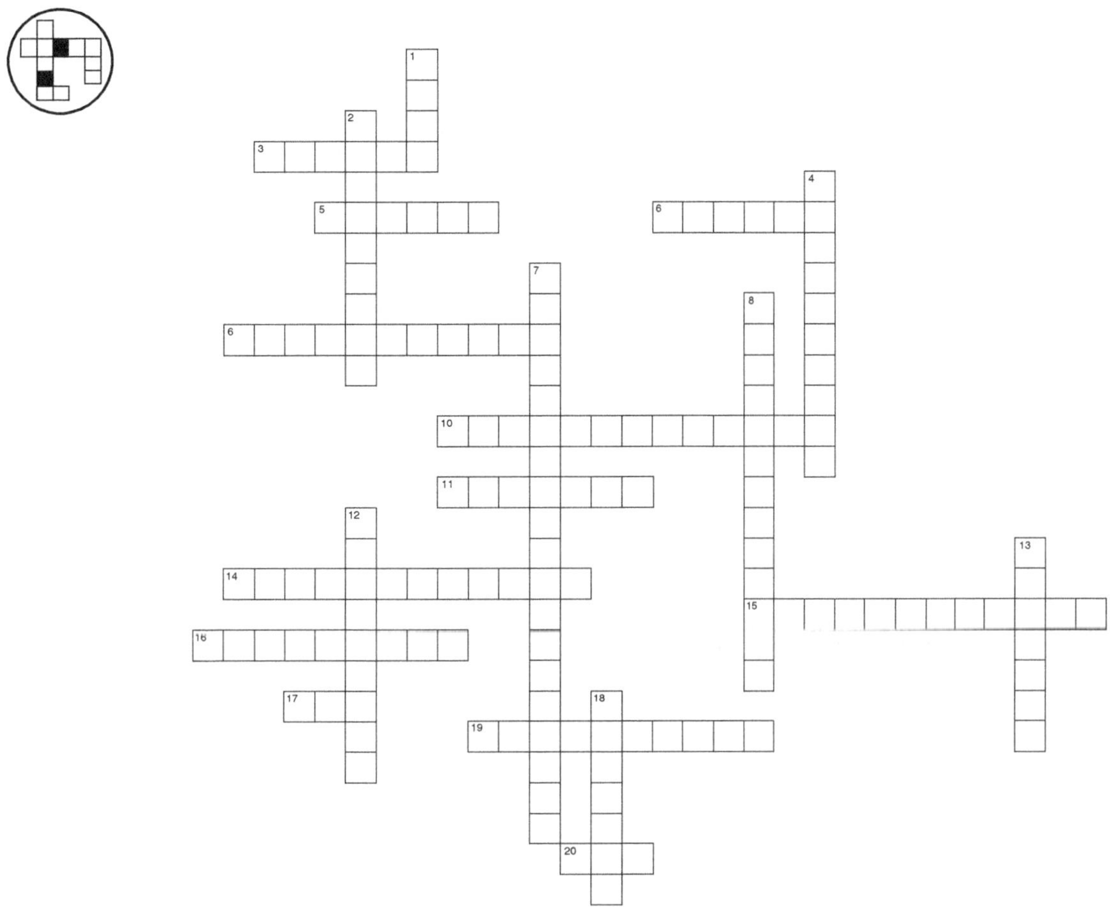

Across

3. The single new cell formed immediately after fertilisation
5. An embryo consisting of 16 cells
6. Ovarian phase occurring after ovulation
9. The process by which the nervous system first forms in the embryo
10. The union of male and female gametes
11. Pregnancy when an embryo implants in one of the Fallopian tubes
14. The reorganisation of the blastocyst into three cell layers
15. Embedding of the embryo into the uterine lining
16. Uterine phase occurring after ovulation
17. Maintains the corpus luteum to ensure progesterone supply during pregnancy
19. Ovarian phase occurring prior to ovulation
20. The day post-fertilisation when implantation usually occurs

Down

1. The fetal period begins in this week
2. The first milk produced by the mother after birth
4. The imaging technique used to view the fetus during pregnancy
7. A continuous layer made of trophoblasts fused together to become a single giant multinucleated cell which forms the basis of the placenta
8. Uterine phase occurring prior to ovulation
12. A substance that is known to cause developmental abnormalities
13. Cell division that occurs in the gametes
18. Cell division that occurs after fertilisation

16 Spot the errors

Find and correct the errors in the following paragraph:

Fertilisation occurs when the egg and sperm combine to create a fertilised egg, also known as an embryo. The egg cell (also known as the oolemma) completes meiosis II during fertilisation, creating a haploid egg cell.

A number of sperm cells may reach the egg and fertilise the egg after undergoing the acrosome reaction, dissolving the sperm and egg membrane and allowing the genetic material from multiple sperm cells and one egg to combine. This creates a new diploid cell. These events mark day 1 of embryonic development.

Multiple-choice questions

17. Oogenesis begins when a female:
- A. is still a fetus
- B. reaches reproductive age
- C. begins menstruation
- D. is under one year of age

18. During implantation:
- A. the risk of failure at this stage is around 5%
- B. endometrial cells divide and surround the blastocyst
- C. trophoblasts erode the endometrium and surround the blastocyst
- D. the endometrium starts to shed as trophoblasts take over the role of nourishing the embryo

19. One of the most important nutrients for normal development of the neural tube in the fetus is:
- A. magnesium
- B. cobalt
- C. folic acid
- D. vitamin C

20. The developing fetus is most sensitive to teratogens during:
- A. the first two trimesters
- B. the entire pregnancy
- C. the final four weeks
- D. the first eight weeks

21. In which order do these vital processes occur?
A. Neurulation, implantation, gastrulation
B. Implantation, gastrulation, neurulation
C. Gastrulation, implantation, neurulation
D. Implantation, neurulation, gastrulation

22. The neural tube is formed from:
A. endoderm
B. mesoderm
C. ectoderm
D. blastocyst

23. The sequence of early embryonic development is:
A. zygote, morula, blastocyst
B. morula, zygote, blastocyst
C. conceptus, zygote, blastocyst
D. polar bodies, zygote, blastocyst

24. The corpus luteum is maintained in the early stages of pregnancy by:
A. FSH
B. LH
C. oestrogen
D. progesterone

25. Pregnancy tests:
A. are based on the detection of progesterone in the urine and provide a result about 14 days after conception
B. are based on the detection of human chorionic corticotropin in the urine and provide a result about 7 days after conception
C. are based on the detection of human chorionic gonadotropin in the urine and provide a result about 11 days after conception
D. are based on the detection of luteinising hormone in the urine and provide a result about 14 days after conception

26. The zona pellucida is important in:
A. gastrulation
B. maintaining sperm motility
C. sperm capacitation
D. preventing polyspermy

27. The part of the sperm cell containing enzymes which break down the zona pellucida is the:
A. acrosome
B. corona
C. pro-nucleus
D. epididymis

CHAPTER 7

The muscular system

1 Muscle types

(a) Label the parts on the following muscle types and identify each muscle type.

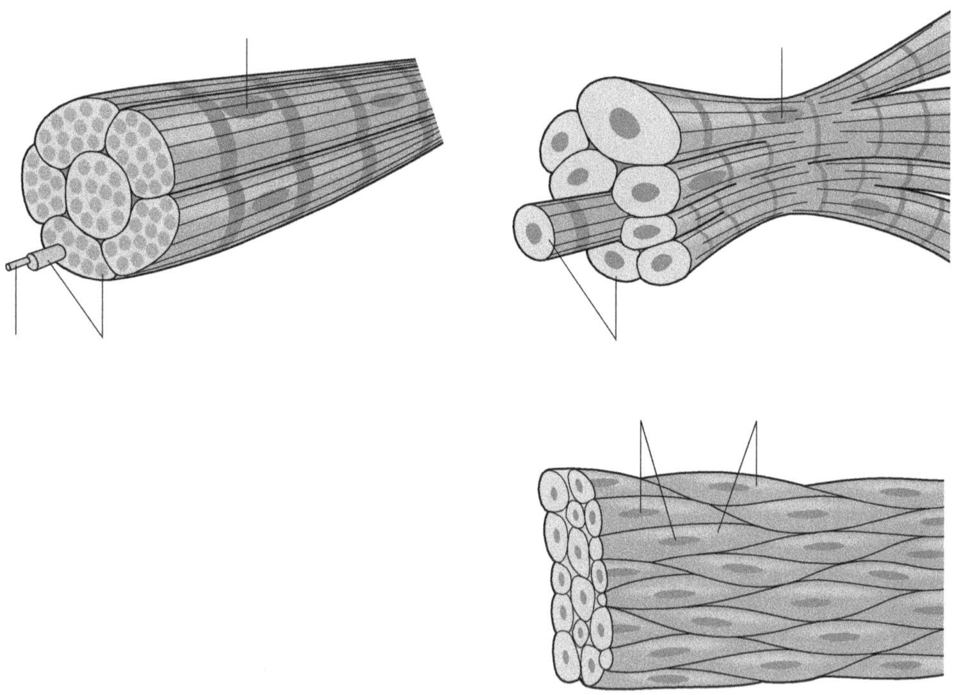

Source: Peate and Nair (2015) / Reproduced with permission of John Wiley & Sons.

(b) Complete the following table:

	Skeletal muscle	Smooth muscle	Cardiac muscle
Location			
Striated/Non-striated			
Control			

(c) Match the pairs.

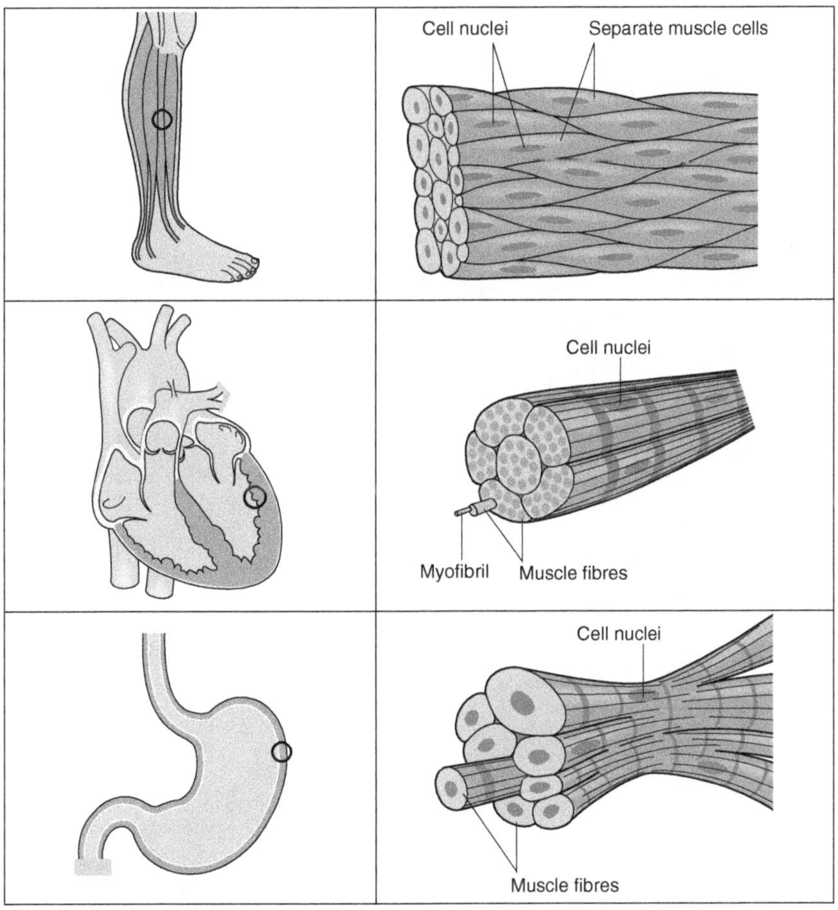

(d) Briefly describe the properties of muscle tissue listed in the following table:

Property	Description
Excitability	
Contractility	
Extensibility	
Elasticity	

2 Time yourself to unscramble these words

SCRA-MBLE

Scrambled	Unscrambled
TEENSTIBLIXIY	
ANTIC	
BRITRIITILAY	
NATIONCORTC	
COMINTOLOO	
ATTUNES	
SIMONY	

3 Skeletal muscle

(a) Identify the unlabelled parts of the skeletal muscle in the following figure and colour in the fascicle.

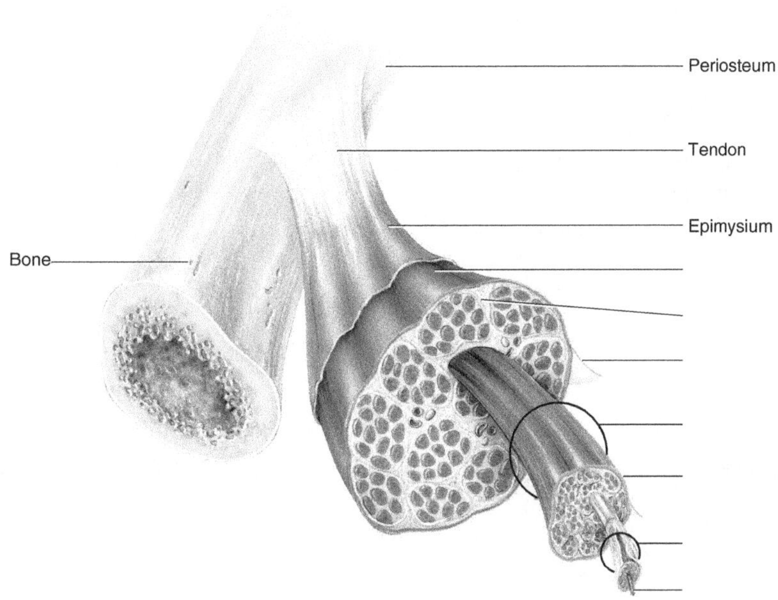

Source: Tortora and Derrickson (2009) / Reproduced with permission of John Wiley & Sons.

(b) Identify the microscopic parts of the skeletal muscle in the following figure:

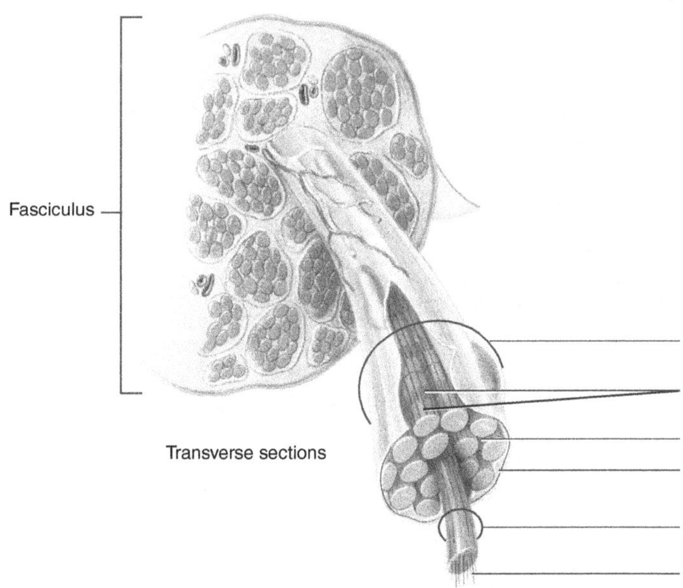

Source: Peate and Nair (2011) / Reproduced with permission of John Wiley & Sons.

(c) Match the pairs.

Whole muscles contain other tissues such as blood vessels, nerves and connective tissue	containing many nuclei and running the full length of the muscle
Each skeletal muscle fibre is a single cell	they have a distinctive banded appearance and lie in parallel bundles
Microscopically, skeletal muscle cells appear cylindrical in shape	In this respect, they can be considered to be organs
Each muscle fibre contains tiny cylindrical structures, myofibrils. These	the A band
The myofibrils play a central role in the muscle contraction mechanism	contain two types of protein filaments
Extending across each of the thick filaments within the sarcomere is a dark area known as	containing myofilaments composed of the proteins actin and myosin, which slide over each other in a ratchet fashion

(d) Place the descriptions in the boxes below into the correct columns in the following table.

Slow oxidative	Fast oxidative-glycolytic	Fast glycolytic

Fibres are dark red in colour due to high level of myoglobin

Also known as type IIa fibres

Fibres are pale in colour due to low level of myoglobin

Metabolise anaerobically

Used for endurance activities

Fatigue resistant

Used for intense activities of short duration

Fibres are large

Fibres are red in colour due to intermediate level of myoglobin

Also known as type I fibres

Metabolise aerobically

Fibres are small

4 Skeletal muscle contraction and relaxation

(a) Identify the nine phases of muscle contraction and relaxation on the figure below. Phases 4 and 7 are completed as an example.

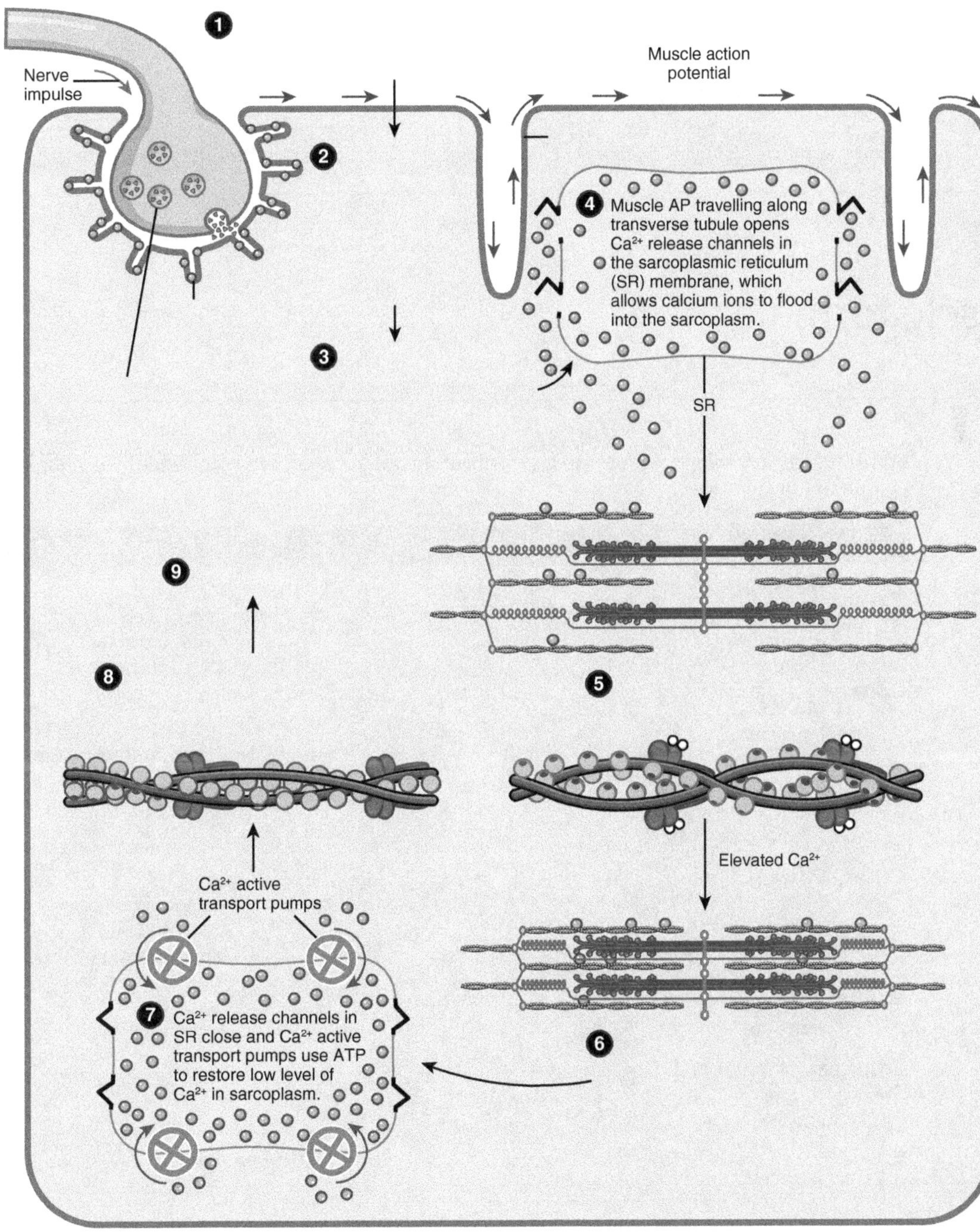

Source: Tortora and Derrickson (2009) / Reproduced with permission of John Wiley & Sons.

(b) Match the pairs.

Acetylcholine when released	a motor unit
When a nerve impulse reaches the axon terminals	and motor end plate contain acetylcholinesterase
The synaptic cleft	acetylcholine is released into the synaptic cleft
The motor neurone and the muscle fibres it controls are known as	causes the electrical potential of the muscle cell membrane to change, triggering contraction of the muscle fibre
The highly branched motor neurone axons mean that	a muscle action potential
Skeletal muscle contracts in response to	one motor neurone can control many muscle fibres

5 Muscle form

(a) Complete the following table. Some elements of the table have been completed. The character/term column is fully complete.

Character/Term	Definition	Example
DIRECTION Transverse Oblique Rectus		Transversus abdominis External oblique Rectus abdominis
SHAPE Trapezius Deltoid Orbicularis Rhomboid Platys-	Trapezoid Triangular Circular Diamond-shaped Flat	
SIZE Major Minor Maximus Minimus Longus Latissimus		Pectoralis major Pectoralis minor Gluteus maximus Gluteus minimus Adductor longus Latissimus dorsi
NUMBER OF ORIGINS Biceps Triceps Quadriceps	Two origins Three origins Four origins	

6 Areas of skeletal musculature

(a) The body's skeletal muscles can be divided into four areas. List these below and mark the areas on the anterior and posterior views of the body in the figure.

____

____

____

____

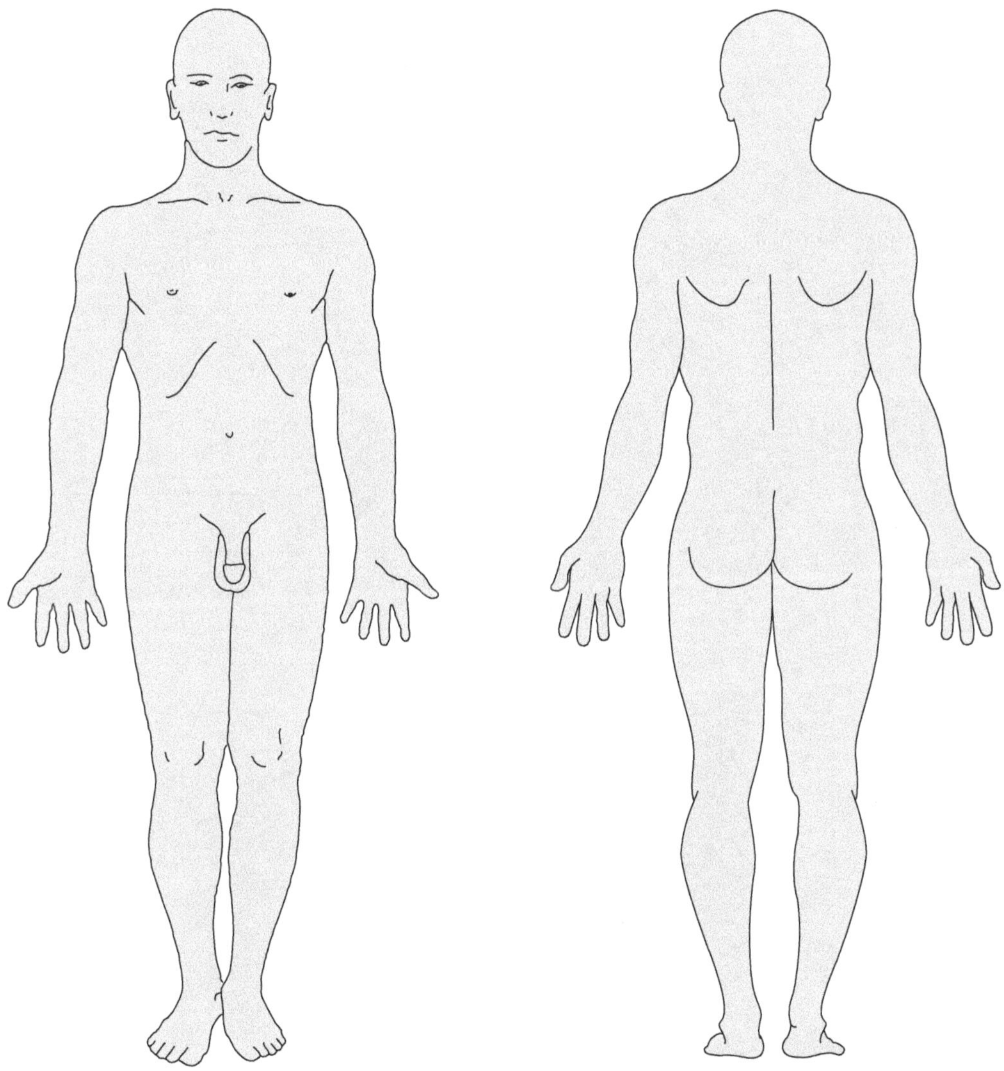

Anterior view Posterior view

7 Naming muscles

(a) Identify the muscles on the following diagrams:

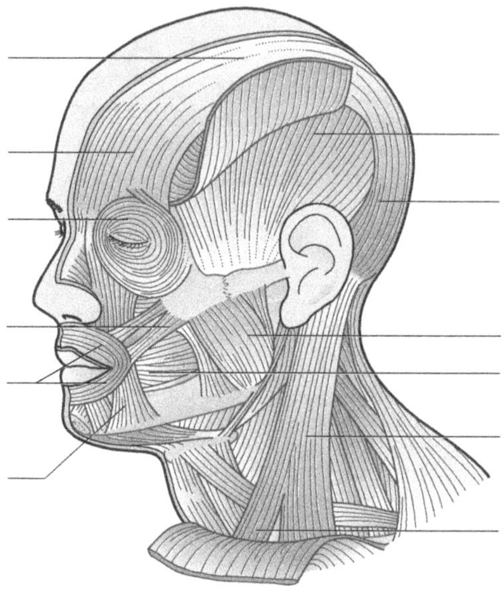

An anterior and lateral view

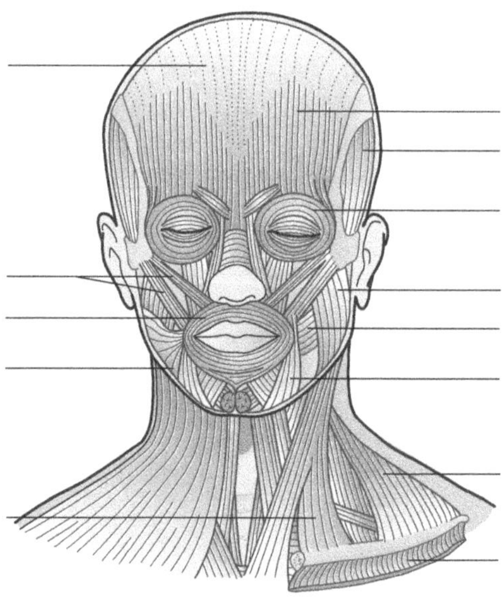

Anterior view

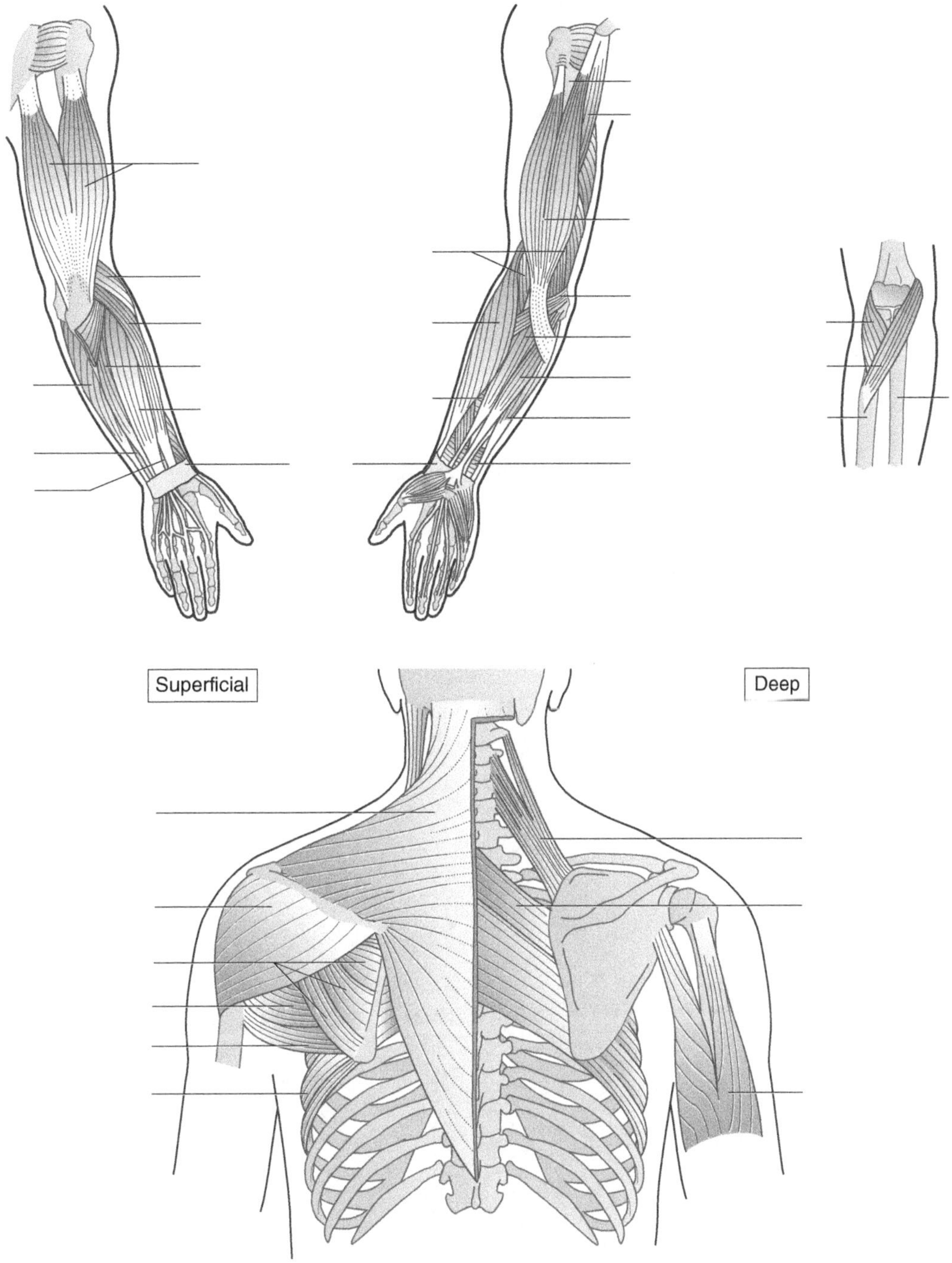

Posterior view

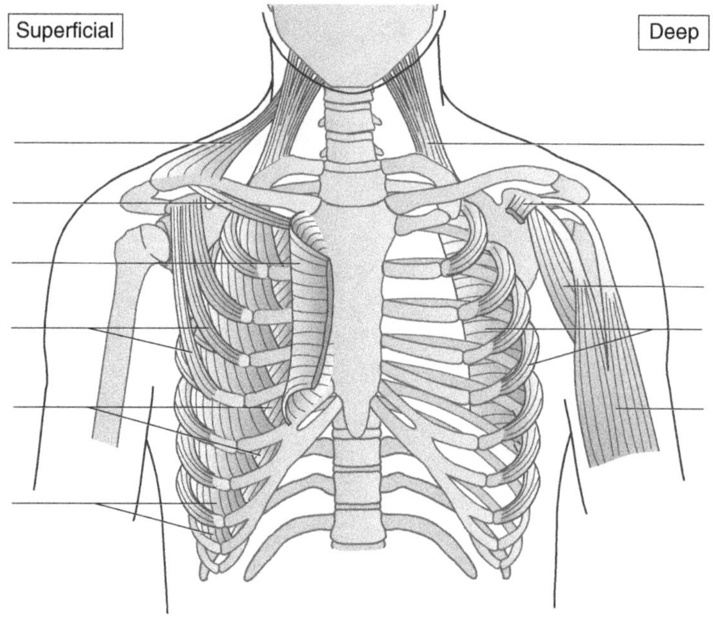

Anterior view

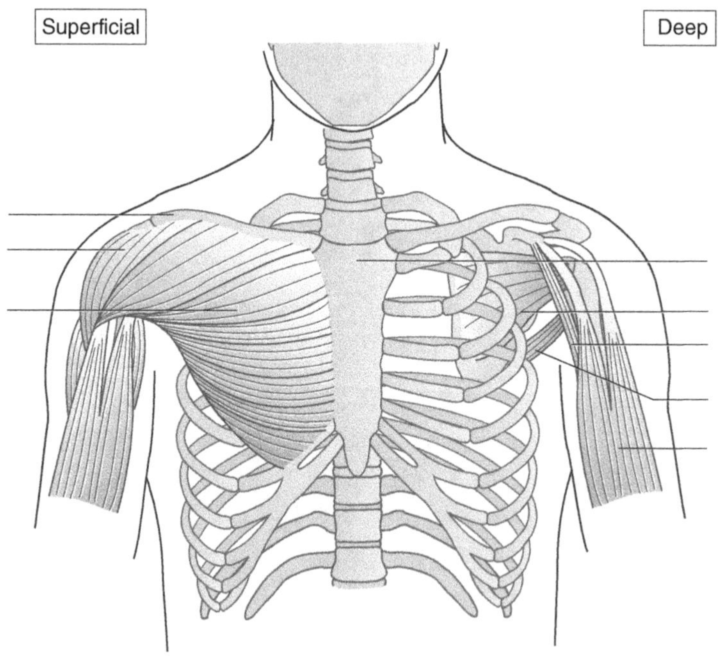

Anterior view

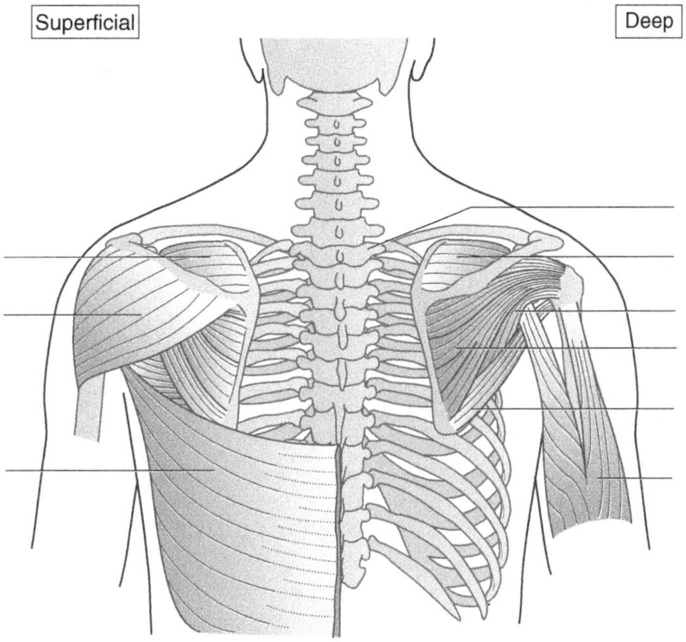

Posterior view

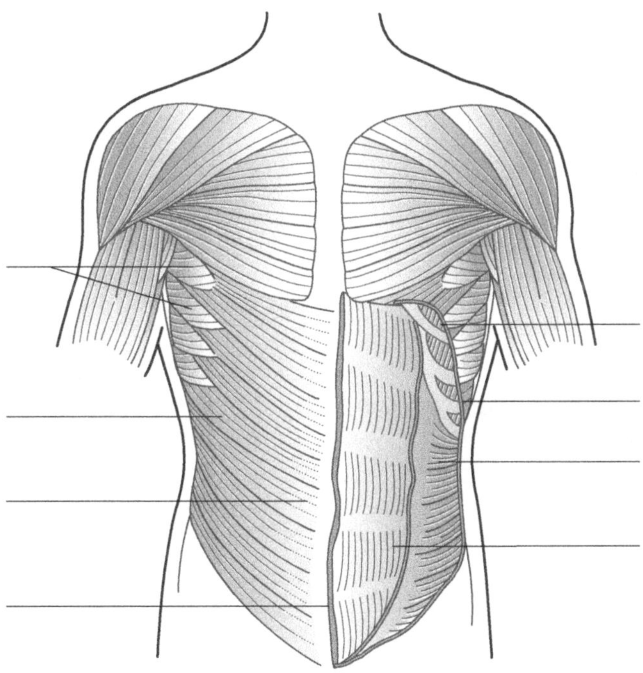

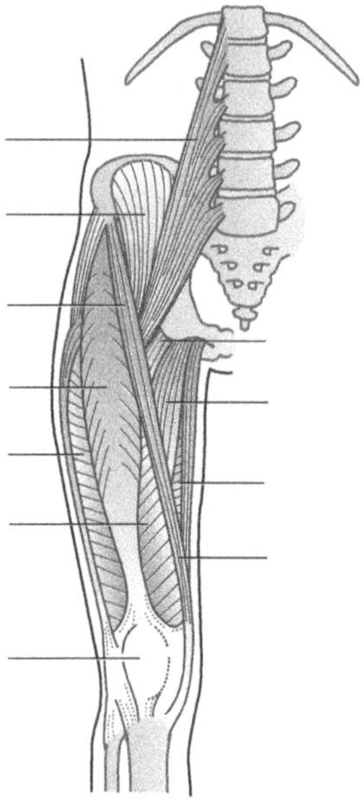

Muscles of the anterior right hip and thigh

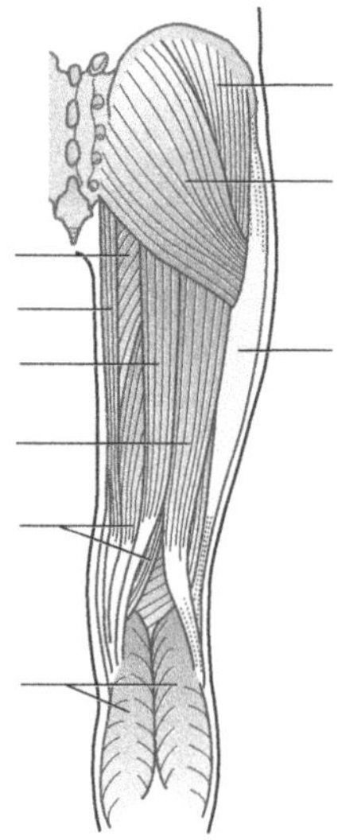

Muscles of the posterior right hip and thigh

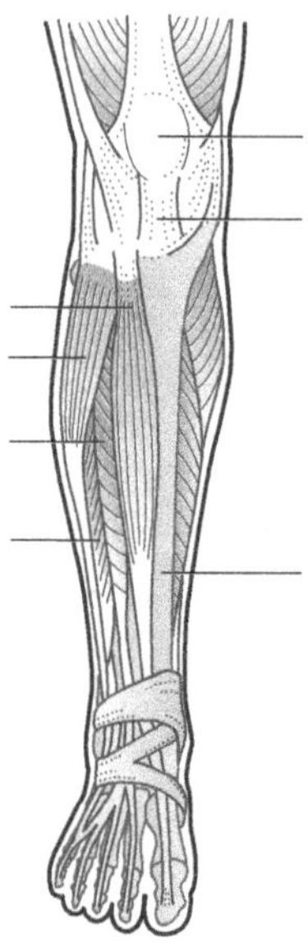

Muscles of the anterior right leg

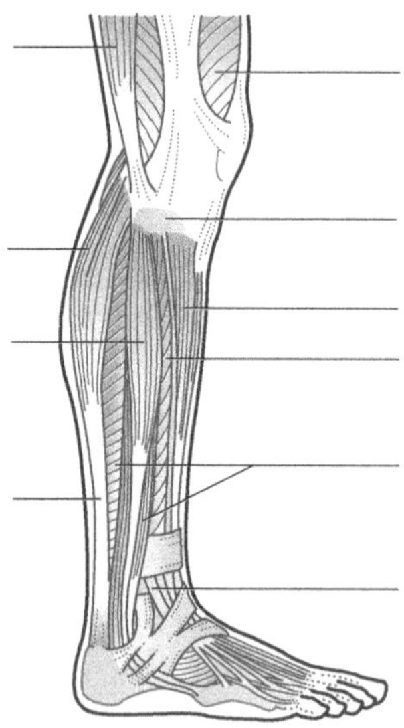

Muscles of the lateral right leg

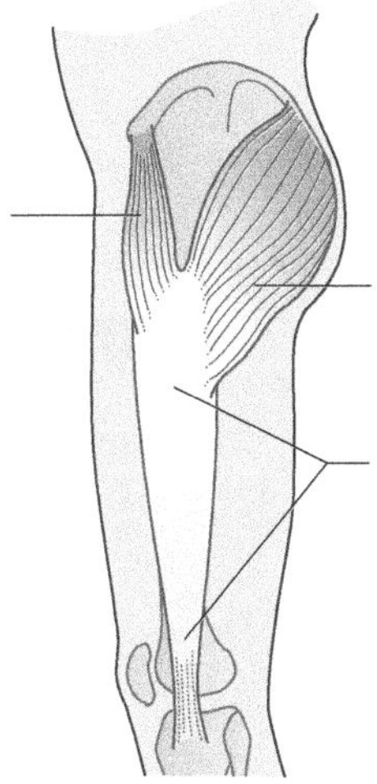

Muscles that move the thigh

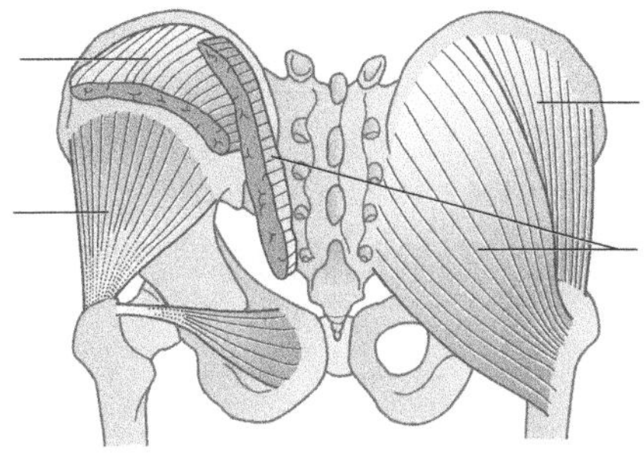

The gluteal muscle group

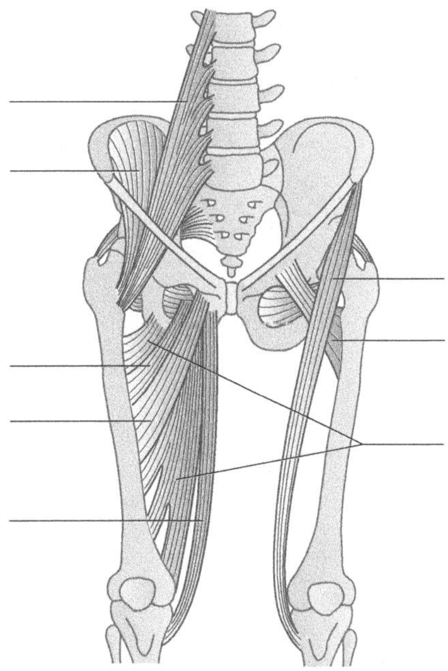

The iliopsoas muscle and the adductor group

Source: Peate and Nair (2011) / Reproduced with permission of John Wiley & Sons.

8 Match the pairs

The skeletal muscles can be	at a minimum of two points to bone or other connective tissue
The skeletal muscles can be	compresses cheeks
The origin of a muscle	at an insertion on the bone that moves
Muscle ends	is on the stationary bone where it begins
The buccinator muscle	divided into four areas
All skeletal muscles are attached	named according to size, shape, location and number of origins, associated bones and the action of the muscle

9 Joint movements

(a) Complete the following table, defining the movements produced at joints by muscle action.

Action	Definition
Extension	
Flexion	
Abduction	
Adduction	
Circumduction	
Supination	
Pronation	
Plantar flexion	
Dorsiflexion	
Rotation	

10 Match the pairs

The opposing muscles are called	agonist and antagonist
An agonist is also called	the muscles mainly responsible for producing an action
Prime movers are	causes muscle movement in the opposite direction
The muscles that produce the opposite actions at a joint are the	a prime mover
The antagonist	antagonist

11 Spot the errors

Identify and correct the errors in the following paragraph:

The process of skeletal muscle contraction begins with a command from a motor neurone, resulting in the release of calcium at the synapse between the motor neurone and the muscle fibre. This results in a muscle action potential, which travels along the T-tubules, causing the release of potassium ions from the endoplasmic reticulum. Potassium ions bind to the protein troponin, found on the myosin fibres, and this uncovers the binding sites for the myosin heads by moving tropomyosin from the sites. The myosin heads then bind to actin, and, with the addition of ATP, swivel, thereby pulling the actin fibres closer to the middle of the sarcomere, shortening the muscle. Muscle can also contract without shortening. In this case, the cross bridges bind and swivel, but although the tension in the muscle increases, the muscle does not shorten. This is known as an isometric contraction.

12 Terminology

Look up the meanings of the prefixes and suffixes in the following terms, write them into the table and then give the meaning of the complete terms.

Sarcoplasm	
Sarco- =	-plasm =
Meaning:	

Myofibril	
Myo- =	-fibril =
Meaning:	

Sarcomere	
Sarco- =	-mere =
Meaning:	

Biceps	
Bi- =	-ceps =
Meaning:	

Deltoid	
Delt- =	-oid =
Meaning:	

13 Snap shot

Intramuscular injection

You have been asked to administer an intramuscular injection under supervision. Your mentor has explained to you that an intramuscular injection is given directly into a selected muscle, and you are being asked to administer it into the gluteus medius (ventrogluteal site) muscle which runs beneath the gluteus maximus from the ilium to the femur. The injection is given into the upper outer quadrant of the buttock. Where in this diagram would you inject?

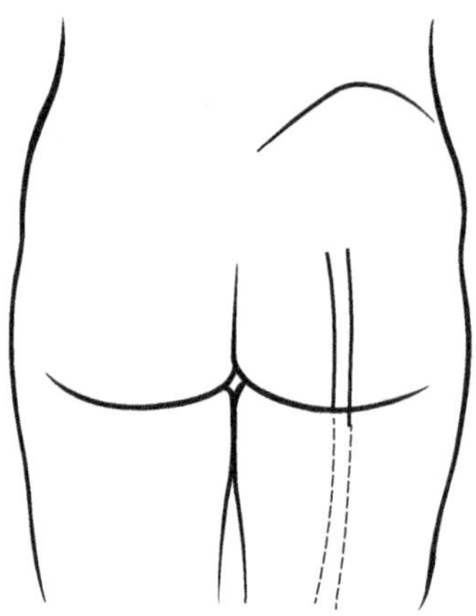

Why is this?

____

____

____

____

____

____

14 Prime movers

(a) Complete the following table by naming the muscle that is the prime mover for each of the movements listed.

Action	Muscle responsible
Pursing lips	
Raising eyebrows	
Rotating palms of the hands upwards	
Pushing the soles of the feet downwards	
Shrugging the shoulders	
Raising the knee	

15 Crossword

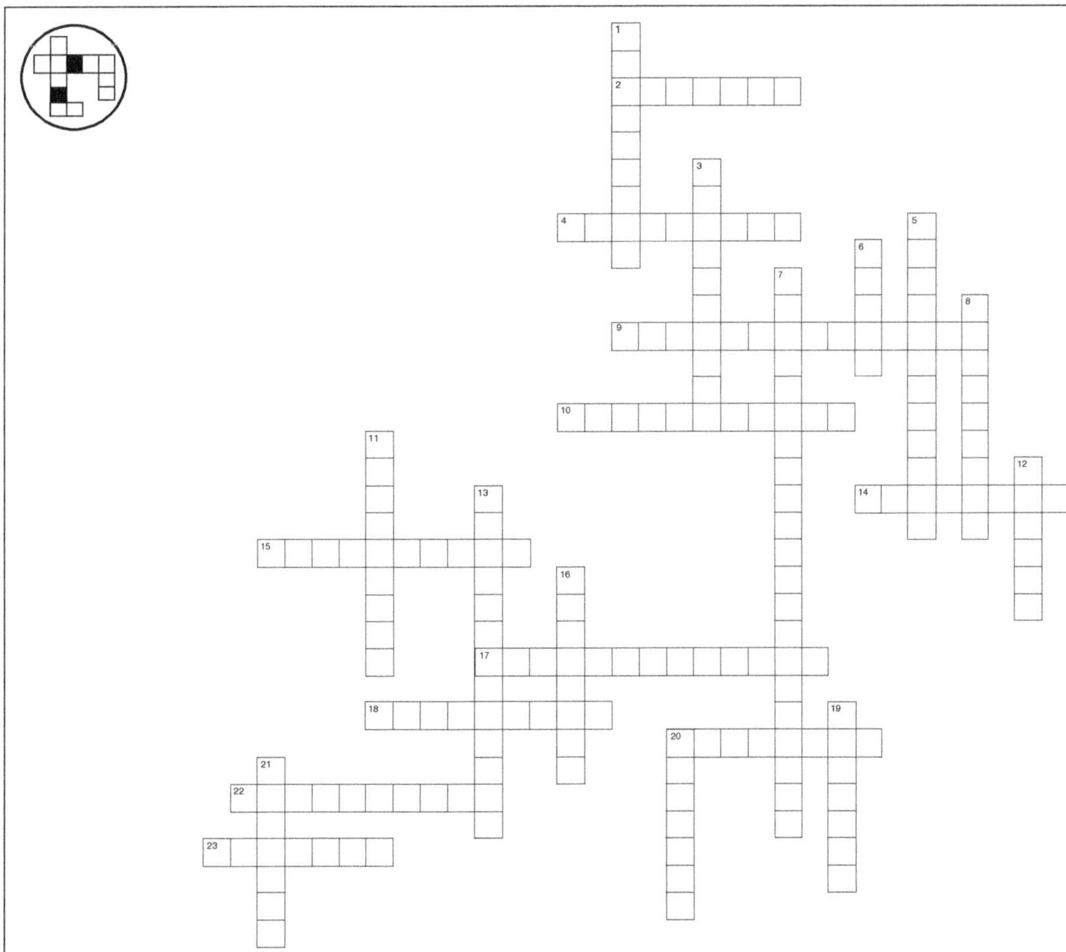

Across

2. Muscle responsible for extension of the elbow joint
4. Fatigue-resistant muscle fibre type for endurance
9. Pushing the sole of the foot downwards
10. Increase in muscle fibre size with weight training
14. Calcium binds to this to uncover cross-bridge binding sites
15. The muscle mainly responsible for producing an action
17. The ability of muscle to shorten when stimulated
18. The contractile unit of the muscle
20. Allow the muscle action potential to reach all parts of a muscle cell almost simultaneously
22. The action of turning the palm of the hand upwards
23. A crucial ion for muscle contraction

Down

1. A motor neurone and the muscle fibres it controls
3. Muscle opposing the agonist
5. The action of rotating the foot at the ankle to point the toes upwards
6. Compressed by the buccinator
7. The organelle that regulates calcium ions in skeletal muscle fibres
8. The attachment point of a muscle to the bone that moves
11. Contraction of a muscle to increase tension but not shorten
12. Works in antagonist pairing with triceps muscle
13. The neurotransmitter released at the neuromuscular junction
16. Chest muscle
19. The force of muscle contraction is transferred to bones by _______
20. Sustained contraction of a skeletal muscle
21. Muscles work by _________ on bones

Multiple-choice questions

16. Which of the following is not a function of the skeletal muscle?
A. Movement
B. Generation of heat
C. Maintenance of posture
D. Calcium homeostasis

17. A shortage of which of the following would cause muscle fatigue?
A. Sodium
B. Chloride
C. Phosphate
D. ATP

18. Muscles are attached to bones by:
A. osteophytes
B. tendons
C. spurs
D. ligaments

19. Skeletal muscles usually operate in ________________ pairs.
A. synergistic
B. dependable
C. reliable
D. antagonistic

20. The end of the muscle that is attached to the bone that moves is the:

A. point of origin
B. insertion
C. detraction
D. tendon

21. The contractile unit of skeletal muscle is the:

A. sarcomere
B. glia
C. neurone
D. actin

22. The striated, or striped, appearance of skeletal muscles is caused by which of the following?

A. Heat
B. Myofibrils
C. Actin
D. ATP

23. What is the energy source for muscle contraction?

A. Vitamin D
B. Calcium
C. ATP
D. None of the above

24. The junction between a motor neurone and a muscle cell is the:

A. neuromuscular junction
B. sinus
C. fistula
D. All of the above

25. The strength of a contraction depends upon the number of:

A. motor units
B. twitches
C. ATP
D. anaerobes

CHAPTER 8

The skeletal system

1 Divisions of the skeleton

On the table below, write in the number of bones in each division of the skeleton and colour the appendicular and axial skeletons using different colours.

Structure	Number of bones	Division of the skeleton	Number of bones	Structure
Axial skeleton • Skull – Cranium – Face • Hyoid • Auditory ossicles • Vertebral column • Thorax – Sternum – Ribs		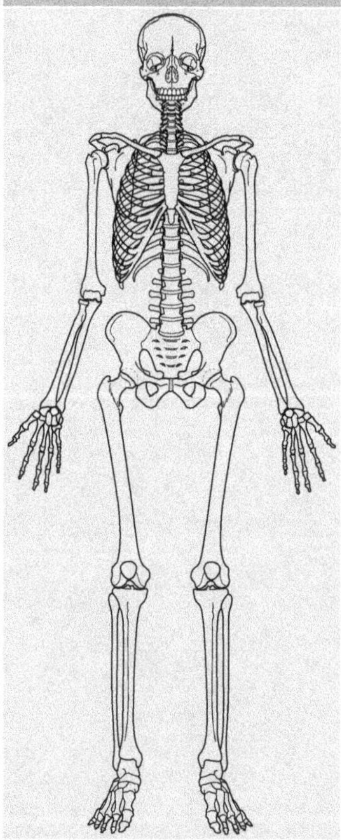		**Appendicular skeleton** • Pectoral (shoulder) girdles – Clavicle – Scapula • Upper limbs – Humerus – Ulna – Radius – Carpals – Metacarpals – Phalanges • Pelvic (hip) girdle – Hip, pelvic, or coxal bone • Lower limbs – Femur – Patella – Fibula – Tibia – Tarsals – Metatarsals – Phalanges
Number of bones	80		126	**Number of bones**
				Total bones in an adult skeleton = 206

Source: Peate et al. (2014) / Reproduced with permission of John Wiley & Sons.

2 Functions of bones

Write notes about the bone functions listed in the following table:

Function	Description
Support	
Movement	
Minerals and lipid store	
Protection	
Blood cell production	

3 Match the pairs

When old bone dies	and more individual bones than adults
Whole bones are made of	the axial skeleton and the appendicular skeleton
The skeleton provides	bones, ligaments, cartilage and tendons
The skeletal system comprises	shape, protection, levers for movement, blood cell production
Infants are born with large amounts of cartilage	a number of different tissues, including bone tissue
The skeleton is divided into two parts for classification purposes	new bone is formed

4 Bone as a tissue

(a) Complete the following table:

Cell	Description	Function
Osteoblasts		
Osteocytes		
Osteoclasts		

(b) Fill in the blanks in the following paragraphs:

Bone tissue is a type of _______________ tissue. Despite its solid appearance, it is a very dynamic tissue, with bone being resorbed and laid down constantly. For example, stress placed on bone stimulates _______________, whereas a lack of stress on bones leads to _______________. The bone matrix contains a large amount of the fibrous protein _______________, with _______________ _______________ salts crystallised onto the fibres to create a material that is hard and strong due to the _______________ but also flexible, due to the _______________. This is important, as it ensures bones are not too brittle.

The density of bone at any point depends on the balance between _______________ and _______________ activity. Because of the _______________ salts, bone represents a large depot of _______________ in the body. When the blood _______________ level drops below normal, _______________ hormone is released into the bloodstream. This stimulates resorption of bone by activating _______________, thereby releasing _______________ ions into the blood.

Because of these unique properties of bone, a _______________ deficiency or low _______________ levels in women will reduce bone _______________, whereas regular _______________ _______________ _______________ will maintain or increase bone _______________.

(c) Match the pairs.

Helps to limit the weight of a bone	Ossification
Allows bones to bend a certain amount without snapping	Osteoporosis
Very low bone density	Spongy bone
Forms strong supportive columns in long bones	Collagen
Replacement of cartilage or membrane with bone	Cortical bone

5 Bone development

(a) Fill in the spaces in the following passage:

Bone formation begins in ___________. The formation involves replacement of another connective tissue with bone, a process known as ___________. For the long bones, it is ____________ that is gradually ___________ in a process known as ___________ ___________. For very flat bones such as the skull, it is a connective tissue membrane that is ___________, in a process known as intramembranous ___________.

(b) Label the following diagram, showing the features of endochondral ossification.

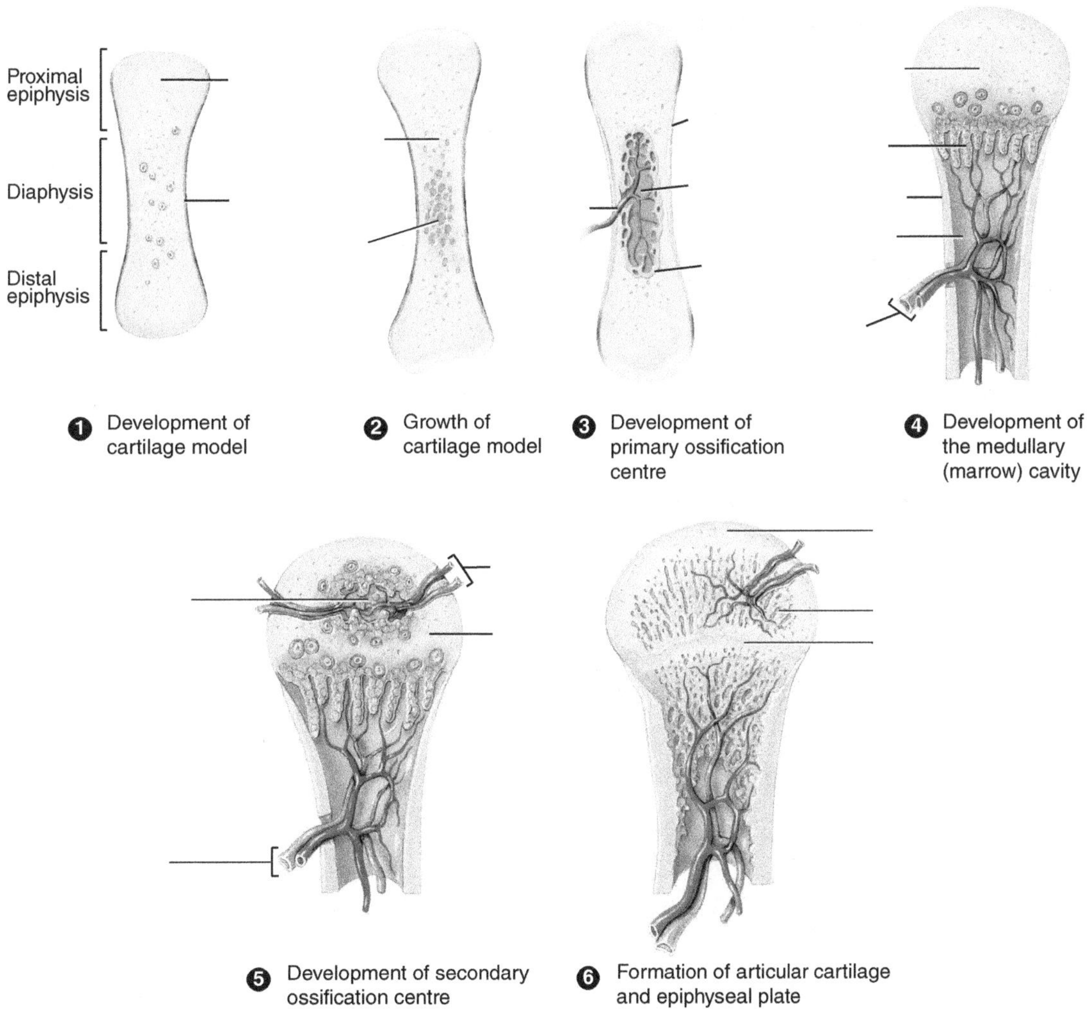

Source: Tortora and Derrickson (2009) / Reproduced with permission of John Wiley & Sons.

(c) Match the pairs.

Endochondral ossification	is cartilage during childhood
The flat bones of the skull, mandible and clavicles	is how the long and short bones are formed
Natural healing of small bone fractures	are formed by a process known as intramembranous ossification
Ossification	occurs by endochondral ossification
The epiphyseal plate	is the conversion of cartilage or another connective tissue to bone

(d) On the diagram below, colour in the growth plates, and above each bone, write the stage of life in which it would be part of the skeleton.

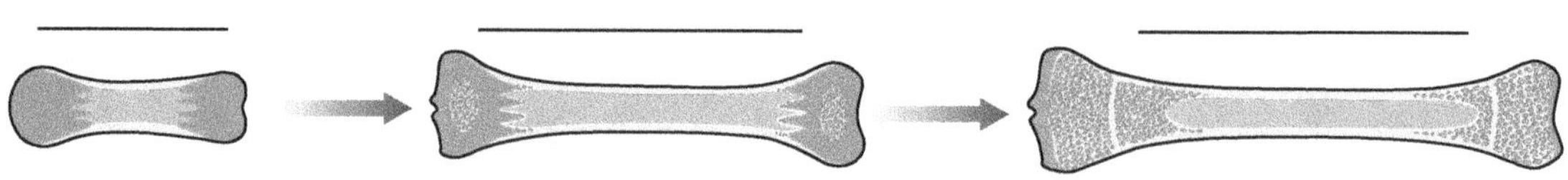

Source: Peate and Nair (2015) / Reproduced with permission of John Wiley & Sons.

6 Time yourself to unscramble these words

Scrambled	Unscrambled
NOODLEDRANCH	
FOSISIACTION	
NILGASTEM	
SYPHIPEALE	
CIRULATETA	
BRUTALEACE	
SYPHISAID	

7 Bone turnover

(a) Spot the errors.
Identify and correct the factual errors in the following paragraph:

The turnover of bone in the skeleton is known as bone remodelling. This has a number of functions – it maintains a healthy skeleton by repairing microfractures and strengthening bone in response to the stresses placed on it, and it plays a central role in cadmium and phosphorous balance in the body. The process of remodelling starts with resorption of bone, carried out by osteocytes, and is followed by deposition of new bone, carried out by osteoclasts. Various factors will tip the balance of the remodelling processes in favour of either net loss or gain of bone. For example, stresses placed on the bones are detected by osteocytes within the bone and will ultimately lead to stimulation of osteoclasts in the same area, causing net addition of bone. Glucocorticoids, such as cortisol, lead to the death of osteoblasts and longer survival of osteoclasts, thereby adding bone.

(b) Place the steps of bone remodelling shown below in the correct order:

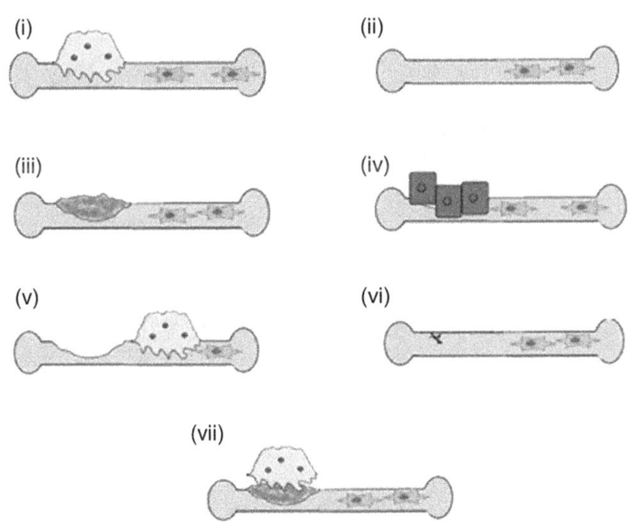

Source: Suzanne Evans (2025).

Correct order: ________________________________

(c) Match the pairs.

Remodelling takes place	it is continuously built, broken down and rebuilt
Bone is dynamic	at different rates in different parts of the body
A fine balance must exist between	the breakdown and buildup of bone
If bone is built up too quickly	remodelling
Weak bone, as a result of too much calcium or bone tissue loss, can result in	an abnormally thick and heavy bone will be formed
Bone resorption and formation is known as	bone that breaks easily

8 Cortical bone

(a) Label the following diagram of the Haversian system, and colour the blood vessels, trabeculae and other components so as to differentiate them.

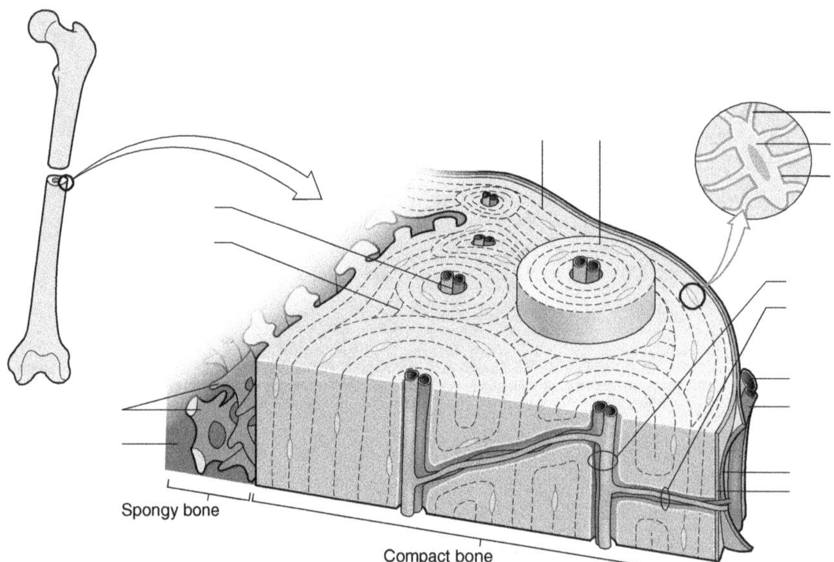

Source: Peate et al. (2014) / Reproduced with permission of John Wiley & Sons.

(b) Match the pairs.

Spongy bone	forms the outer edges of bones
Bone marrow	is dense and compact
Cortical bone	is porous and light
Cortical bone	are the struts of bone that give spongy bone strength
Trabeculae	is found in the ends and interior of long bones

9 Fracture repair

Fill in the missing stages of bone fracture repair.

Fracture occurs

↓

____

↓

Chondroblasts form fibrocartilage at the site of fracture

↓

____

↓

Bone remodelling occurs

↓

____

↓

Spongy bone is converted to compact bone

10 Bone types, bone shapes

(a) Fill in the classifications based on shape for the bones shown below:

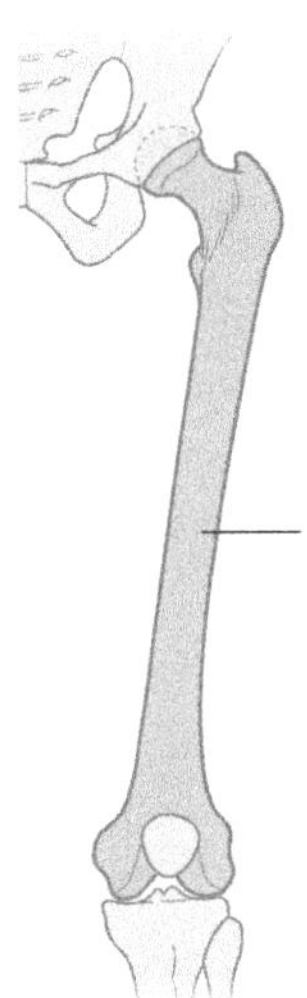

____________bone

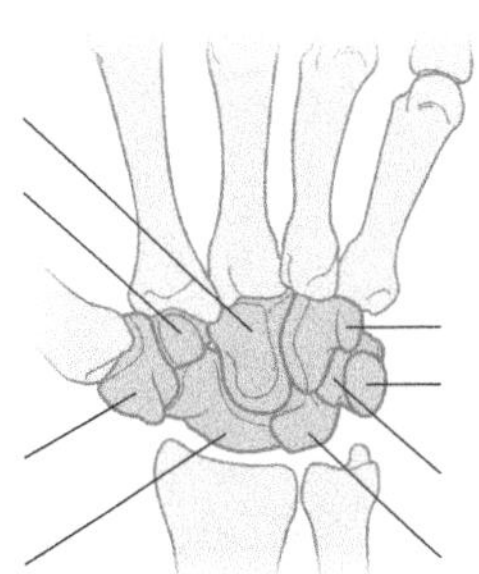

________________bones

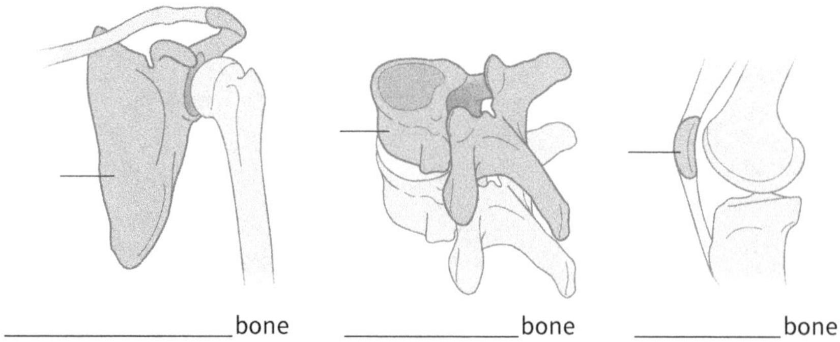

(b) Name the labelled bones on the skeleton shown here:

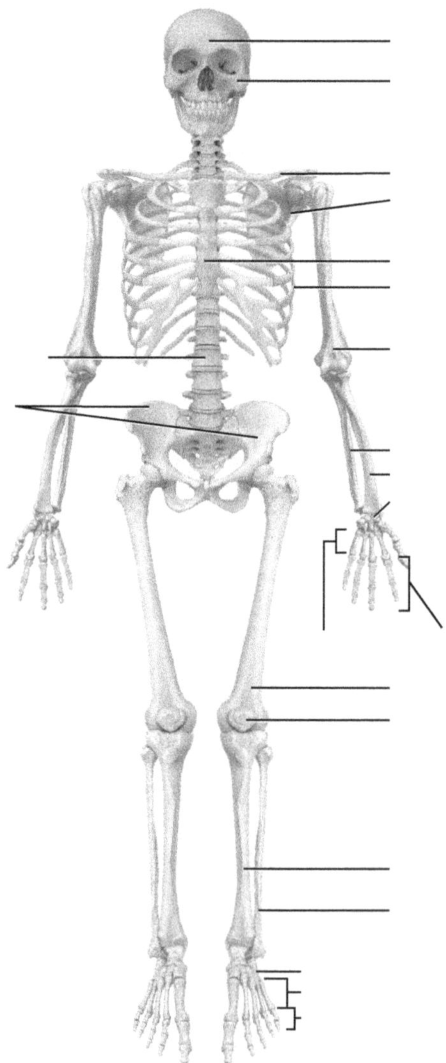

Source: Peate and Nair (2015) / Reproduced with permission of John Wiley & Sons.

11 Joints

Complete the following table, showing the various types of joints.

	Name of joint type	Examples
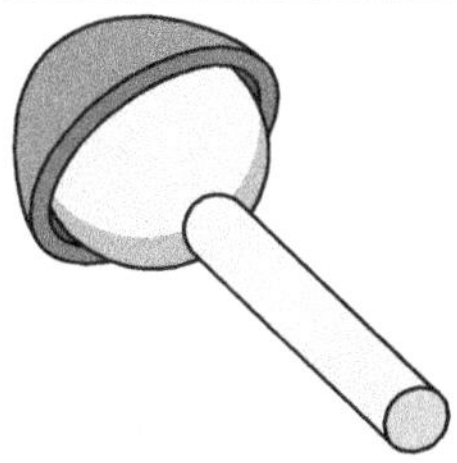		
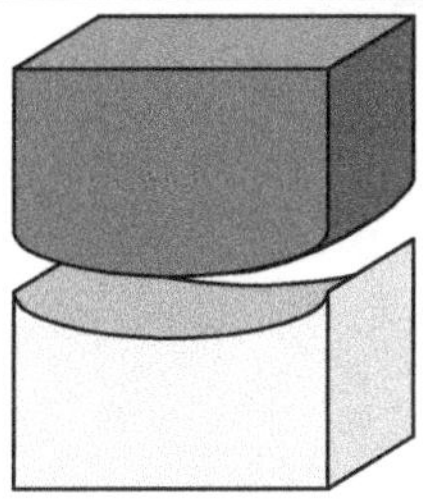		
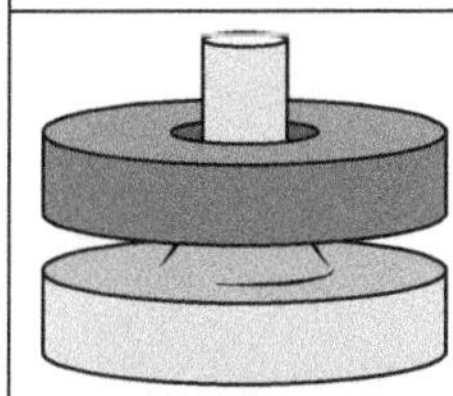		
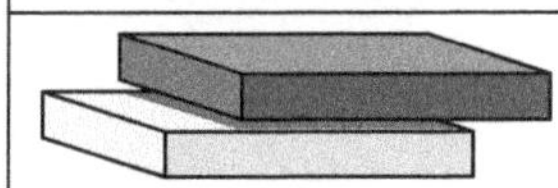		
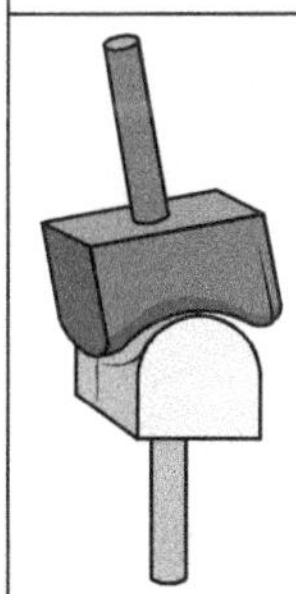		
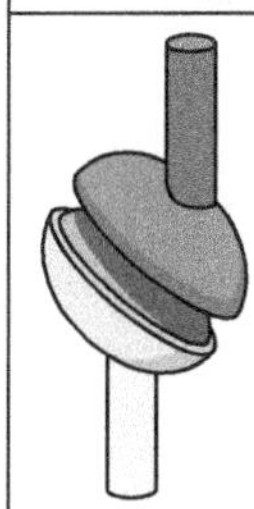		

Source: Peate and Evans (2026) / Reproduced with permission of John Wiley & Sons.

12 Cartilage, tendons and ligaments

Colour and label the tendons, ligaments and cartilage on the following diagrams. Identify the type of cartilage in each case.

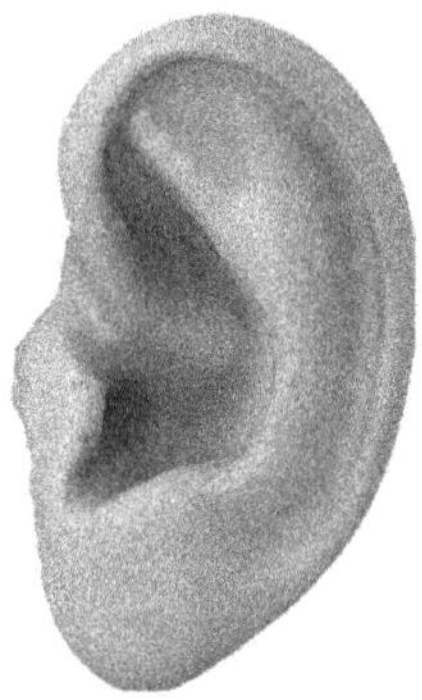

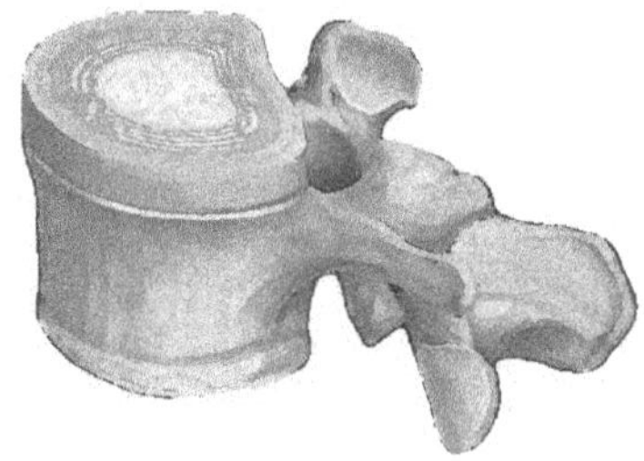

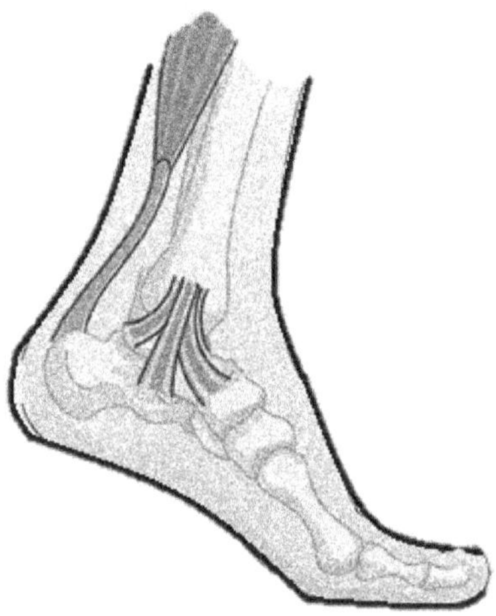

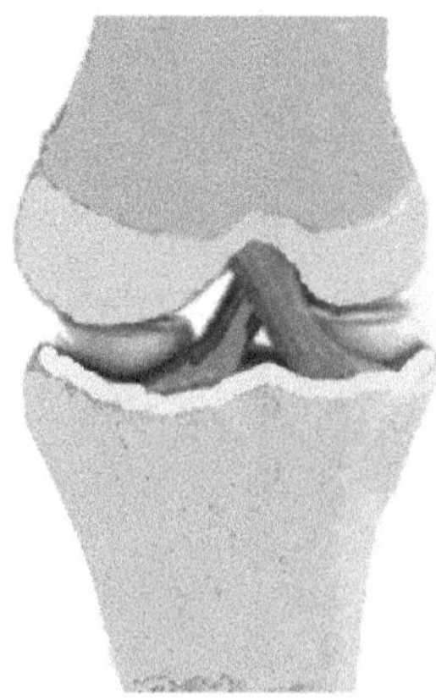

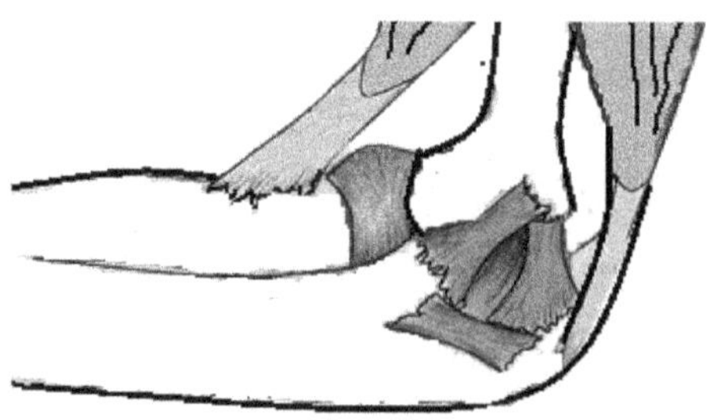

13 Terminology

Look up the meanings of the prefixes and suffixes in the following terms, write them into the table and then give the meaning of the complete terms.

Arthritis	
Arthr- =	-itis =
Meaning:	

Periosteum	
Peri- =	-osteum =
Meaning:	

Synovium	
Syn- =	-ovium =
Meaning:	

Perichondrium	
Peri- =	-chondrium =
Meaning:	

Osteopenia	
Osteo- =	-penia =
Meaning:	

Osteoporosis	
Osteo- =	-porosis =
Meaning:	

14 Clinical notes

(a) Interpret the following notes and write them in a form that a patient could more easily understand, then answer the follow-up questions.

Pt. ♀ 67 yo, fall at home. Pain R wrist. Pt lucid & oriented to time & place.
Medical Hx HTN, CHF, asthma. Smoker, no regular exercise.
Meds: Diuretic, Steroid puffer.
Diag.: Colle's fracture
DEXA T score −2.9
Rx: Bisphosphonate, Vit.D & Ca.

(b) What is a Colle's fracture?

(c) What does a T score of −2.9 mean?

(d) What action do bisphosphonate drugs have on bone?

(e) What effect would an anti-inflammatory steroid have on bone?

(f) Besides the medications that have been added, what additional advice would be appropriate for this patient?

15 Snap shot

Preventing osteoporosis

Lifestyle factors such as diet and exercise influence how healthy the bones are.
Regular exercise is an essential activity in helping people to prevent osteoporosis. The role of the nurse is multifaceted, and one aspect of this role is to help people live healthy lives and prevent potential problems. What advice would you give to an adult with regards to taking exercise?

16 Crossword

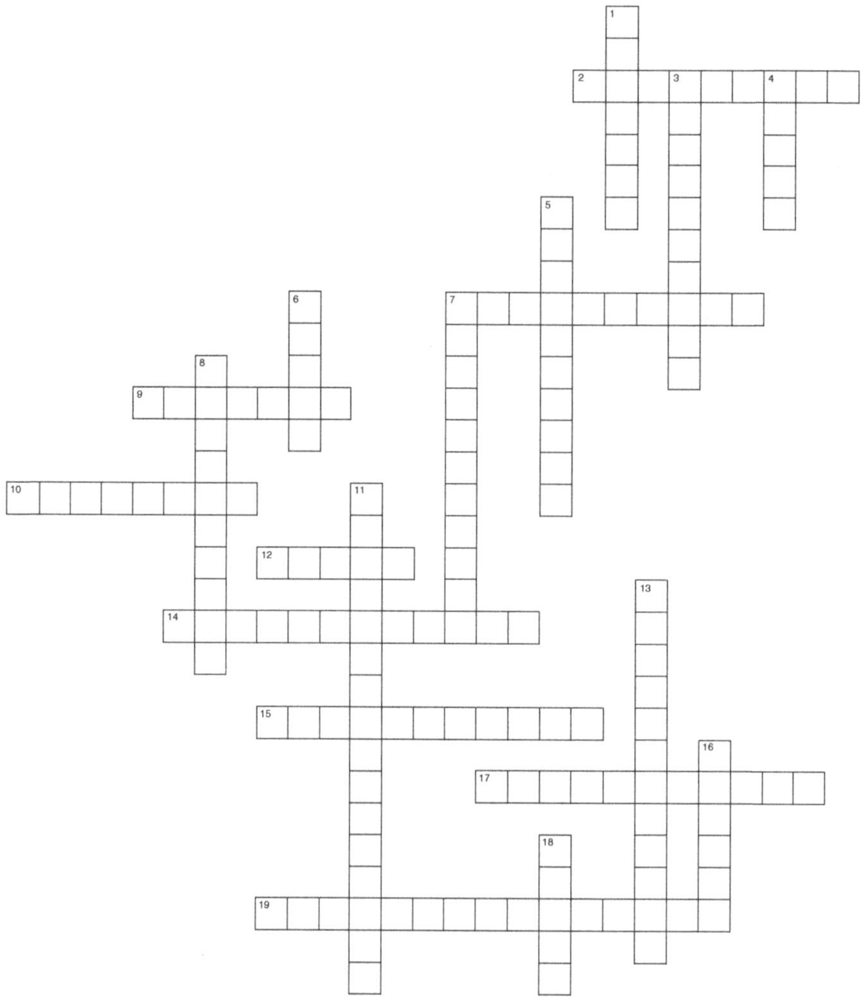

Across

2. Infants are born with a skeleton template made of this material that later becomes ossified
7. Bone cells with long processes
9. Bones of the wrist
10. Bones of the middle ear
12. Bony protection for the brain
14. Function of red bone marrow
15. Bone resorption and formation
17. Cells that remove bone
19. The type of ossification that occurs during the formation of the flat bones

Down

1. Cartilage type with a smooth glassy, friction-reducing surface
3. Inflammation of tendons
4. The hyoid bone is part of the _____ skeleton
5. Lower than normal bone density
6. Bony protection for the spinal cord
7. Cells that build bone
8. A type of bone tissue found in the epiphyses of long bones
11. Lipids are stored in the bone here
13. Conversion of a connective tissue to bone
16. The bone that rotates around the ulna during pronation of the hand
18. The number of types of cell present in bone

Multiple-choice questions

17. What is an osteophyte?
A. A bone cell
B. A small bony outgrowth
C. A bone cancer cell
D. A lymph cell

18. Where is the lateral malleolus located?
A. The hip
B. The tibia
C. The fibula
D. The cranium

19. What is the clavicle also known as?
A. The rib
B. The breastbone
C. The collar bone
D. The pelvis

20. What does kinesiology mean?
A. The study of light
B. The study of brain
C. The study of energy
D. The study of movement of the body

21. What are joints that permit free movement known as?
A. Diarthroses
B. Haemarthroses
C. Synarthroses
D. Amphiarthroses

22. When do muscle cells use the anaerobic process of glycolysis?
A. When the number of mitochondria is high
B. During intense physical activity, when oxygen delivery to the mitochondria is not enough to meet demand
C. When slow-twitch muscles are working
D. When there is a buildup of lactic acid in the cell

23. How do cardiac muscles differ from skeletal muscle fibres?
A. They have a greater reliance on anaerobic metabolism
B. They are larger than skeletal muscles
C. They can undergo tetanus
D. They do not require neural stimulation to contract

24. The muscular system:
A. can work independently of other body systems
B. contains approximately 700 muscles that can be voluntarily controlled
C. will hypertrophy if not used regularly
D. does not play a role in controlling body temperature

25. Cardiac muscle can contract without neural stimulation because it has the following property:
A. Plasticity
B. Excitability
C. Pacesetting
D. Automaticity

CHAPTER 9

The circulatory system

1 Formed elements of blood

Label and colour the formed elements of blood in the following diagram:

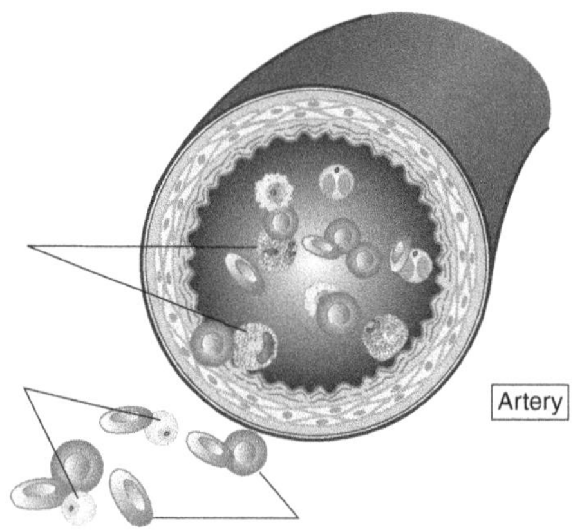

2 Blood composition

Fill in the missing blood components and their percentage values on the diagram below, and colour the formed elements of blood.

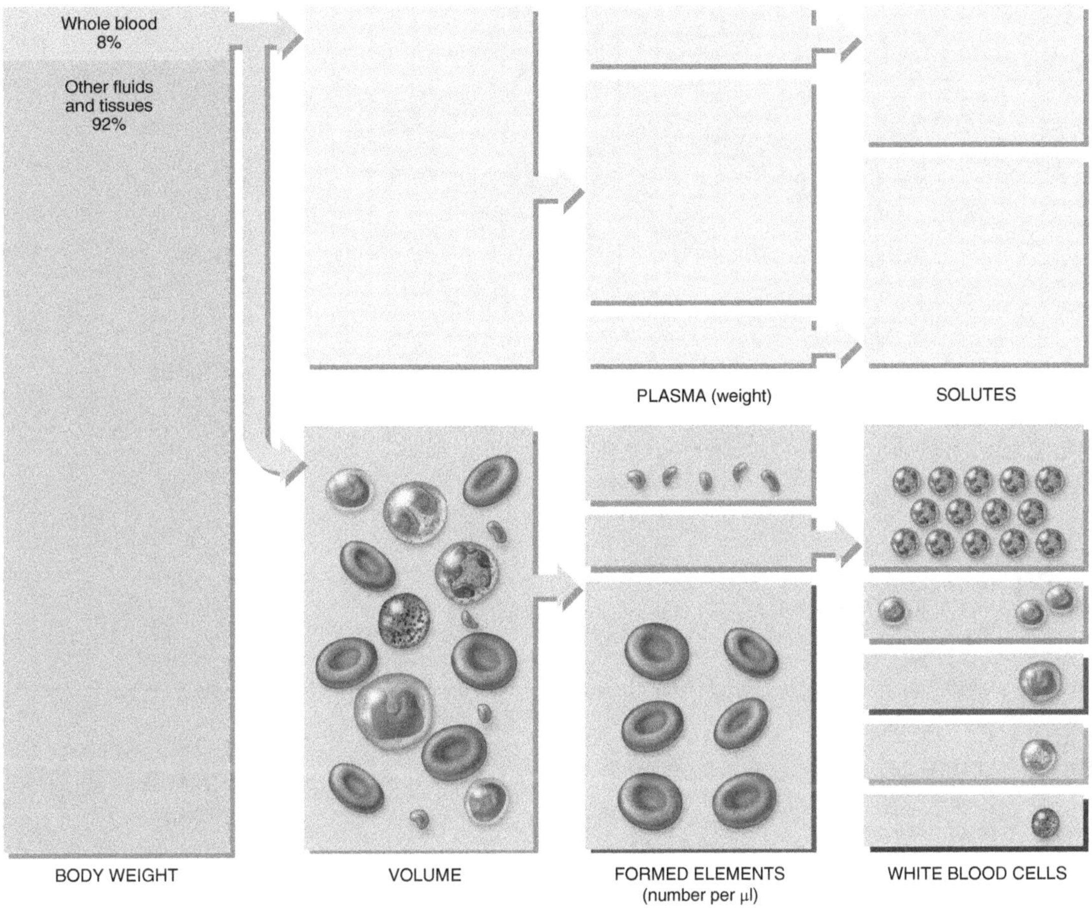

Source: Tortora and Derrickson (2009) / Reproduced with permission of John Wiley & Sons.

3 Separation of blood conpnents

Label the elements of whole blood that can be seen in the test tube after centrifugation, shown in the following diagram. Add the percentage that each value contributes to the total volume.

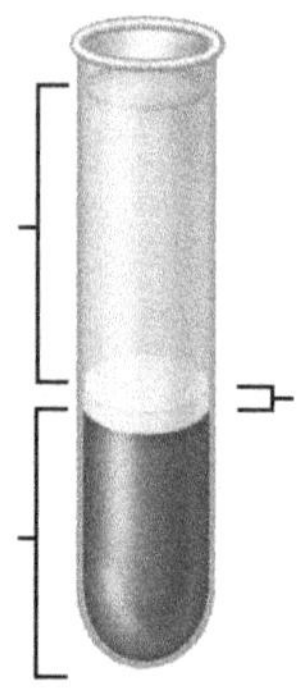

Source: Tortora and Derrickson (2009) / Reproduced with permission of John Wiley & Sons.

4 Match the pairs

Blood is a fluid	red blood cells, white blood cells, platelets
The formed elements	connective tissue
The fluid portion of blood	the buffy coat
The layer between plasma and erythrocytes in a centrifuged sample of blood	plasma
The buffy coat consists of	haematocrit
The percentage of blood volume occupied by red blood cells	white blood cells and platelets

5 Time yourself to unscramble these words

Scrambled	Unscrambled
CHATTIAMORE	
SLEEPTALT	
EYESTRYCORTH	
AMSLAP	
GHARAHOREEM	
STEELMEN	
PHYML	

6 Functions of blood

Describe the functions of blood in the following table:

Function	Description
Transportation	
Thermoregulation	
pH balance	
Removal of waste products	
Blood clotting	
Defence	

7 Naming the formed elements

(a) Fill in the names of the blood cells on the diagram of haemopoiesis and colour each cell type to highlight their structural differences.

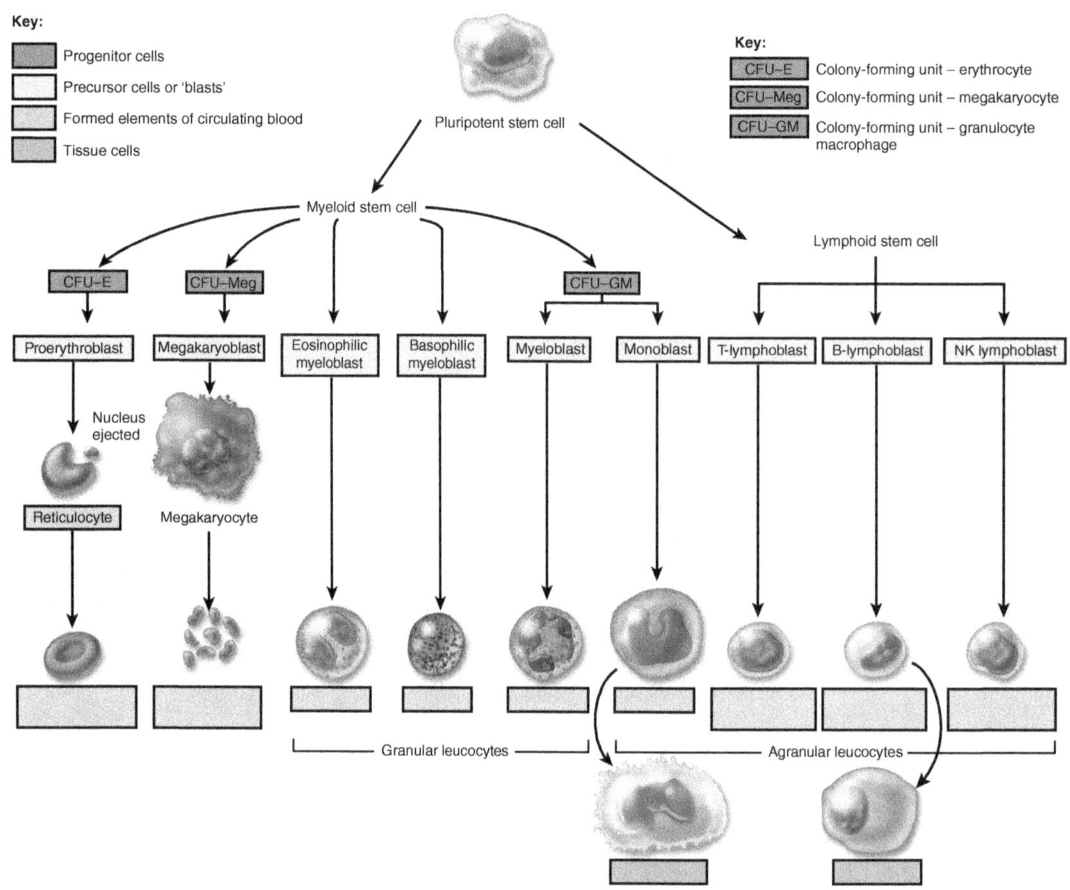

Source: Tortora and Derrickson (2009) / Reproduced with permission of John Wiley & Sons.

(b) Fill in the blank words in the following passage:

The circulatory system includes the ____________, the ____________, the blood ____________ and the ____________ system. The blood vessels carry blood throughout the ____________ system. Blood consists of ____________ elements and a fluid portion, known ____________.
Blood is a ____________ tissue, and its formed elements are ____________ ____________, ____________ ____________ and ____________. The process by which formed elements develop is called ____________. In the last three months of gestation and throughout life, the ________________ is the primary centre for haemopoiesis.

8 Match the pairs

Blood helps to maintain the body temperature by	erythrocytes
By the mechanism of clotting	in order to produce blood cells
The process by which formed elements of blood develop is known as	haemopoiesis
Multipotent stem cells divide into myeloid and lymphoid stem cells in the bone marrow	loss of blood cells and body fluids is halted
Myeloid stem cells further subdivide in the bone marrow producing	in the thymus and may then migrate to other lymph tissues
T-lymphocytes continue their development	distributing heat produced by chemical activity of cells evenly, throughout the body

9 Erythropoiesis

Complete the following diagram showing the steps of erythropoiesis:

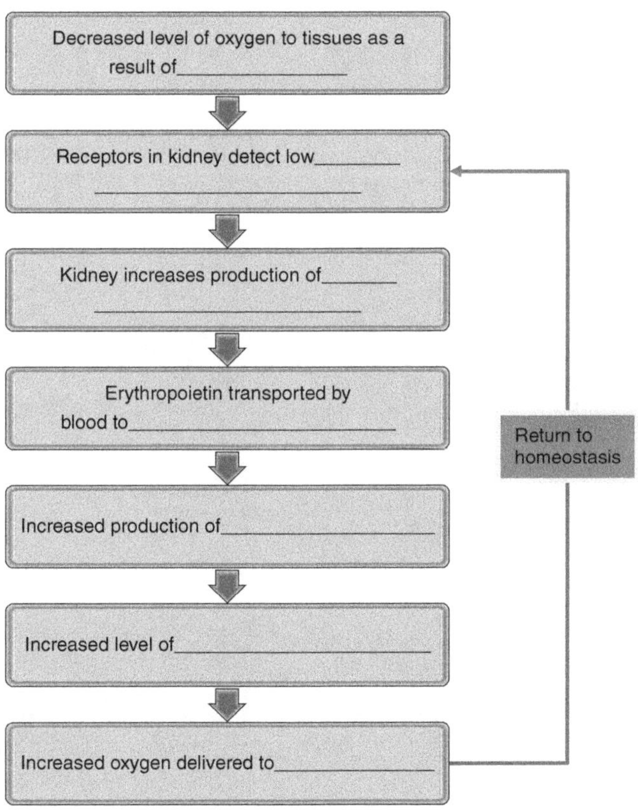

10 Haemoglobin

Colour and label the haemoglobin molecule shown here:

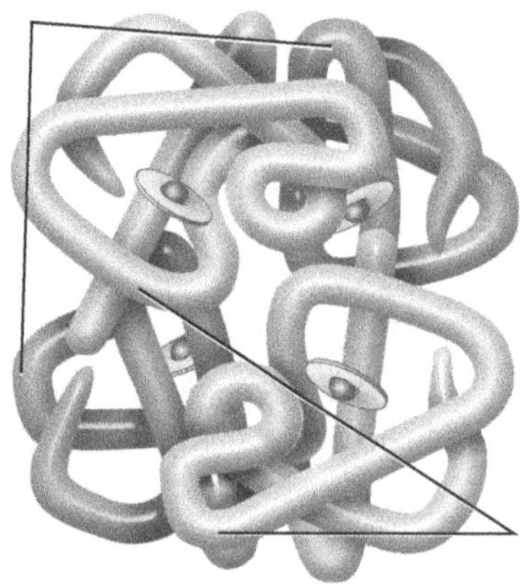

11 Identifying blood cells

Label the blood cells shown and name each cell.

(a) ______________________________

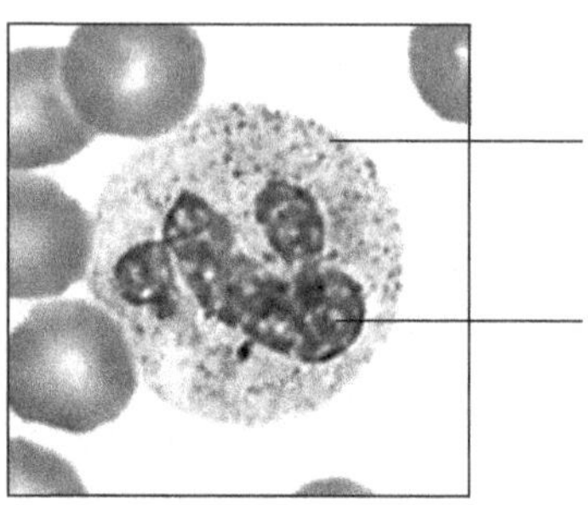

(b) ______________________________

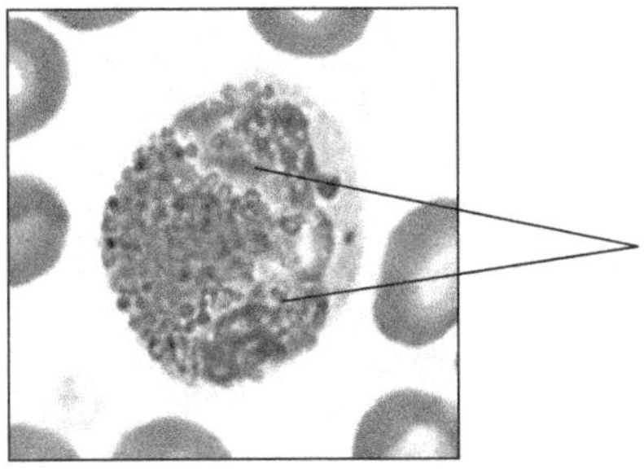

(c) ______________________________

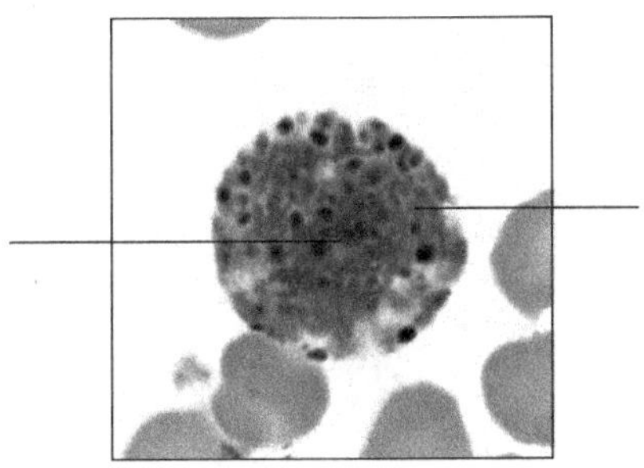

(d) ______________________________

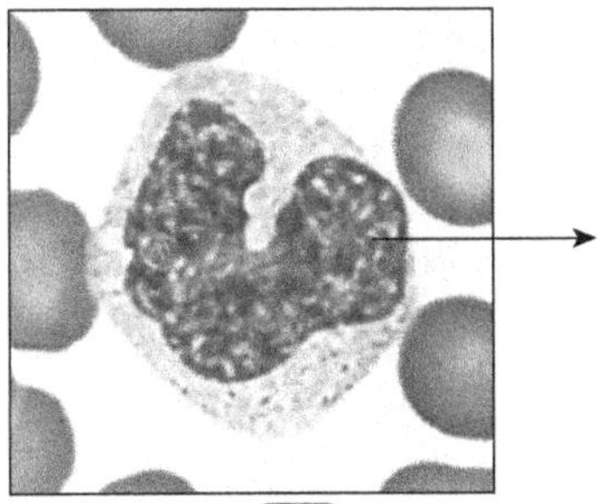

LM all 1600x

(e) ______________________________

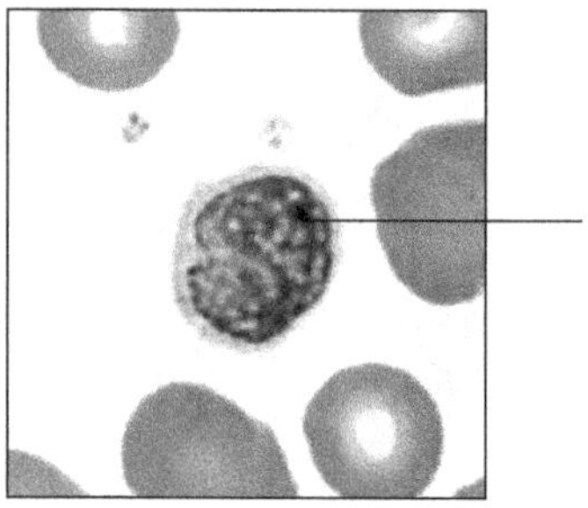

Source: Tortora and Derrickson (2009) / Reproduced with permission of John Wiley & Sons.

12 Identifying leucocyte types

Colour in and name the various types of white blood cells shown here:

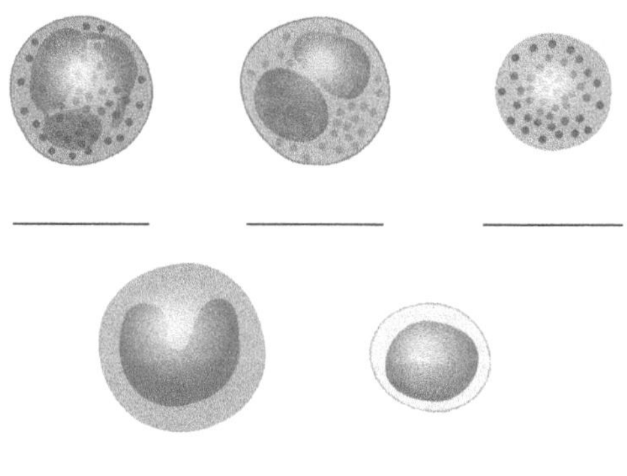

Source: Peate and Nair (2011) / Reproduced with permission of John Wiley & Sons.

13 Haemostasis

(a) Fill in the empty boxes in the following diagram showing the two remaining major steps of haemostasis:

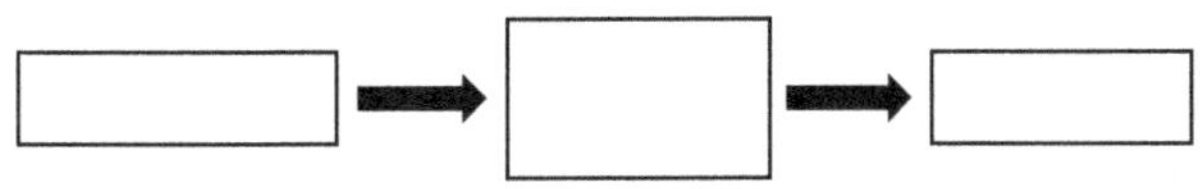

(b) Complete the boxes in the following diagram showing the coagulation process:

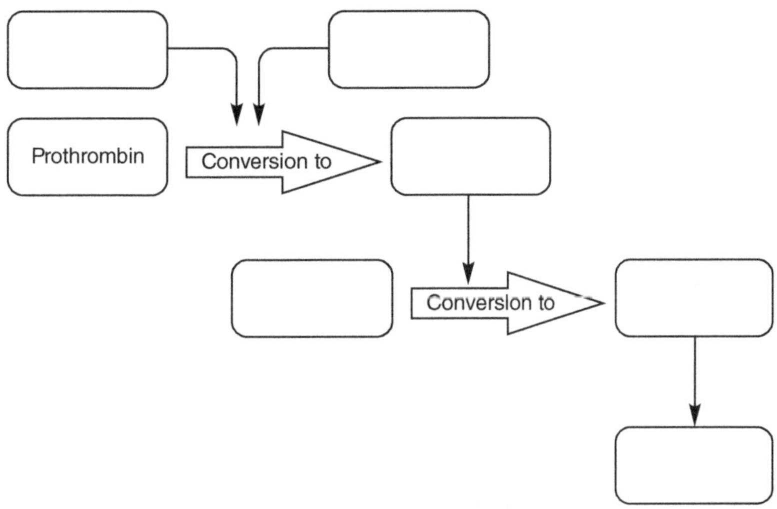

14 Blood types

(a) Fill in the antibodies present in the plasma of each blood type shown here.

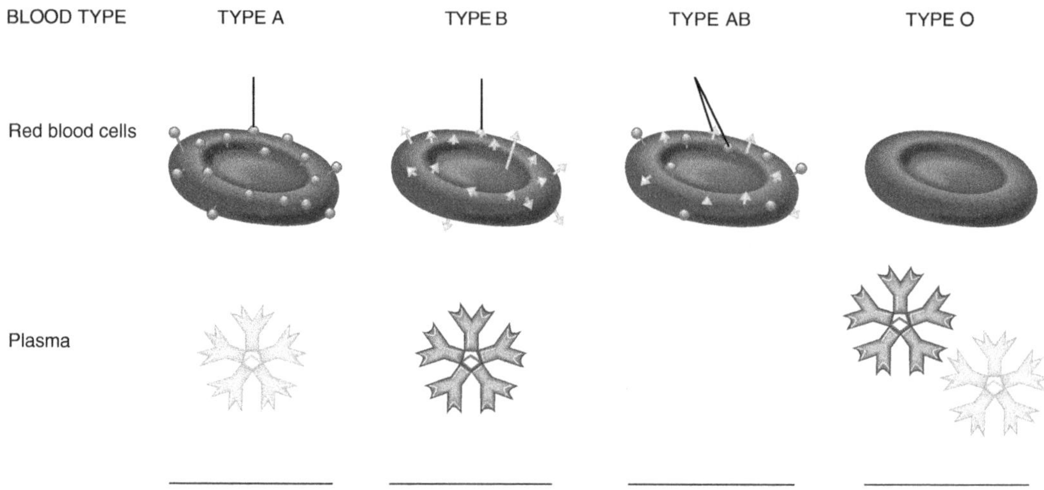

Source: Tortora and Derrickson (2009) / Reproduced with permission of John Wiley & Sons.

(b) Complete the following table:

Blood type	Antigens on red cells	Antibodies in plasma	Can donate blood to	Can receive blood from
A				
B				
AB				
O				

15 Match the pairs

The most abundant blood cells	antigens
Location of blood cell production	megakaryocytes
Iron-containing portion of haemoglobin	erythrocytes
Precursor cells for platelets	bone marrow
Red cell surface markers	haem

16 Blood vessel types

(a) Colour in the vessels in the following diagram to show oxygenated versus deoxygenated blood and label the vessels.

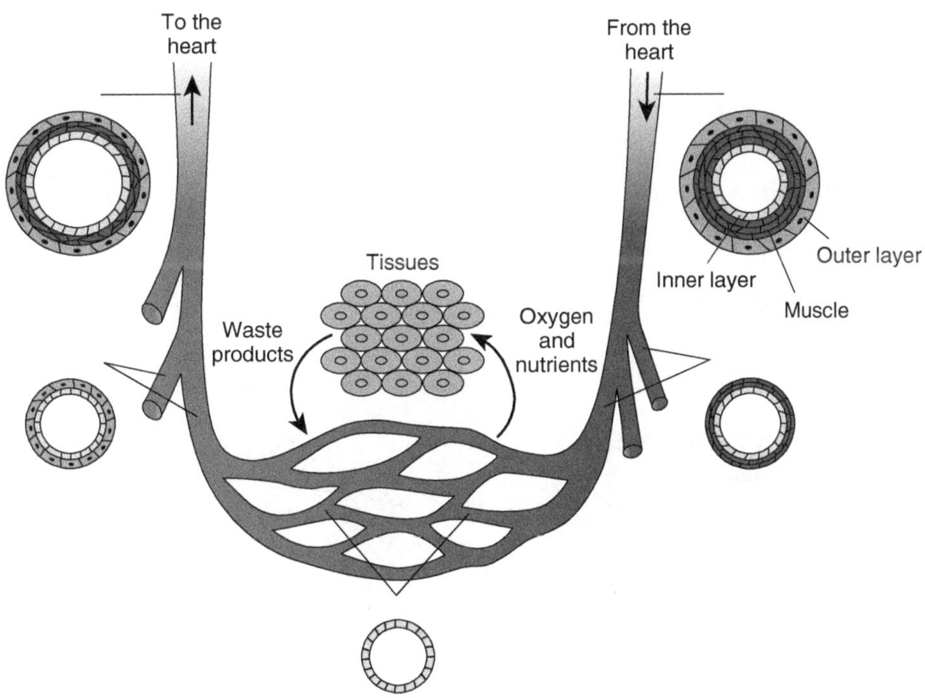

Source: Peate and Nair (2011) / Reproduced with permission of John Wiley & Sons.

(b) Identify the vein and the artery in the following diagram and label the features of both.

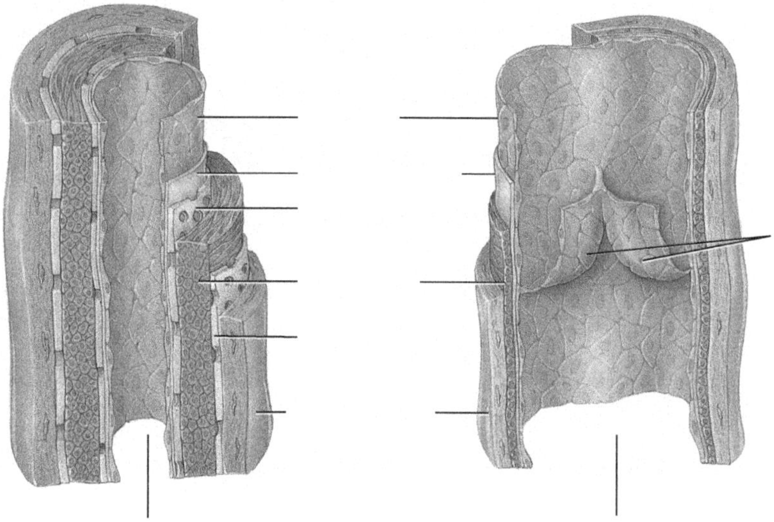

(c) Label the diagram of a capillary here:

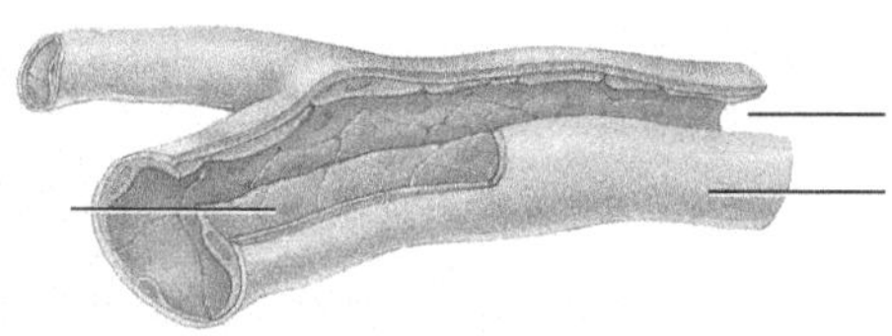

Source: Tortora and Derrickson (2009) / Reproduced with permission of John Wiley & Sons.

(d) Identify the artery and vein in the following diagram and label the wall layers.

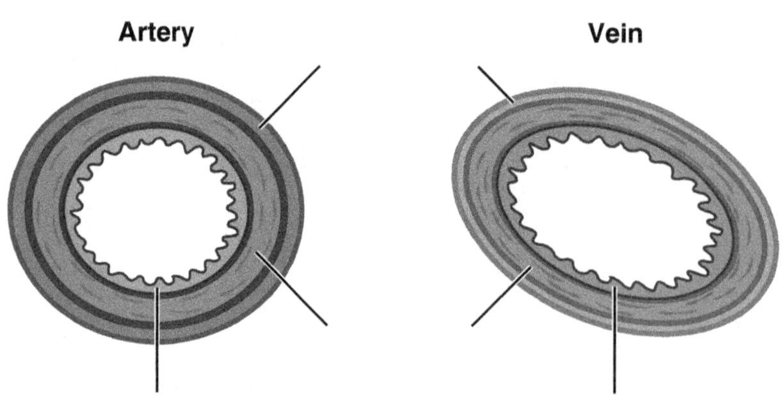

Source: Peate and Nair (2011) / Reproduced with permission of John Wiley & Sons.

(e) List the differences in both structure and function between arteries and veins in the following table:

Arteries	Veins

17 Blood vs lymphatic vessels

(a) Colour the following diagram to distinguish between blood and lymph vessels, and between arterial and venous vessels, and label the diagram.

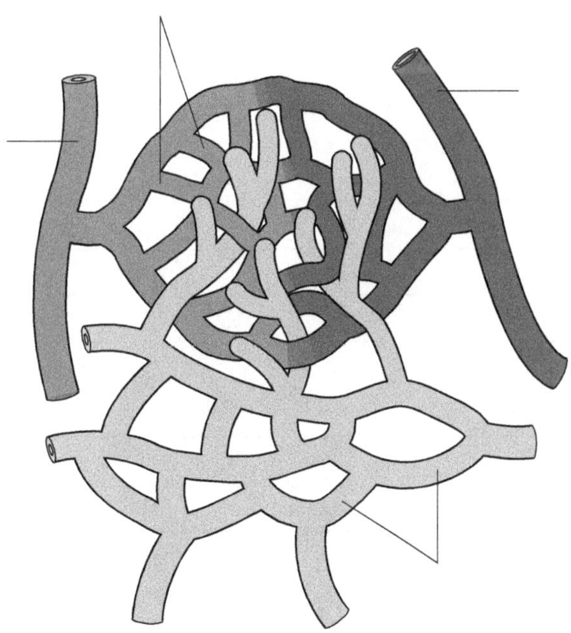

Source: Peate and Nair (2011) / Reproduced with permission of John Wiley & Sons.

(b) Match the pairs.

Arteries	lymphatic capillaries
Veins	enable the exchange of water, nutrients and chemicals between the blood and the tissues
Capillaries	carry blood from the capillaries back towards the heart
Capillaries are	carry the blood away from the heart
Small, closed-end lymphatic vessels	filter out harmful substances from the lymph
Lymphocytes in lymph nodes	tiny, thin-walled vessels between arteries and veins that supply the tissues

18 Terminology

Look up the meanings of the prefixes and suffixes in the following terms, write them into the table and then give the meaning of the complete terms.

Haemolysis	
Haemo- =	-lysis =
Meaning:	

Erythropoietin	
Erythro- =	-poietin =
Meaning:	

Haemoglobin	
Haemo- =	-globin =
Meaning:	

Leukocyte	
Leuko- =	-cyte=
Meaning:	

Haemopoiesis	
Haem- =	-poiesis=
Meaning:	

Neutrophil	
Neutro- =	-phil =
Meaning:	

19 Snap shot

Varicosities

Usually, blood collected from superficial venous capillaries is directed upward and inward via one-way valves into superficial veins. These then drain via perforator veins that pass through muscle fascia into deep veins. A leaking valve allows a retrograde flow back into the vein. Unlike deep veins, which are thick walled and confined by fascia, the superficial veins cannot withstand high pressure and eventually become dilated and tortuous. When one valve fails, it puts additional pressure on its neighbours, which can result in retrograde flow, and ultimately varicosity of the whole local superficial venous network.
On the following diagram, identify where varicosities can occur.

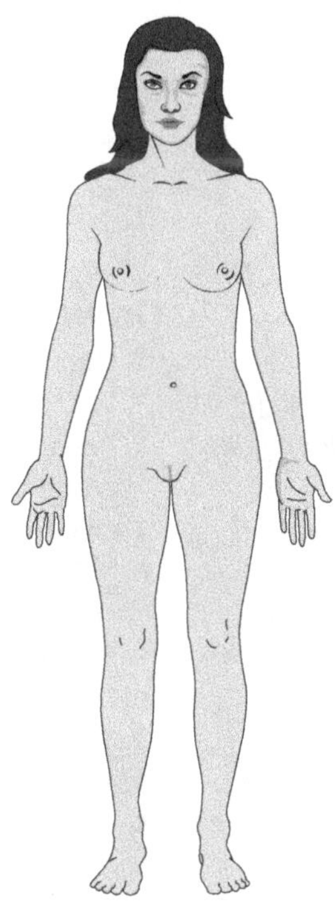

20 Crossword

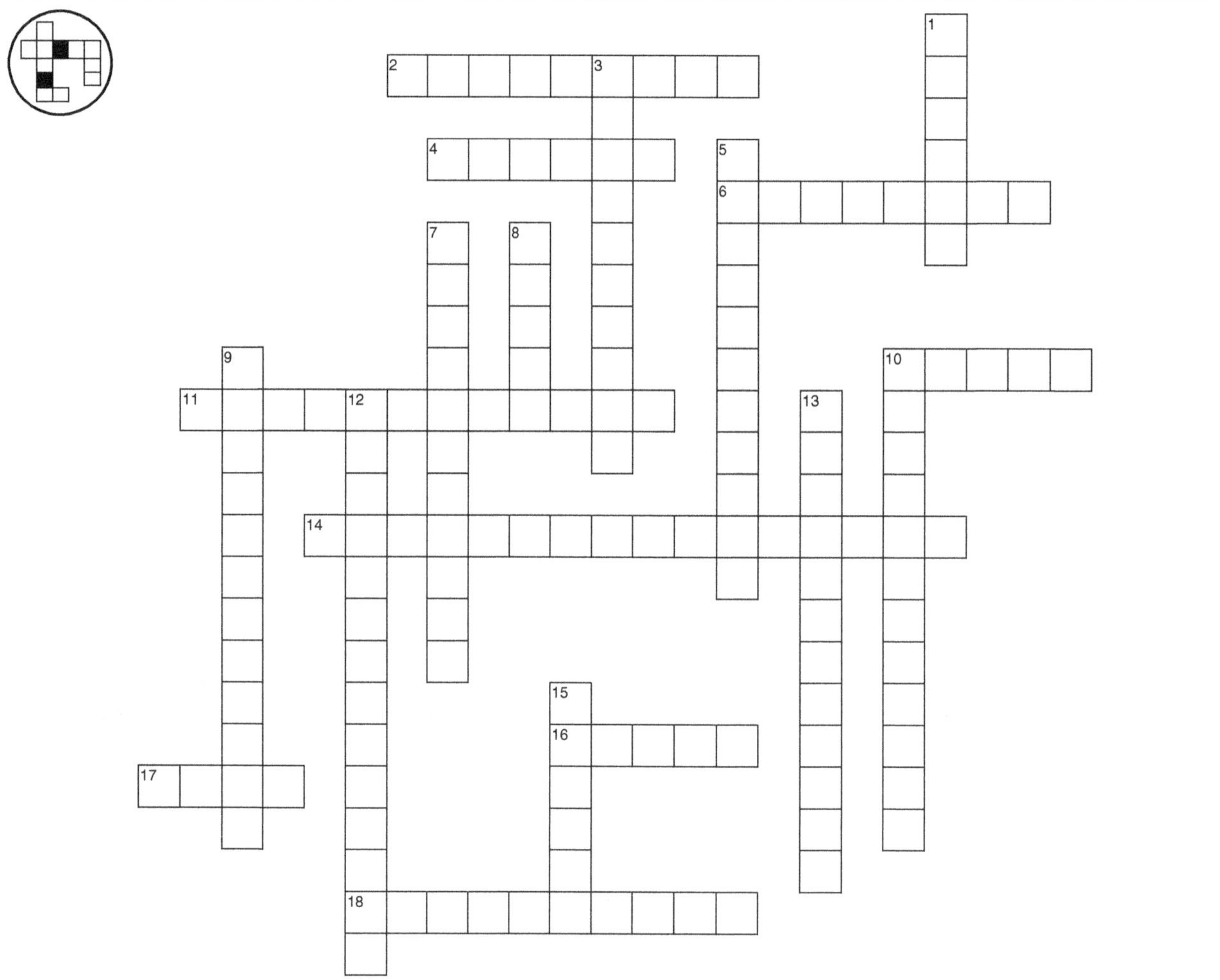

Across

2. Cell fragments found in the buffy coat
4. The T-lymphocytes continue their development here
6. Markers located on the surface of the red blood cells that can trigger an immune response
10. Arteries transport blood away from this organ
11. Platelets
14. Contraction of smooth muscle of the vessel wall
16. Tissue fluid that is returned to the venous circulation, after being cleaned in nodes and flowing through specialised vessels
17. Iron-containing portion of haemoglobin molecule
18. Process of white blood cells migrating from the blood vessel

Down

1. Organ that destroys old, worn-out red blood cells
3. White blood cells
5. Percentage of the blood volume occupied by red blood cells
7. Oxygen-carrying protein
8. 'Coat' between the plasma and erythrocytes in a centrifuged sample of whole blood
9. Platelets release these vasoconstrictors
10. Process by which blood cells are formed
12. The cells from which platelets are derived
13. Red blood cells
15. The fluid portion of blood

Multiple-choice questions

21. The erythrocyte:
A. is phagocytic
B. transports oxygen
C. prevents blood coagulation
D. destroys antibodies

22. The neutrophil:
A. is a cytotoxic T-cell
B. is a granulocytic phagocyte
C. secretes chyme
D. deactivates plasmin

23. Thrombin:
A. activates fibrinogen
B. is responsible for the formation of the complement
C. i inactivated by vitamin B12
D. is inactivated by prothrombin

24. What statement is true regarding the administration of type A+ blood to a type O– recipient?
A. The blood types are compatible; no haemolytic reaction is expected
B. People with O– blood are allergic to type A+ blood
C. The blood types are incompatible; haemolysis will occur
D. Those with type O– blood can safely receive type A+ blood

25. Erythropoietin:
A. is synthesised by the kidneys
B. stimulates the bone marrow to make red blood cells
C. is released by the kidney in response to hypoxaemia
D. All of the above

26. What is most likely to cause jaundice?
A. Anaemia
B. An increase in erythropoietin
C. A deficiency of the extrinsic factor
D. Haemolysis

27. Which of the following is a true statement?
A. The reticulocyte is an undeveloped thrombocyte
B. The neutrophil is a phagocytic granulocyte
C. The neutrophil, basophil and eosinophil are elements of the megakaryocyte
D. A deficiency of reticulocytes causes hypoprothrombinaemia

28. Hypoprothrombinaemia along with a prolonged prothrombin time is:
A. a cause of spontaneous bleeding
B. indicative of pernicious anaemia
C. a result of heparin therapy
D. a consequence of thrombocytopenia

29. Hyperbilirubinaemia:
A. can be caused by haemolysis
B. causes jaundice
C. can cause kernicterus
D. All of the above

CHAPTER 10

The cardiac system

1 Location of the heart

Label the following diagram, showing the organs of the thorax:

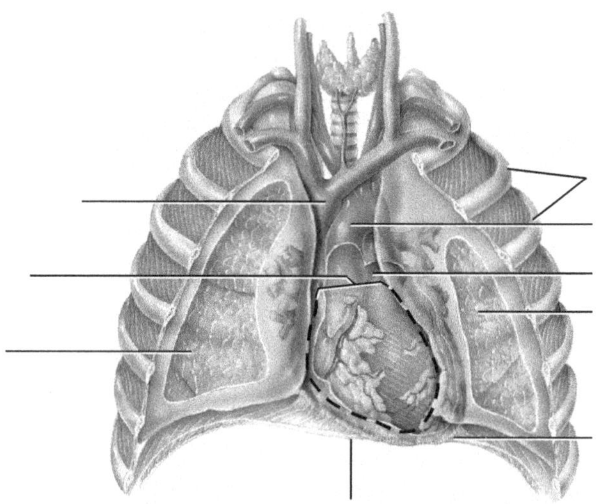

Source: Tortora and Derrickson (2009) / Reproduced with permission of John Wiley & Sons.

2 Anatomy of the heart

(a) Label and colour the components of the heart shown here:

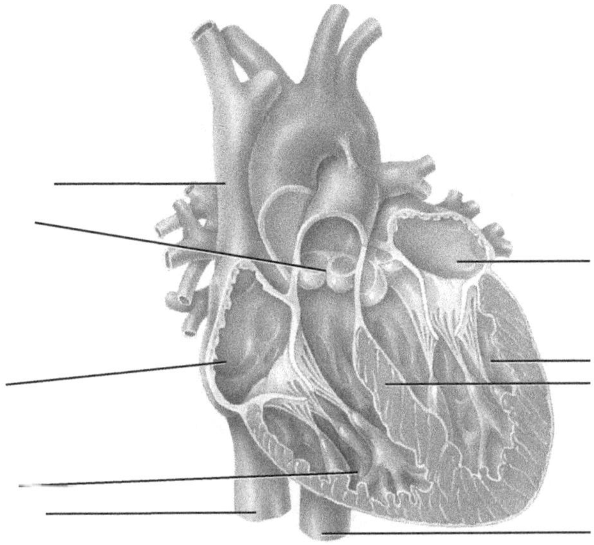

(b) Label and colour in the various layers of the heart wall shown here:

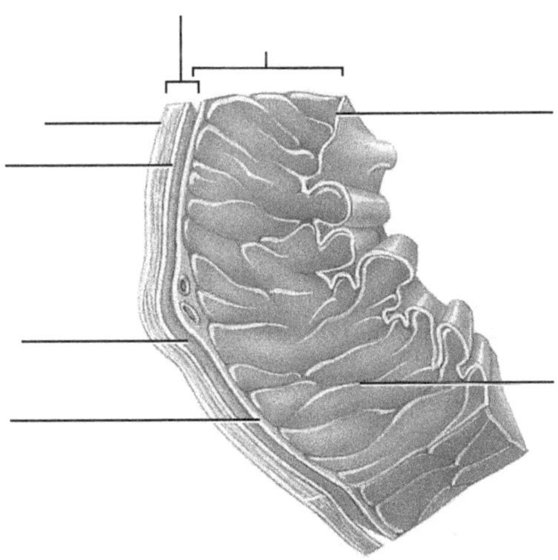

Source: Tortora and Derrickson (2009) / Reproduced with permission of John Wiley & Sons.

(c) Match the pairs.

The apex of the heart is below	this reduces friction as the heart moves during its cycle of contraction and relaxation
Between the parietal and visceral pericardium is a thin film of pericardial fluid	the base of the heart, lying on the diaphragm
The bulk of muscle in the heart is	prevent the backward flow of blood from the ventricles into the atria
The atria are	divides the ventricles
The atrioventricular valves	the myocardium
The interventicular septum	the smaller chambers of the heart

SCRA-MBLE

(d) Time yourself to unscramble these words.

Scrambled	Unscrambled
ARATI	
SERVENTICL	
DECARUMRIPI	
DECORUMNADI	
DACOMRUMIY	
DISCUTRIP	
DISCUBIP	

3 The coronary circulation

(a) Label the following diagram showing the coronary arteries:

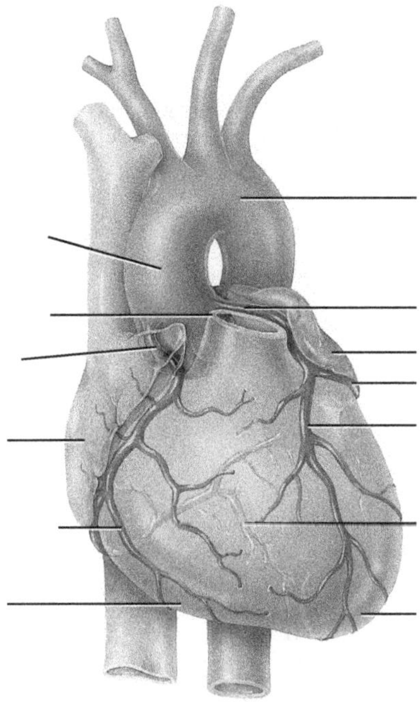

Source: Tortora and Derrickson (2009) / Reproduced with permission of John Wiley & Sons.

(b) Complete the following table to indicate the areas of the heart supplied by the various branches of the coronary arteries.

Artery	Major branches	Area of the heart supplied
Left anterior descending (LAD)	Diagonals Septals	
Circumflex artery	Oblique marginal	
Right coronary artery (RCA)	Posterior descending artery	

4 Blood flow through the heart

(a) Label the following diagram to show the components represented by the boxes, then using two different colours (red arrows for oxygenated blood and blue arrows for deoxygenated blood), indicate the flow of blood through the heart.

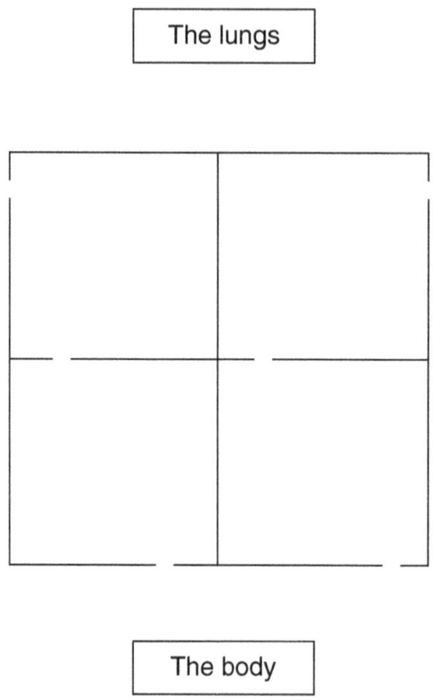

(b) Label the following diagram to show how the blood flows through the various structures of the heart.

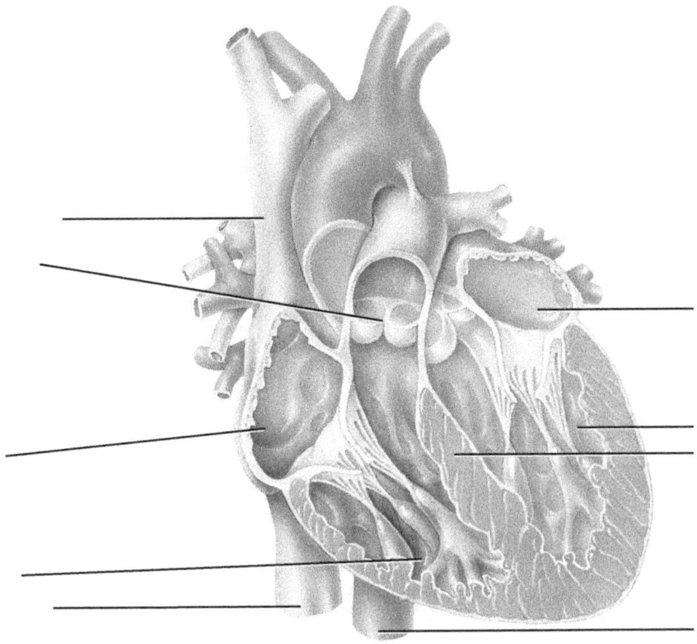

Source: Tortora and Derrickson (2009) / Reproduced with permission of John Wiley & Sons.

(c) Time yourself to unscramble these words.

Scrambled	Answer
CRUFMECLIX	
YARNCROO	
MYSTICES	
YONEXTAGED	
SEVONU	
TRAILARE	

5 Match the pairs

The heart receives	the atrium and the ventricle, as well as their associated valves
The heart receives a plentiful supply of blood ensuring the constant supply of	approximately 5% of the body's blood supply
The endocardium is	oxygen and nutrients and the efficient removal of waste products
The circumflex artery supplies the	supplied with blood directly from the inside of the heart chambers
The heart is best thought of as two pumps	back and side of the left ventricle
The pumps are made up of two chambers	the right and the left pumps

6 Conducting system of the heart

Label the following diagram and draw in the electrical conduction pathways of the heart:

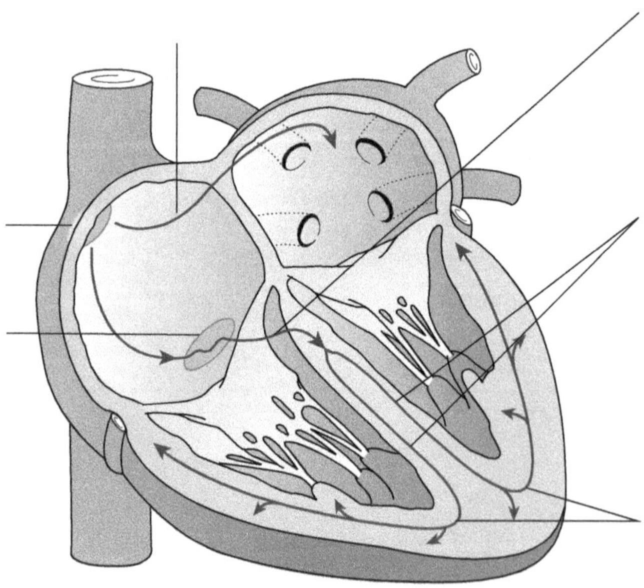

Source: Peate et al. (2014) / Reproduced with permission of John Wiley & Sons.

7 The electrocardiogram

(a) Label the waves of the normal ECG shown here.

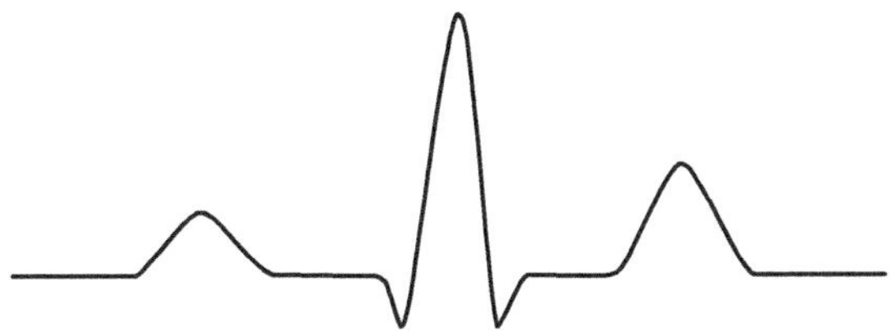

(b) Complete the following table:

ECG letter(s)	Electrical activity	Mechanical activity
P		Atrial contraction
QRS		
T	Ventricular repolarisation	

8 Hormones acting on the heart

Fill the actions on the heart of the hormones listed below:

Hormones	Action
Epinephrine	
Norepinephrine	
Thyroxine	

9 Match the pairs

The cardiac cycle refers to	in the carotid sinus and the aortic arch, sensitive to the amount of stretch in these blood vessels
Systole corresponds to	the autonomic nervous system and hormone activity
Diastole corresponds to	the volume of blood the heart pumps out in 1 minute
'Cardiac output' is a term meaning	the relaxation of a heart chamber (atrium or ventricle)
Heart rate is controlled by two main mechanisms:	the contraction of a heart chamber (atrium or ventricle)
Baroreceptors are specialised mechanical receptors located	the mechanical activity of the heart

10 Snap shot

Taking a patient's pulse

Pulse rate assessment is an essential activity that requires a skilled, competent and confident person to undertake the task safely and effectively. The nurse needs to understand how the pulse rate is maintained, factors impacting upon the pulse and how to measure the pulse rate effectively and safely. Having taken a pulse, the nurse must also understand what the various measurements may mean, how to record the pulse rate and how to report any abnormality, ensuring that the person is provided with care that is safe and responsive to their needs.

On this diagram, identify the sites that may be used to assess a person's pulse.

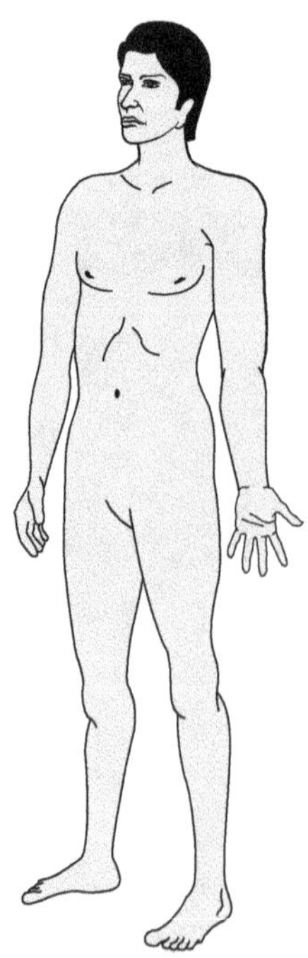

11 Definition of terms

Define the following terms:

Term	Definition
Asystole	
Bradycardia	
Tachycardia	
Arrhythmia	
Sinus rhythm	
Fibrillation	

12 Crossword

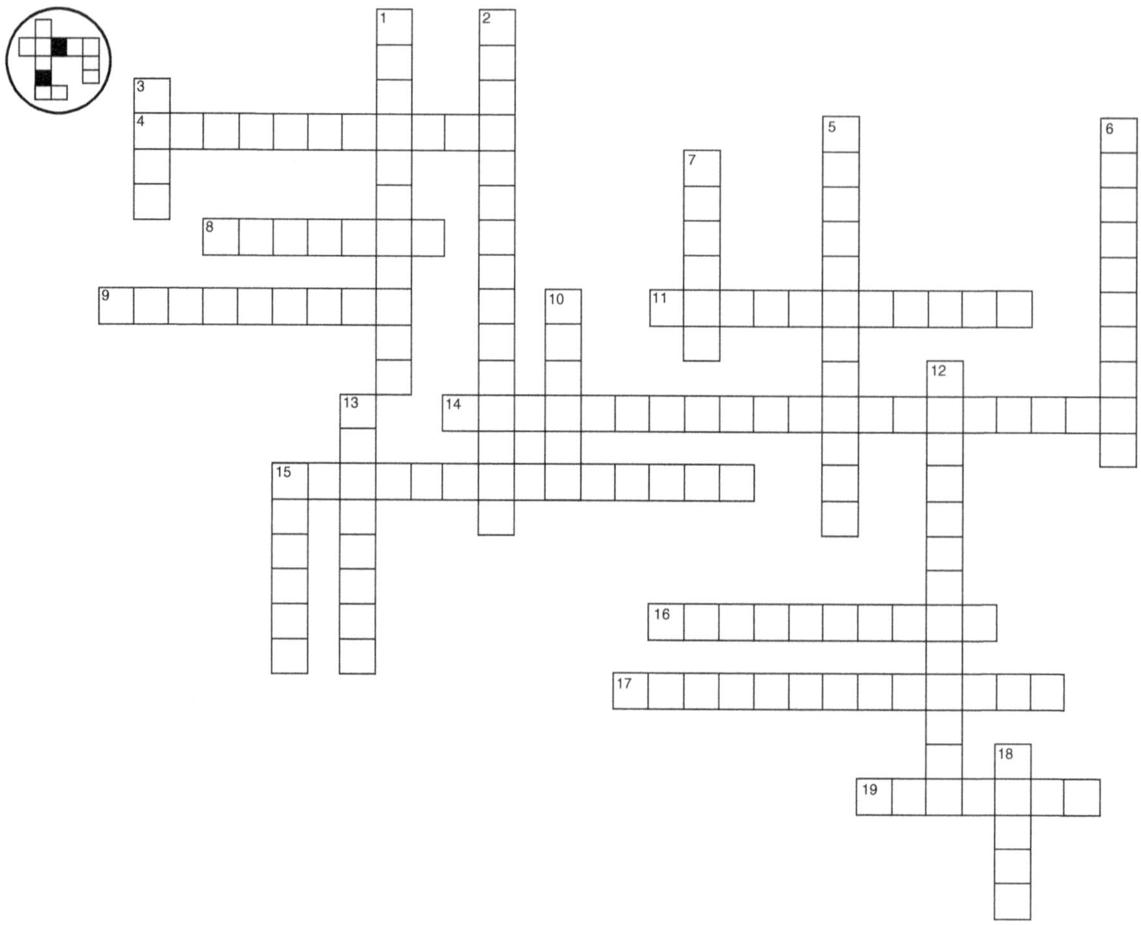

Across

4. The epithelium lining the interior of the heart chambers

8. The stretch placed on cardiac muscle fibres prior to their contraction

9. The pressure that the ventricles have to overcome to eject blood when they contract

11. Tough double-layered membrane surrounding the heart

14. The electrical conduction through this area is slowed to ensure that atria and ventricles do not contract together

15. The origin of electrical activity for a cardiac cycle

16. The blood flowing through the pulmonary veins is ___

17. The product of stroke volume and heart rate

19. The portion of the cardiac cycle when heart chambers are contracting

Down

1. This would be induced by parasympathetic effects on the heart

2. After flowing through the pulmonary valve, the blood enters the ________

3. The ventricle with the thickest wall

5. Cardiac cells are able to generate an action potential without a stimulus – a property known as ___________

6. The artery that supplies blood to the posterior and lateral wall of the left ventricle

7. When the left ventricle starts to relax, the aortic valve _____

10. Pain due to inadequate blood flow to the heart muscle

12. Specialised mechanical receptors located in the carotid sinus and the aortic arch

13. Blood flows into the heart through this vessel

15. The dividing wall between the ventricles

18. The largest blood vessel in the body

13 Terminology

Myocardium	
Myo- =	-cardium =
Meaning:	

Electrocardiogram		
Electro-=	-cardio=	-gram=
Meaning:		

Thrombolysis	
Thrombo- =	-lysis =
Meaning:	

Myocardial Infarction	
Myocardial =	Infarction =
Meaning:	

Coronary
Meaning:

Tachycardia	
Tachy- =	-cardia =
Meaning:	

14 Clinical case notes

Write the following notes out in a form that could be understood by a patient and then answer the follow-up questions.

(a) A&E presn. 58 yo ♂, acute crushing chest pain. Anxious and diaphoretic. Aspirin 160 mg admin. ECG indic.STEMI. Emergency PCI.

(b) What would be the purpose of giving the patient aspirin?

(c) What is a STEMI?

(d) What is PCI?

Multiple-choice questions

15. Which of the following areas conducts the cardiac impulse the fastest?
   A. Sino-atrial node
   B. Atrioventricular node
   C. Purkinje fibres
   D. Atrial bands

16. Which of the following statements is correct about cardiac output?
   A. Cardiac output is determined by the heart rate and pulse
   B. Stimulation of the sympathetic nerves decreases cardiac output
   C. Vagal discharge increases cardiac output
   D. Cardiac output is determined by heart rate and stroke volume

17. Which statement is true of ventricle diastole?
   A. Blood is ejected from the ventricles
   B. The semilunar valves are open
   C. The atrioventricular valves are closed
   D. The ventricles are filling

18. Which of the following is the function of a valve?
   A. To control the direction of blood flow through the heart
   B. To regulate the amount of carbon dioxide bound to haemoglobin
   C. To regulate strength of cardiac contraction
   D. To direct the progression of the cardiac impulse

19. Which of the following is true concerning the structures of the electrical conduction system?
   A. The AVF node is the pacemaker
   B. In normal sinus rhythm, the electrical signal arises within the SA node
   C. The Purkinje fibres spread the electrical signal from the right atrium to the left atrium
   D. None of the above

20. Which of the following is bradycardia?
   A. Heart rate below 60 beats per minute
   B. No cardiac output
   C. Heart rate over 100 beats per minute
   D. None of the above

21. Pacemaker cells in which of the following areas cycle at the highest rate?
   A. Left coronary artery
   B. SA node
   C. Ventricular myocardium
   D. AV node

22. The coronary arteries:
   A. branch from the aorta just after the aortic valve
   B. prevent the right atrium from filling with blood
   C. have maximum blood flow when the ventricles are contracted
   D. None of the above

23. What is ventricular systole?

A. Atrial depolarisation

B. Cardiac arrest

C. Ventricular filling

D. Ventricular contraction

24. Oxygenated blood flows through the:

A. coronary veins

B. pulmonary veins

C. pulmonary arteries

D. None of the above

CHAPTER 11

The gastrointestinal system

1 Processes taking place in the gastrointestinal tract

Complete the following table, describing the key processes that take place in the gastrointestinal tract.

Function	Description
Ingestion	
Propulsion	
Digestion	
Absorption	
Elimination	

2 Structures of the gastrointestinal system

Label the following diagram and colour in the oesophagus, stomach, small intestine and large intestine.

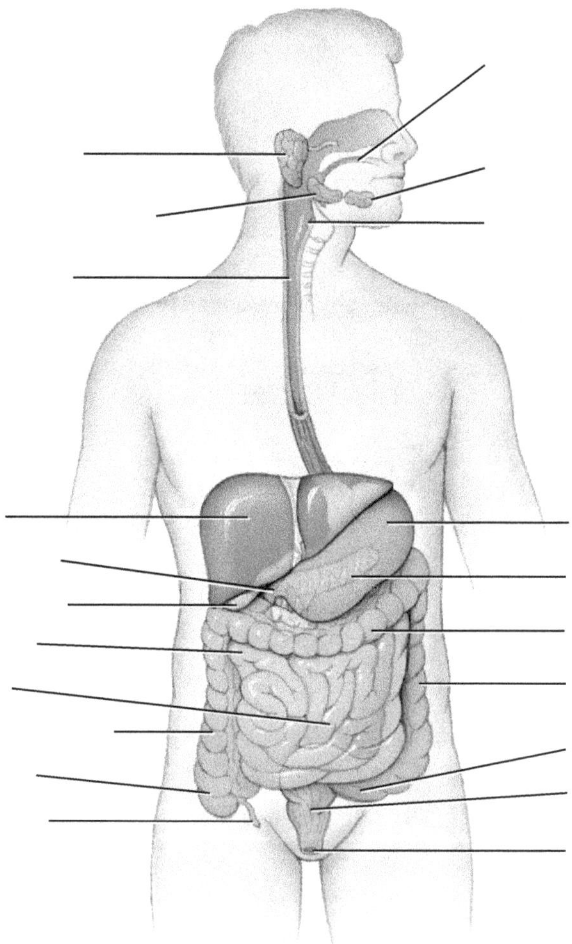

Source: Tortora and Derrickson (2009) / Reproduced with permission of John Wiley & Sons.

3 The oral cavity

(a) Label the following diagram:

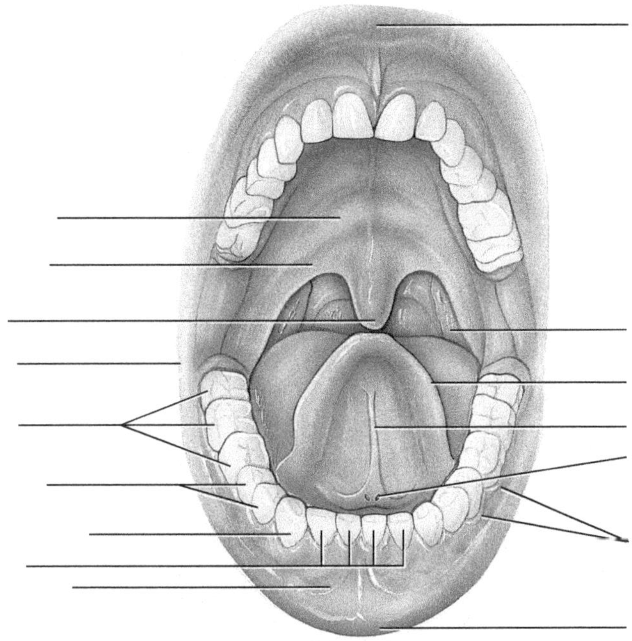

(b) Label and number the teeth in the following diagram and colour the various types of teeth:

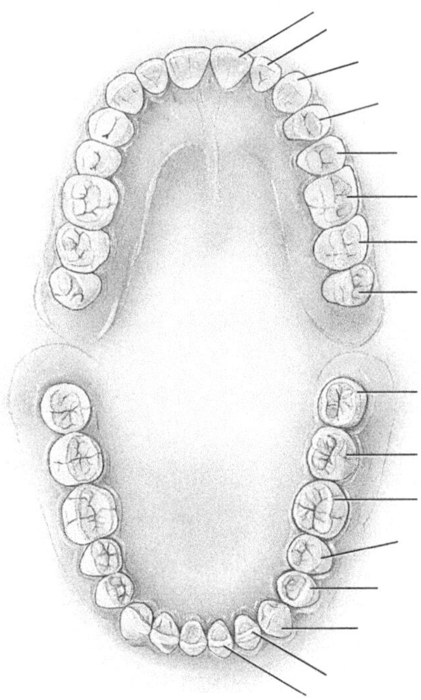

Source: Tortora and Derrickson (2009) / Reproduced with permission of John Wiley & Sons.

4 Salivary glands

(a) Label the three main salivary glands in the following diagram, and colour them in.

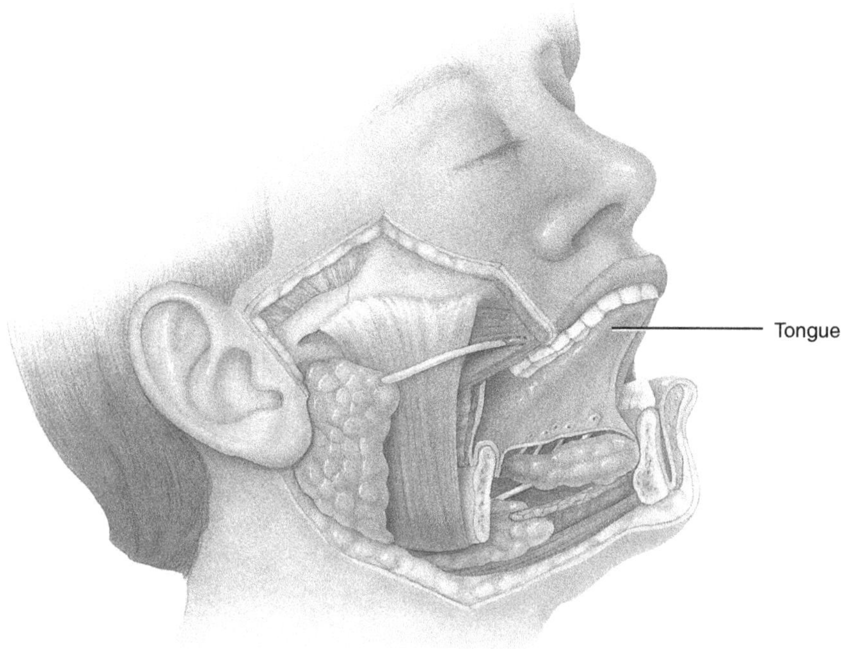

Source: Tortora and Derrickson (2009) / Reproduced with permission of John Wiley & Sons.

(b) Complete the following table:

Saliva contains:
The functions of saliva are:
The pH of saliva is:
The volume of saliva produced daily by a healthy individual is:

5 Swallowing

(a) Label the following diagram of the structures of the mouth and throat and colour in the epiglottis and the tongue:

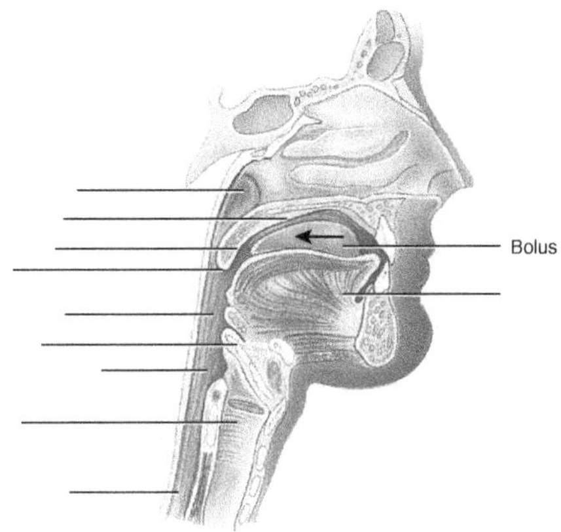

Source: Tortora and Derrickson (2009) / Reproduced with permission of John Wiley & Sons.

(b) What happens during the initial phase of swallowing shown in (a)?

(c) What phase of swallowing is shown in the following diagram, and what happens during this phase?

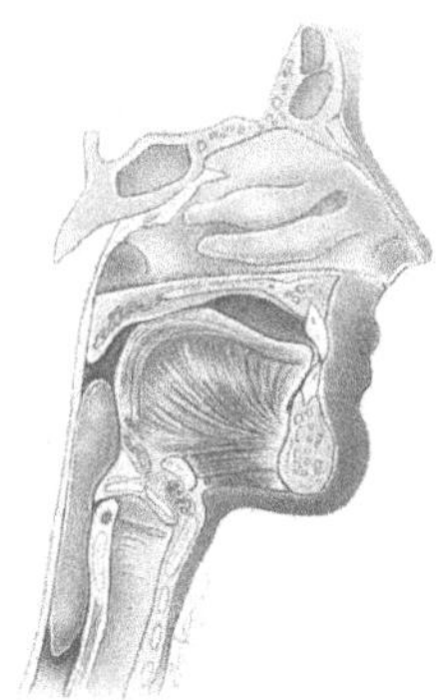

Source: Tortora and Derrickson (2009) / Reproduced with permission of John Wiley & Sons.

(d) Label the following diagram:

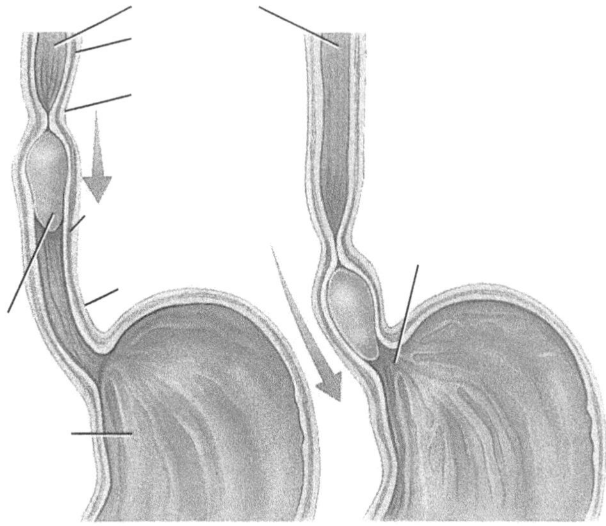

Source: Tortora and Derrickson (2009) / Reproduced with permission of John Wiley & Sons.

6 Match the pairs

The tongue is a large	located anterior to the ears
The palate	stimulates saliva secretion in response to the sight, smell or taste of food
The parotid glands are the largest of the salivary glands and are	and enters the oesophagus
The activity of the parasympathetic fibres	oral, nasal and laryngeal parts
The pharynx consists of	forms the roof of the mouth and consists of hard and soft parts.
The food bolus leaves the oropharynx	voluntary muscular structure which occupies much of the oral cavity

7 Time yourself to unscramble these words

SCRA-MBLE

Scrambled	Unscrambled
LUPISPORON	
LAXIAML	
VASAIL	
LAMESAY	
YESYMOLZ	
GASHOSOUPE	
XNYRAHP	
USLOB	

8 Layers of the gastrointestinal tract

Label the following diagram of the layers of the gastrointestinal tract and colour the layers:

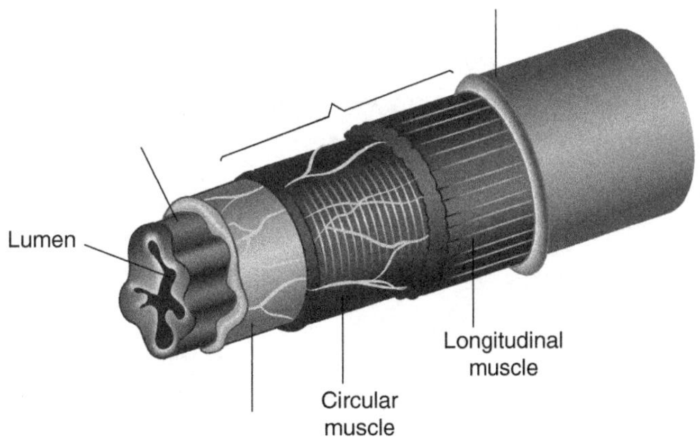

9 The stomach

(a) Label the following diagram showing the parts of the stomach:

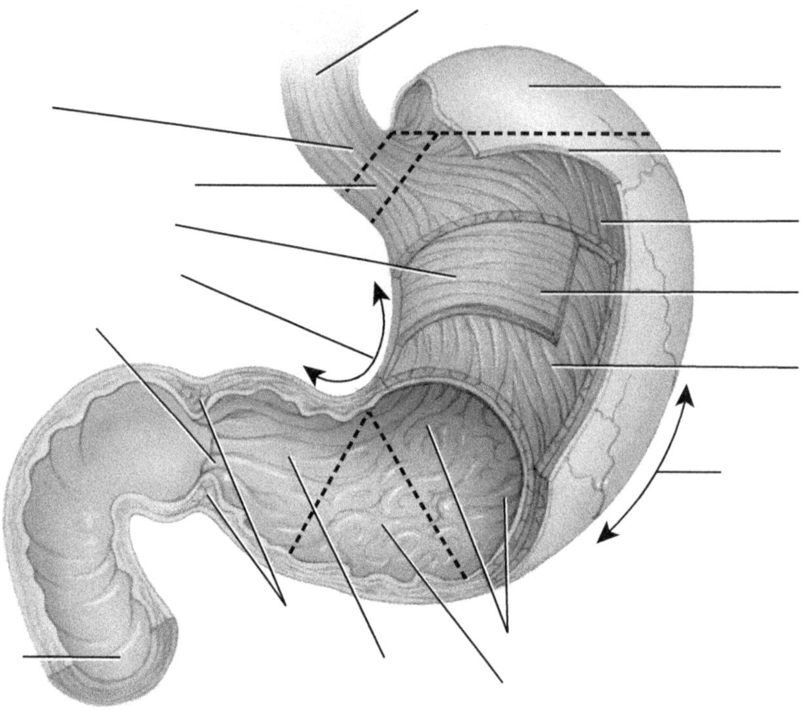

Source: Tortora and Derrickson (2009) / Reproduced with permission of John Wiley & Sons.

(b) Complete the following table with the function of the various cells found in the gastric mucosa:

Component	Functions
Surface mucous cells	
Mucous neck cells	
Parietal cells	
Chief cells	
Enteroendocrine cells (G cells)	

(c) Label the following diagram and identify the surface mucous cell, mucous neck cells, parietal cell, chief cell and G cell. Then list the secretion of each cell.

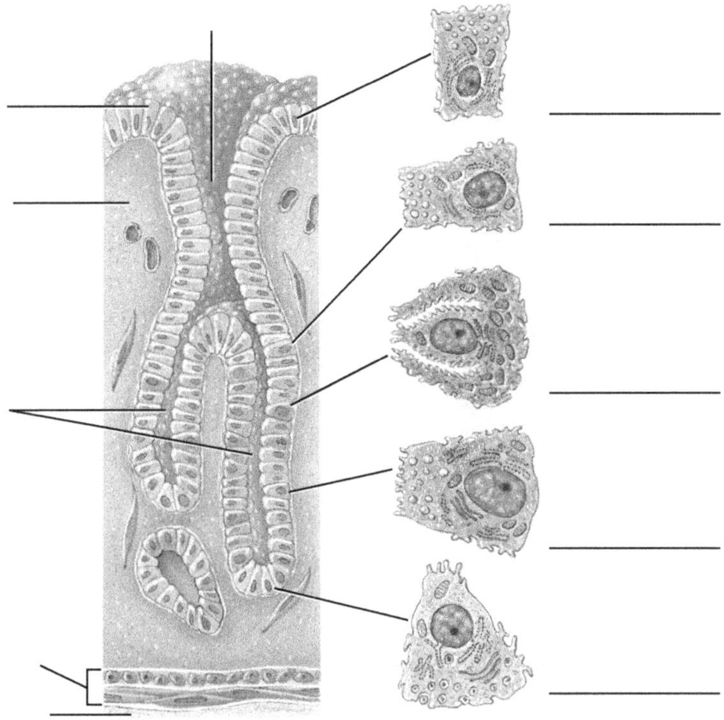

Source: Tortora and Derrickson (2009) / Reproduced with permission of John Wiley & Sons.

10 Match the pairs

The stomach is a muscular organ	the lower oesophageal sphincter
The stomach receives food through	to churn the food and enhance digestion
Food enters the stomach through	the oesophagus
The stomach secretes acid	Rugae
Ridges of mucosa that line the stomach are called	found on the left side of the upper abdomen
The stomach muscles contract periodically	to destroy infectious organisms

11 Small intestine

(a) Label the following diagram showing the sections of the small intestine and the adjacent structures, and colour the sections of the small intestine to show their location:

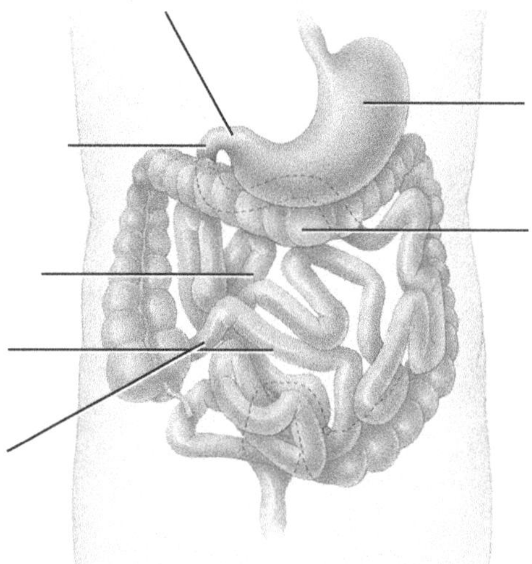

Source: Peate and Nair (2014) / Reproduced with permission of John Wiley & Sons.

(b) Complete the following table with the main roles and a brief description of each section of the small intestine:

Section	Function/description
The duodenum	
The jejunum	
The ileum	

12 Large intestine

Label the following diagram showing the large intestine:

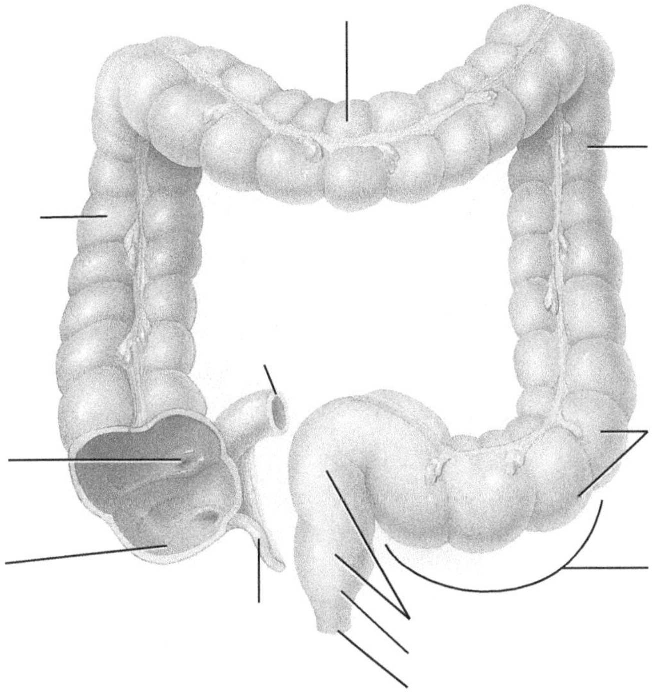

Source: Peate and Nair (2014) / Reproduced with permission of John Wiley & Sons.

13 Match the pairs

The small intestine consists of	four sections
The first section of the small intestine is called	anal canal
The large intestine consists of	three sections
The large intestine mucosa contains large numbers of goblet cells that secrete mucus to	water, some vitamins, minerals, electrolytes and drugs
The simple columnar epithelium changes to stratified squamous epithelium at the	the duodenum
The large intestine absorbs	ease the passage of faeces and protect the walls of the colon

14 The accessory organs of digestion

(a) Complete the labels on the diagram below and colour the accessory organs:

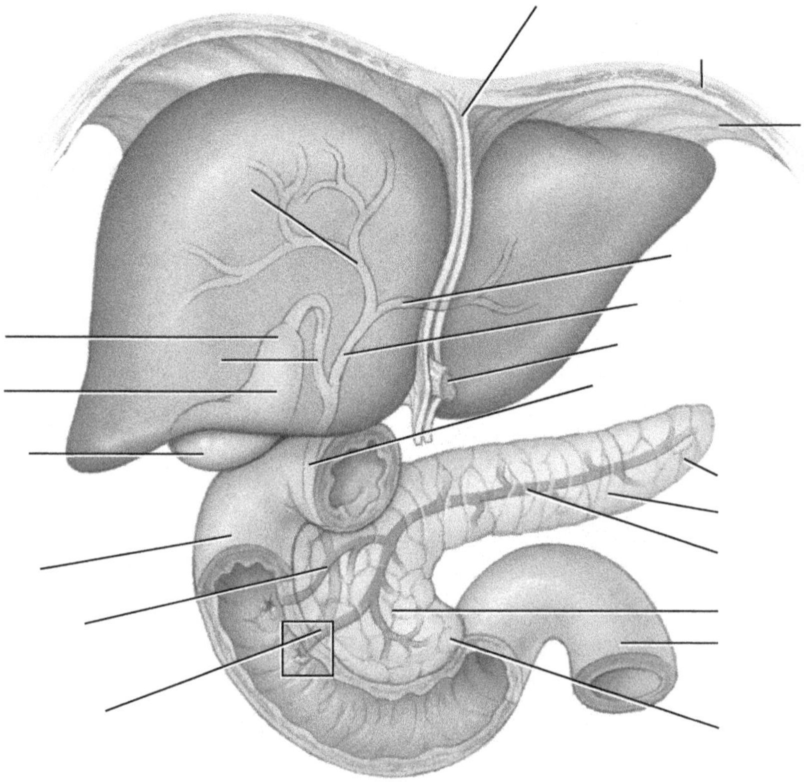

Source: Peate and Nair (2014) / Reproduced with permission of John Wiley & Sons.

(b) Fill in the blanks in the following passage:

Bile is produced in the ____________. The main function of bile is to ____________ ____________ to make them easier for enzymes to digest them. An adult ____________ will produce up to 1 litre of bile per day, but since it is only needed after a meal, it is stored in the ____________ ____________. It is also concentrated there, by the removal of ____________. The release of bile from the gall bladder after a meal is stimulated by the hormone ____________, which is secreted from the ____________ ____________ when chyme containing fats arrives in the ____________.
Bile is composed of ____________ salts, ____________ and pigments such as ____________. The emulsification of ____________ produces by bile provides the ____________-digesting enzyme ____________ with a much larger surface area to work on.

(c) Complete the following table, describing the major functions of the liver:

Function	Description
Synthesis of proteins (plasma protein, clotting factors)	
Detoxification and metabolism of drugs, hormones and toxins	
Conversion of excess glucose to glycogen and glycogen storage	
Processing of haemoglobin to extract iron for re-use, storage of iron	
Conjugation of bile	
Production of bile	
Synthesis of cholesterol and cholesterol-carrying proteins	

(d) Label the following diagram of the pancreas and colour in the ducts:

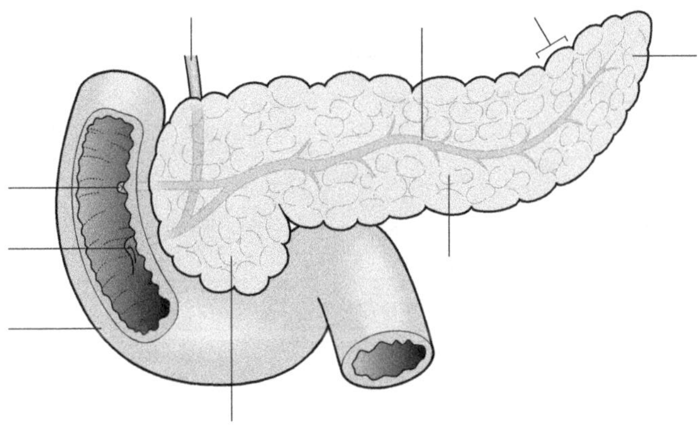

Source: Peate and Nair (2015) / Reproduced with permission of John Wiley & Sons.

(e) List the secretions of the pancreas in the following table:

	Exocrine pancreas	Endocrine pancreas
Products secreted		
Secretion stimulated by		

(f) Match the pairs.

The liver is located	the release of pancreatic juice
The liver is involved in lipid metabolism, lipogenesis and	the endocrine and exocrine products
The gall bladder functions as a	synthesis of cholesterol
When the walls of the gallbladder contract, bile is expelled into the cystic duct and down into the common bile duct before entering the duodenum via the	reservoir for bile
The cells of the pancreas are responsible for making	hepatopancreatic ampulla
Parasympathetic vagus nerve stimulation promotes	in the right upper quadrant

15 Terminology

Diarrhoea	
Dia- =	-rrhoea =
Meaning:	

Cholecystokinin		
Chole- =	-cysto- =	-kinin =
Meaning:		

Cholecystitis		
Chole-=	-cyst-=	-itis =
Meaning:		

Oesophagus	
Oeso- =	-phagus =
Meaning:	

Bariatric	
Bar- =	-iatric =
Meaning:	

Hypochondriac	
Hypo- =	-chondriac =
Meaning:	

16 Snap shot

Drug-induced gastric irritation

Whilst medications are given to promote a person's health and well-being, there are many types of medication that can cause the patient harm (this is known as iatrogenic).

Elizabeth Hernandez is a 68-year-old lady who has osteoarthritis and has been taking a medication called Arthrotec (diclofenac and misoprostol). The dose is diclofenac 50 mg/misoprostol 200 mg: one tablet orally three times daily. Arthrotec is used to treat osteoarthritis and rheumatoid arthritis in people at high risk for developing stomach or intestinal ulcers.

Diclofenac is a non-steroidal anti-inflammatory drug (NSAID). It works by reducing the production of prostaglandins, physiologically active lipids that have a range of effects, including inflammation and pain at sites of damage, but also reduction of gastric acid secretion and stimulation of protective mucus secretion in the stomach.

Misoprostol replaces the prostaglandin effect that is missing from the stomach after NSAID use. It reduces gastric acid secretion and replaces mucus and bicarbonate.

In order to prevent gastric ulcers occurring, what advice should the nurse give to Ms Hernandez?

17 Crossword

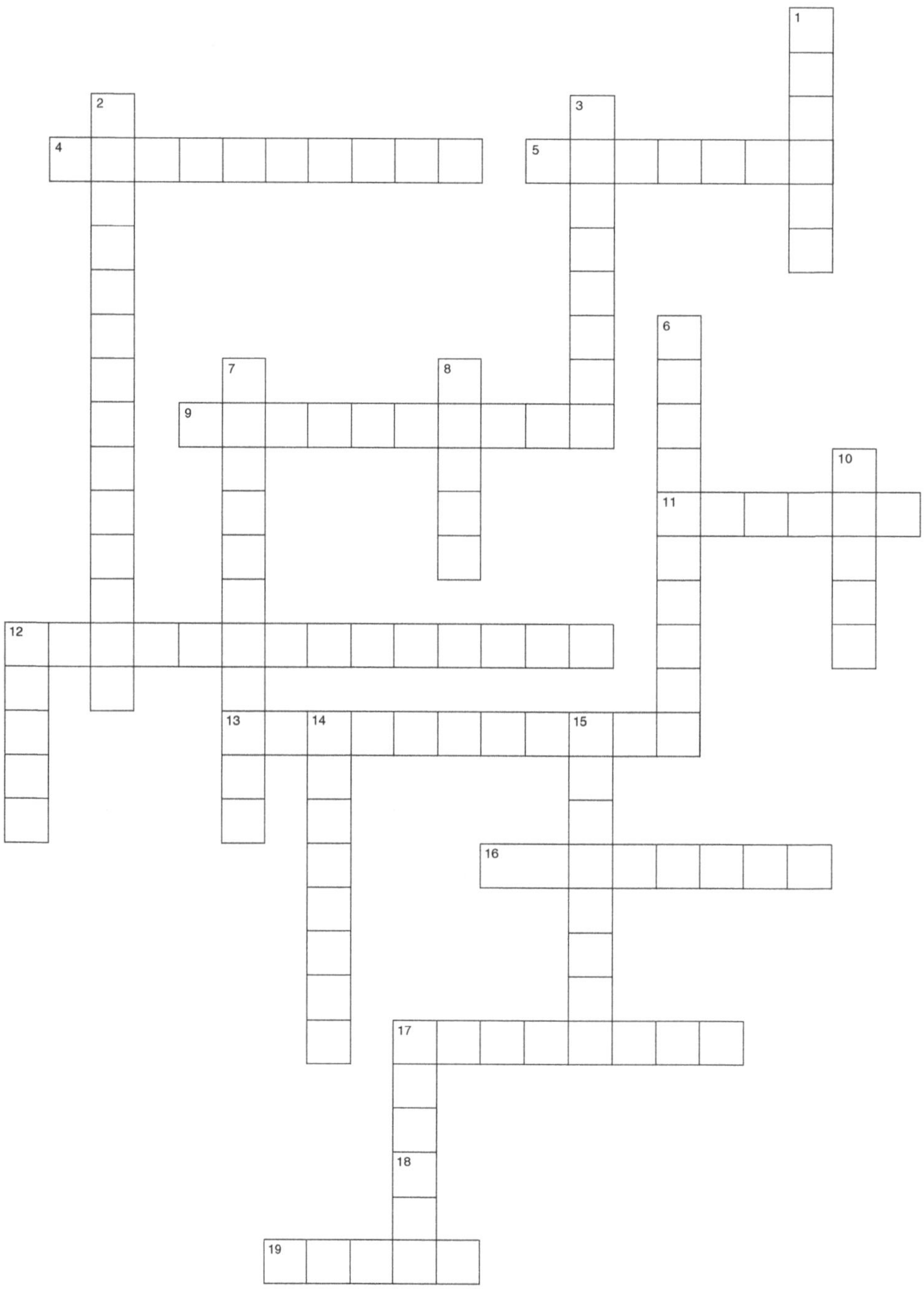

Across

4. Proteins are digested and absorbed as ___________
5. Lymphatic capillary of the small intestine
9. The type of anaemia caused by vitamin B12 deficiency
11. Stores faecal matter until defaecation
12. Glucose is one of these
13. The bile breakdown product that gives faeces its colour
16. The first section of the duodenum
17. Cells producing hydrochloric acid and intrinsic factor
18. Drug that prevents water absorption in the colon would be expected to cause this
19. The products of digestion are absorbed and transported directly to the __________

Down

1. Cells that secrete mucus
2. Where most products of digestion are absorbed
3. Accessory organ of digestion which secretes digestive enzymes and hormones
6. Process that follows digestion
7. Rhythmic contractions of the gastrointestinal (GI) tract that travel in waves along the tract
8. The ascending colon is on the ________ side of the body
10. Ridges of mucosa on the inner surface of the stomach
12. Carbohydrate digestion starts here
14. The anal sphincter under voluntary control
15. Component of saliva with antibacterial action
17. Forms the roof of the mouth

Multiple-choice questions

18. The oesophagus:
A. secretes vitamin D
B. secretes intrinsic factor necessary for the absorption of vitamin B_{12}
C. is a hollow tube carrying food from the pharynx to the stomach
D. is where chyme is formed

19. Which of the following is true concerning the stomach?
A. It digests all fats
B. It is lined with microvilli
C. It is attached distally to the jejunum and proximally to the oesophagus
D. It delivers chyme to the duodenum

20. Which of the following is NOT descriptive of bile?
A. Aids in the digestion of fat
B. Acts as an emulsifier
C. Is classified as a lipase
D. Is stored by the gall bladder

21. The role of bicarbonate in the digestive system is:
A. to control the pH in the stomach
B. to bind to sugars to aid their digestion
C. to neutralise gut contents entering the duodenum
D. none of the above

22. Which of the following is not a function of the liver?
A. Synthesis of blood-clotting factors
B. Production of bile
C. Secretion of cholecystokinin and secretin
D. Storage of fat-soluble vitamins

23. What is emulsification?

A. The chemical digestion of fat into fatty acids and glycerol
B. Absorption of fatty acids into the lacteal
C. Mechanical breakdown of large fat globule into smaller fat globules
D. Conversion of fat into a water-soluble form

24. The pancreas:

A. secretes a mix of digestive enzymes
B. secretes bile
C. is dependent on the spleen
D. empties its digestive enzymes into the ileum

25. The duodenum is most concerned with:

A. the secretion of vitamin B_{12}
B. digestion and absorption
C. the production of clotting factors and plasma proteins
D. None of the above

26. The valve that prevents regurgitation of stomach contents into the oesophagus is the:

A. cardiac sphincter
B. pyloric sphincter
C. ileocaecal valve
D. rugae

27. GI contents pass from the transverse colon into the:

A. ascending colon
B. descending colon
C. sigmoid colon
D. anal canal

CHAPTER 12

The renal system

1 Structures of the renal system

Label the parts of the renal system on this diagram:

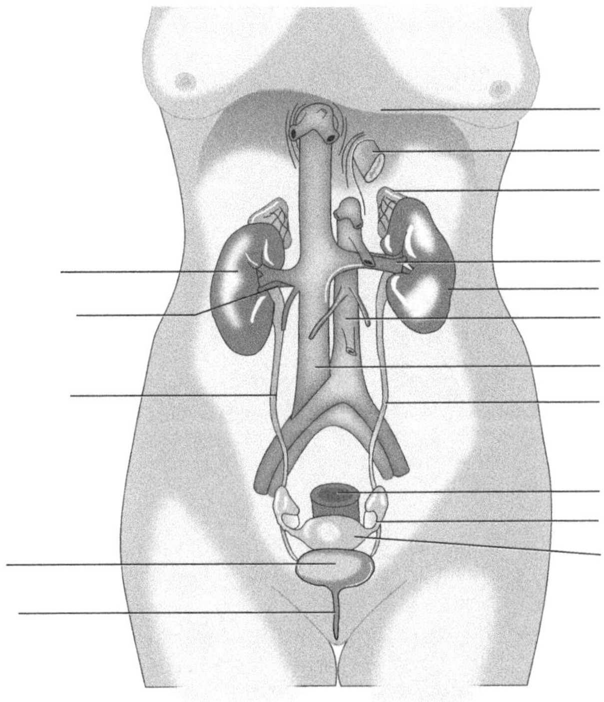

Source: Tortora and Derrickson (2009) / Reproduced with permission of John Wiley & Sons.

2 The kidney

(a) In the following table, summarise the functions of the kidney.

Function	Description

(b) Label the diagram of a kidney shown here:

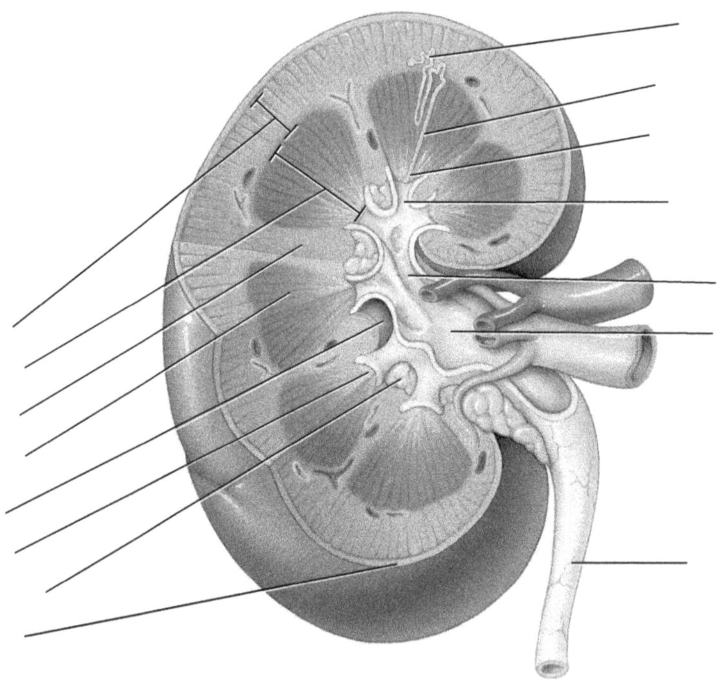

Source: Tortora and Nair (2009) / Reproduced with permission of John Wiley & Sons.

(c) Label the two major vessels and colour the blood vessels supplying the kidney in the following diagram using different colours for the veins and arteries.

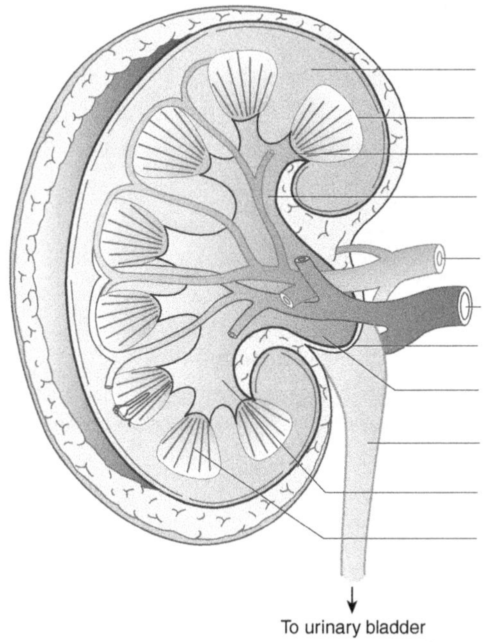

Source: Peate and Nair (2011) / Reproduced with permission of John Wiley & Sons.

(d) Label the blood vessels in the following diagram:

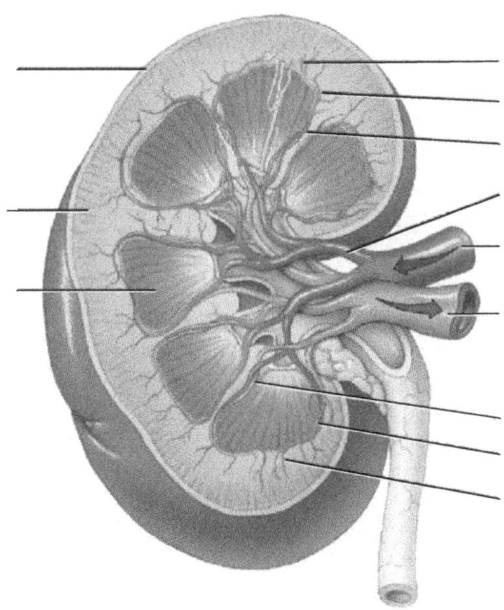

(e) Match the pairs.

The kidneys play an important role in	an abundance of blood vessels and tubules of the nephrons
The kidneys have	is the outermost part of the kidney
Hormones secreted by the kidneys include	maintaining homeostasis
The renal cortex	an endocrine function
The renal pelvis	forms the expanded upper portion of the ureter
The medulla has	renin and erythropoietin

SCRA-MBLE

(f) Time yourself to unscramble these words.

Scrambled	Answer
DELLAMU	
SPLIVE	
LIFTRATION	
BAPTISRONREO	
PHOTOTYRERIEIN	
TREEUR	
CASAFI	
SLYCACE	

3 Nephrons – the functional units of the kidney

(a) Label the sections of the nephron in the following diagram, and colour each in a different colour:

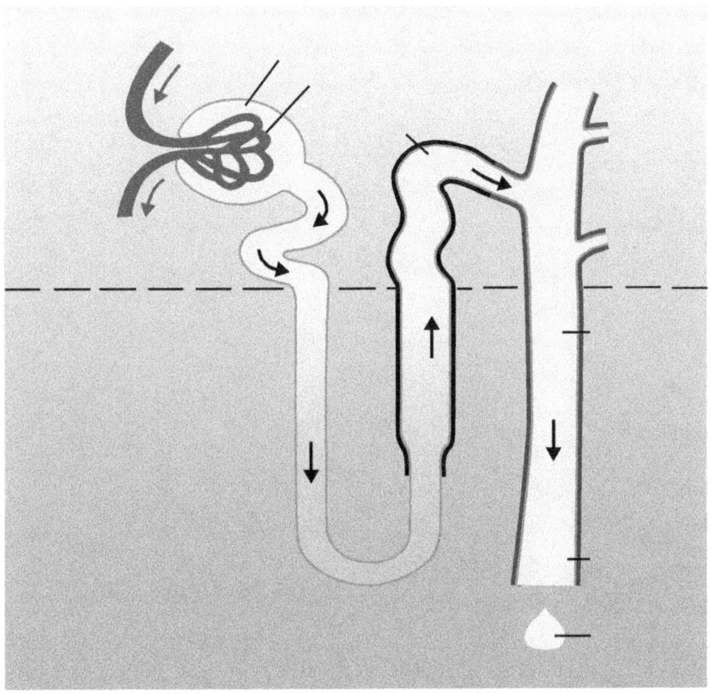

(b) Label the diagram of the Bowman's capsule here:

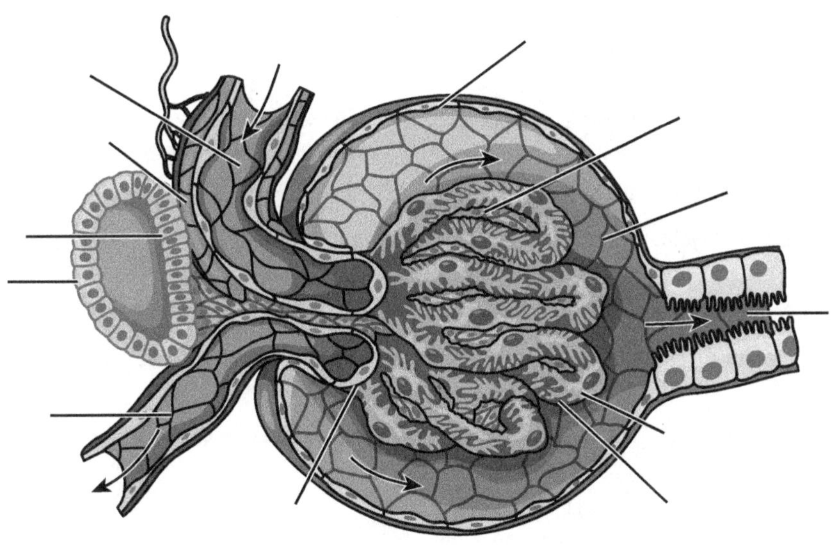

Source: Tortora and Derrickson (2009) / Reproduced with permission of John Wiley & Sons.

(c) Fill in the blanks:

The three processes occurring in the nephron that ultimately lead to the production of urine are ____________________, ____________________ and ____________________.

(d) Fill in the following table with a brief description and the function of each of the listed components of the nephron:

Component	Description/function
Proximal convoluted tubule	
Loop of Henle	
Distal convoluted tubule	
Collecting duct	

(e) Match the pairs.

Microscopic structures, the functional units of the kidney are	is highly permeable to water, but not to ions or urea. Water moves out of the tubule by osmosis
The descending limb of the loop of Henle	are reabsorbed in the proximal convoluted tubule
The distal convoluted tubule	allows the kidney to produce urine that is more concentrated than the tissue fluids
The thin ascending limb of the loop of Henle	nephrons
Salt, water and glucose	actively transports sodium and chloride ions out of the tubule
The loop of Henle	is the site of secretion of certain ions and reabsorption of water under the control of ADH
The thick ascending limb of the loop of Henle	is permeable to ions but not water. Sodium and chloride ions diffuse out of the tubule

4 Hormones acting on the kidney

Complete the following table, showing hormones acting on the kidney and their functions:

Hormone	Secreted by	Trigger for release	Effects
Aldosterone			
Atrial natriuretic peptide	Atria of the heart		
Brain natriuretic peptide	Ventricles of the heart		
Antidiuretic hormone			
Parathyroid hormone			

5 Endocrine functions of the kidneys

Complete the following table, showing hormones produced by the kidney and their functions:

Hormone	Secreted by	Trigger for release	Effects
	Kidney		
	Kidney		

6 Match the pairs

The kidneys	arises from the abdominal aorta at the level of first lumbar vertebra
Kidneys synthesise hormones such as	stimulates the production of red blood cells
Kidneys produce erythropoietin, which	water
Healthy kidneys keep bones strong by producing	maintain fluid balance, electrolyte balance and the acid–base balance of the blood
Renal artery	renin and angiotensin
Urine is 96%	the hormone calcitriol

7 Bladder, ureters and urethra

(a) Label the following diagram of the bladder and associated structures, and colour the various layers of the bladder wall.

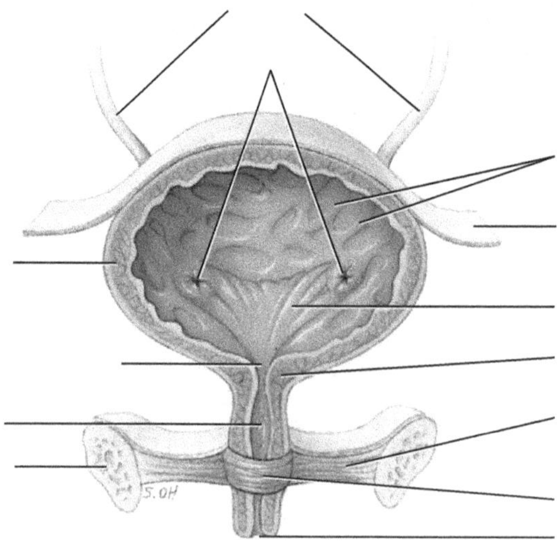

Source: Tortora and Derrickson (2009) / Reproduced with permission of John Wiley & Sons.

(b) Label the diagram of the male urethra and associated structures and colour in the ureters, bladder and urethra.

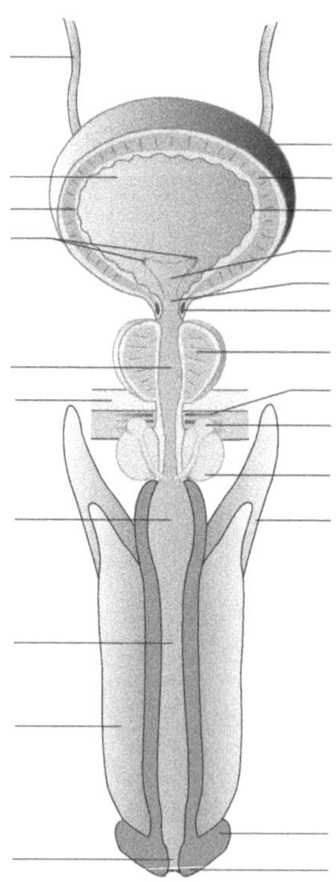

Source: Peate and Nair (2011) / Reproduced with permission of John Wiley & Sons.

(c) Match the pairs.

The urinary bladder is	a muscular tube that drains urine from the bladder to the outside of the body
In the male the bladder lies	called the trigone
In the female the bladder lies	anterior to the rectum
The inner floor of the bladder includes a triangular section	anterior to the vagina and inferior to the uterus
The ureters are	tubular organs which run from the renal pelvis to the posterolateral base of the urinary bladder
The urethra is	a hollow muscular organ located in the pelvic cavity posterior to the symphysis pubis

8 Terminology

Erythropoietin		
erythro- =	-poiet =	-in =
Meaning:		

Angiotensin	
Angio- =	-tensin =
Meaning:	

Natriuresis	
Natri- =	-uresis =
Meaning:	

Nephrotoxic	
Nephro- =	- toxic =
Meaning:	

9 Spot the errors

Identify and correct the errors in the following paragraph:

The kidney performs its functions through the actions of over 1 million neurones, which are the functional units of the kidney. Three processes occur in these function units, leading to the production of urine. During these processes, waste products of metabolism are removed, along with excess acid and excess water, if required. These processes are filtration, recycling and excretion, and they occur at different points along the nephron. Filtration of the blood occurs at the glomerulus, which is a knot of small veins through which the blood is filtered under pressure. The inflow and outflow of the blood to the glomerulus can be adjusted to increase or decrease the pressure inside it, thereby increasing or decreasing the degree of filtration. At this point, most of the contents of the blood are filtered, apart from blood cells and proteins too large to go through the blood vessel walls.

The second process, recycling, is the movement of substances from the distal convoluted tubule and collecting duct back into the blood. Substances such as glucose and amino acids are returned to the bloodstream in this way. Ions, particularly potassium ions, which are the most abundant ions in the extracelluar fluid and therefore the strongest contributor to the osmotic pressure of the plasma, are also returned to the bloodstream. The number of ions returned to the blood versus the number excreted in the urine is determined by the system that controls blood volume – the renin–angiotensin–adrenaline system. This system controls blood volume because the more ions retained, the more water is also retained in the blood stream.

10 Snap shot

Urinalysis

Andy Coulston is 38 years of age and has been to the general practice. He was complaining of pain when he 'passed water': he said it is like 'peeing razor blades'. After taking Andy's history and examining him, the practice nurse asked him to provide a urine specimen so she could carry out a dipstick analysis.
What is urinalysis and why was it performed? What might test results reveal?

11 Crossword

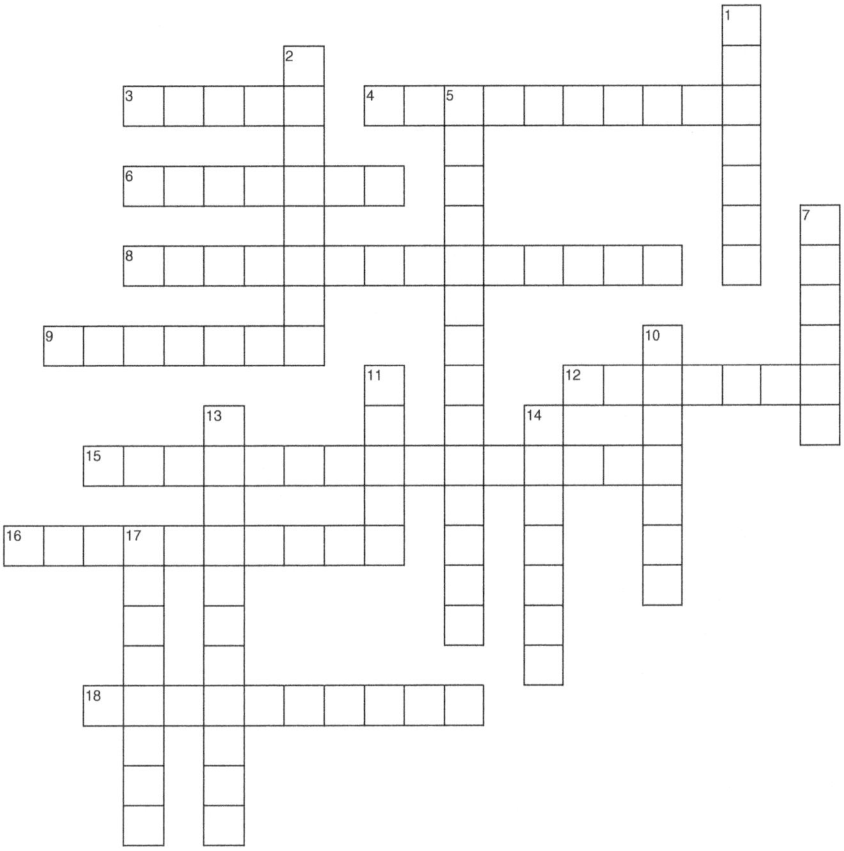

Across

4. Blood in the urine
5. Before flowing down the ureters, urine collects here
8. Hormone that increases water reabsorption from the collecting duct
10. Hypoxia would stimulate the release of ____________ from the kidneys
15. Form of vitamin D activated in the kidney
16. Sodium reabsorption in the distal convoluted tubule is increased by this hormone
18. Normally completely reabsorbed in the proximal convoluted tubule
19. When the kidney releases renin, the expected result will be a/an __________in blood pressure

Down

1. Significant amounts of this in the urine is an indicator of glomerular damage
2. Outer layer of kidney
3. Urination
6. Blood leaving the glomerulus flows into the ____________ arterioles
7. The structure responsible for concentrating the urine
9. The kidneys maintain acid-based balance by secreting these into the tubule
11. Atrial natriuretic peptide causes sodium reabsorption to ____________
12. The main nitrogenous waste excreted by the kidneys
13. The ascending loop of Henle is impermeable to __________
14. Aldosterone increases the excretion of _______________
17. The muscle of the bladder

Multiple-choice questions

12. What is micturition?
A. Vomiting
B. Excretion
C. The bladder's ability to store urine
D. The act of urination

13. The kidneys filter around ____ litres of blood and produce around ______ litres of urine per day.
A. 180; 0.2-0.5
B. 1800; 1-2
C. 1800; 0.2-0.5
D. 180; 1-2

14. Which is the first tubular structure to receive the glomerular ultrafiltrate?
A. Collecting duct
B. Distal convoluted tubule
C. Loop of Henle
D. Proximal convoluted tubule

15. The active pumping of Na^+ from the proximal convoluted tubule into the peritubular capillaries:
A. concentrates the urine
B. prevents diuresis
C. is responsible for the passive reabsorption of water
D. occurs only when a person is dehydrated

16. Which of the following is not true of aldosterone?
A. It is a mineralocorticoid
B. It is the 'salt-retaining' hormone
C. It is a glucocorticoid
D. It promotes tubular reabsorption of sodium and water

17. The renal pelvis:
A. is found close to the bladder
B. forms the expanded upper portion of the ureter
C. determines the amount of urine passed
D. determines the pore size of the glomeruli

18. What would a drug blocking the renal reabsorption of Na^+ be expected to cause?
A. Muscle weakness
B. A diuresis
C. Retention of water
D. An increase in blood volume

19. Why is glucose not usually excreted in the urine?
A. Glucose is not usually filtered
B. All filtered glucose is usually reabsorbed
C. Glucose in the urine is metabolised to uric acid
D. None of the above

20. The kidneys would respond to an increase in blood pressure by:

A. increasing renin release
B. retaining sodium
C. producing a larger volume of urine
D. none of the above

21. Oliguria:

A. can be caused by bladder dysfunction
B. can be caused by hypotension
C. is a response to an antiemetic
D. most often accompanies a decline in serum creatinine

CHAPTER 13

The respiratory system

1 Structures of the respiratory system

1. Label the following diagram of the respiratory system:

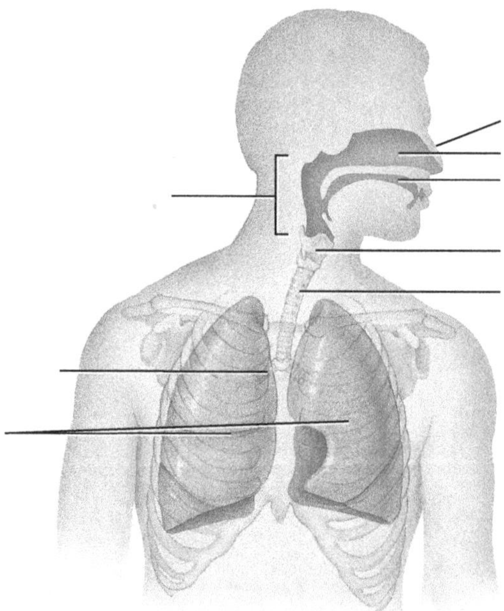

Source: Tortora and Derrickson (2009) / Reproduced with permission of John Wiley & Sons.

2 The upper respiratory tract

Label the following diagram of the upper respiratory tract:

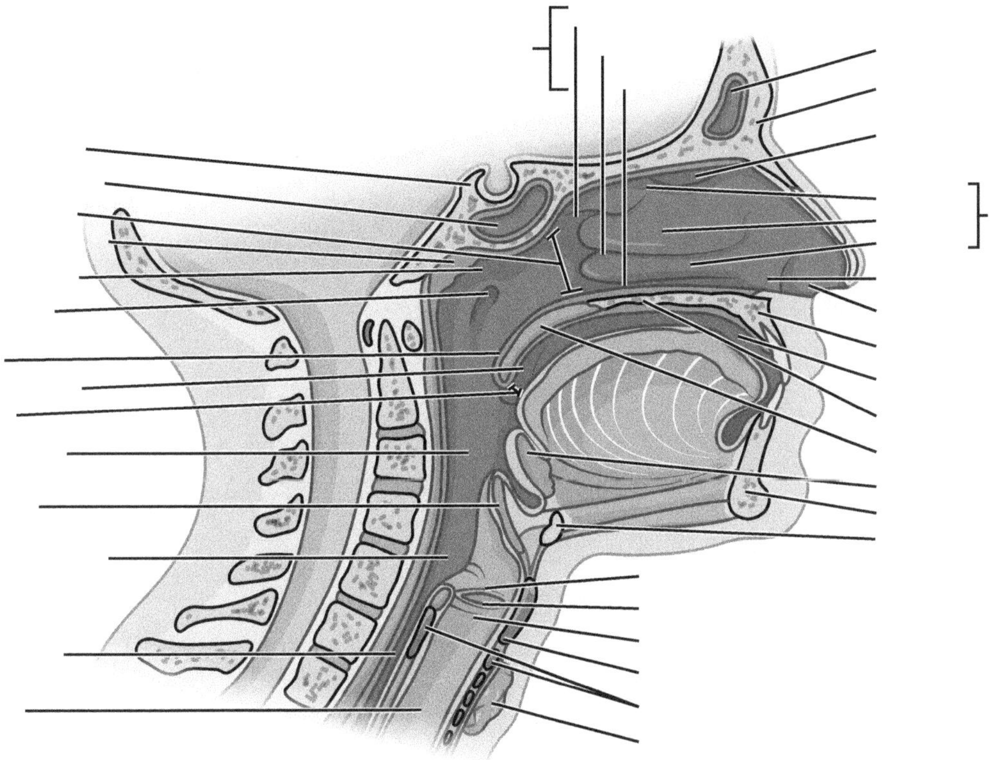

Source: Peate and Nair (2014) / Reproduced with permission of John Wiley & Sons.

3 The larynx

Label and colour the components of the larynx shown in the following diagram:

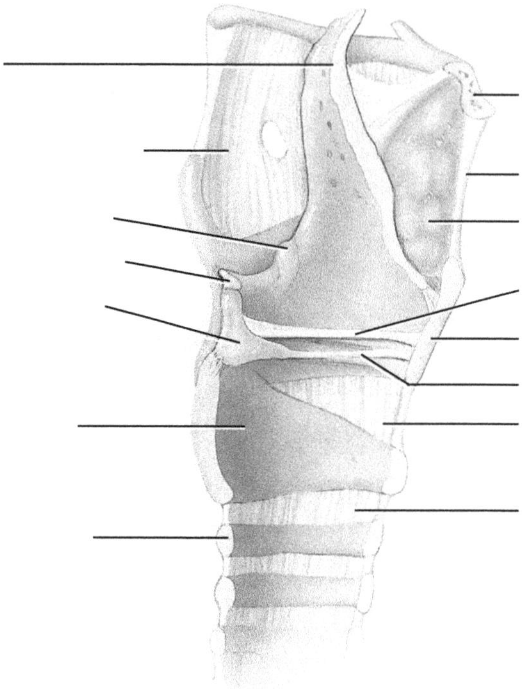

Source: Tortora and Derrickson (2009) / Reproduced with permission of John Wiley & Sons.

4 The trachea and bronchial tree

Label the following diagram of the bronchial tree and colour the cartilage:

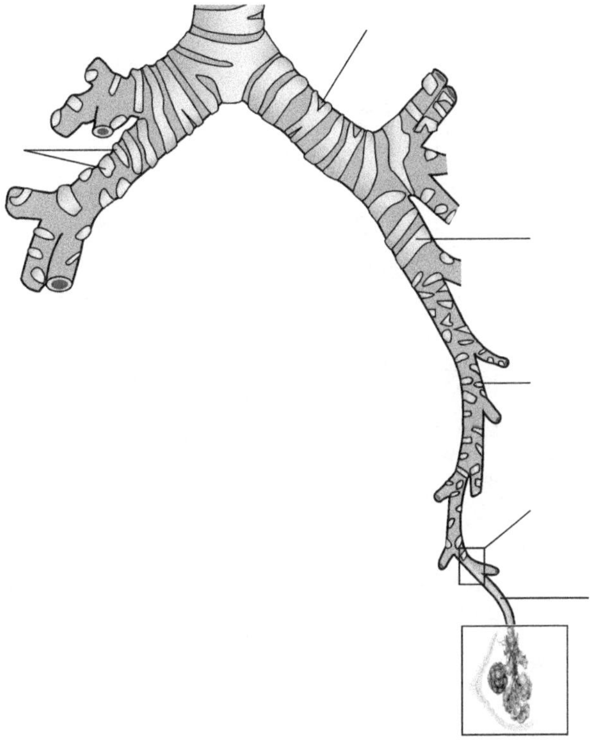

Source: Peate and Nair (2011) / Reproduced with permission of John Wiley & Sons.

5 The lungs

Label the following diagram of the lower respiratory tract:

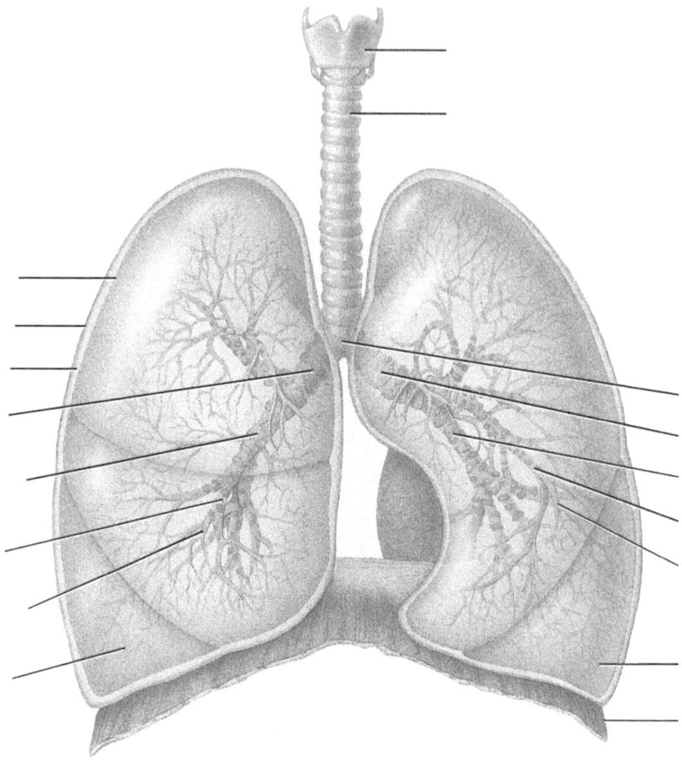

Source: Peate and Nair (2014) / Reproduced with permission of John Wiley & Sons.

6 Match the pairs

As cells use oxygen	warms, filters and moistens the inhaled air
The organs of the upper respiratory tract are the	three lobes in the right lung and two in the left
The upper respiratory tract	carbon dioxide is produced as waste
Nine pieces of cartilage, three single pieces and three pairs,	mouth, nose, nasal cavity and pharynx
The trachea	form the larynx
The lungs are divided into lobes,	extends from the laryngopharynx to the carina

7 Time yourself to unscramble these words

Scrambled	Unscrambled
CHEATAR	
SHURCONB	
NARXYPH	
NARCIA	
RULEAP	
CGARATILE	
SHOENCROBIL	
VEILOLA	

8 Phases of respiration

(a) Fill in the following table showing the four phases of respiration with brief descriptions of each:

Phase	Description
Ventilation	
External respiration	
Gas transport	
Internal respiration	

(b) Mark where the four phases of respiration would be occurring on the diagram below:

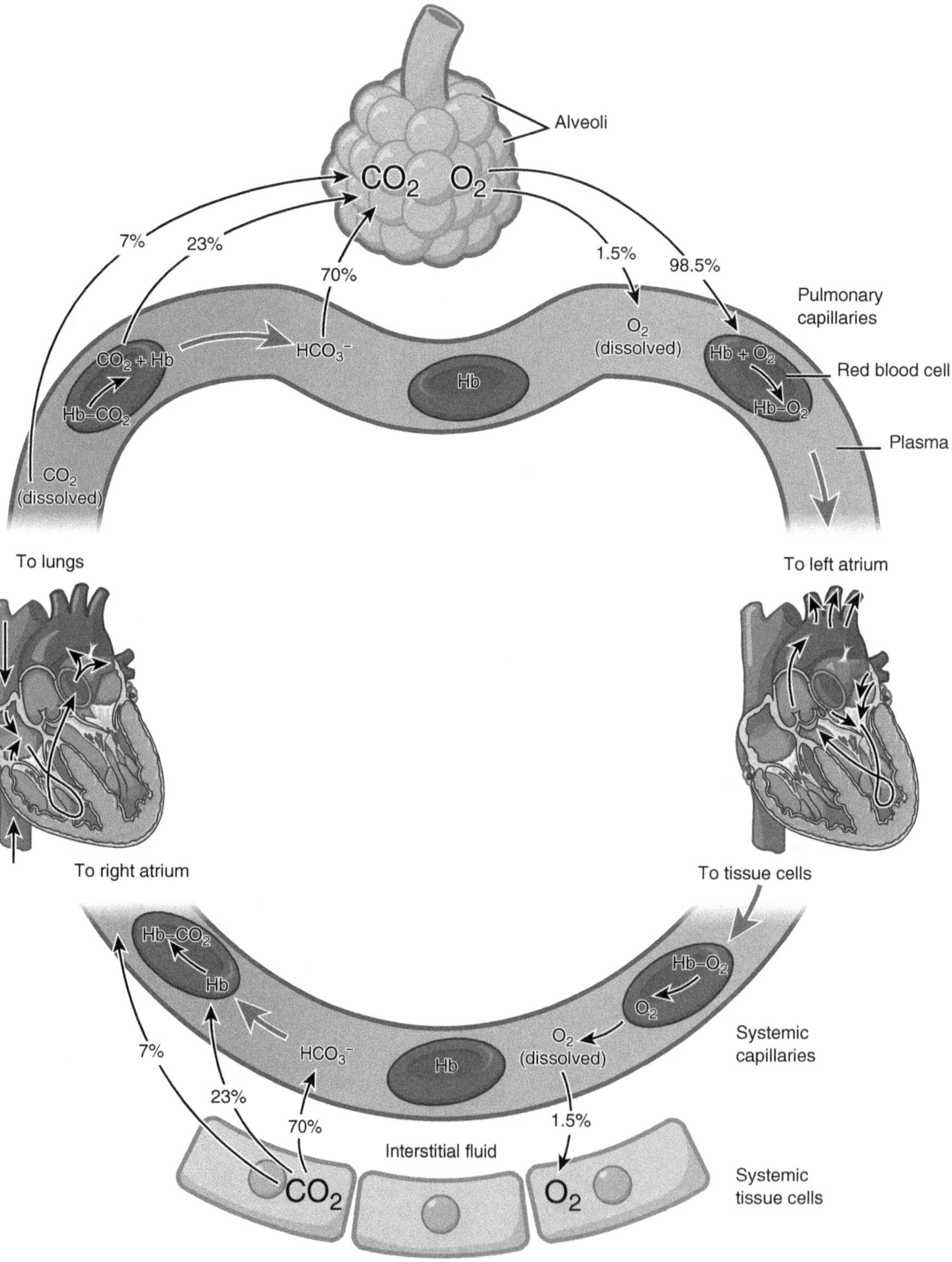

Source: Tortora and Derrickson (2017) / Reproduced with permission of John Wiley & Sons.

9 Ventilation

(a) Label the following diagram showing the chest and ribs during inhalation and exhalation:

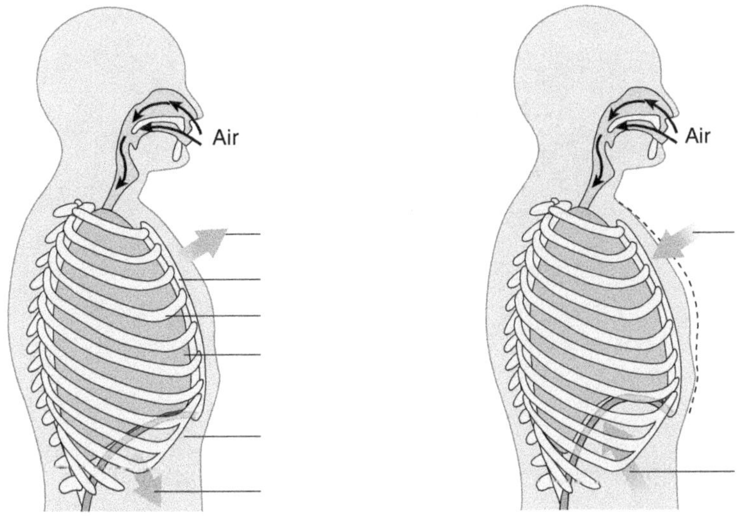

Source: Peate and Nair (2011) / Reproduced with permission of John Wiley & Sons.

(b) Label the muscles involved in ventilation in the following diagram:

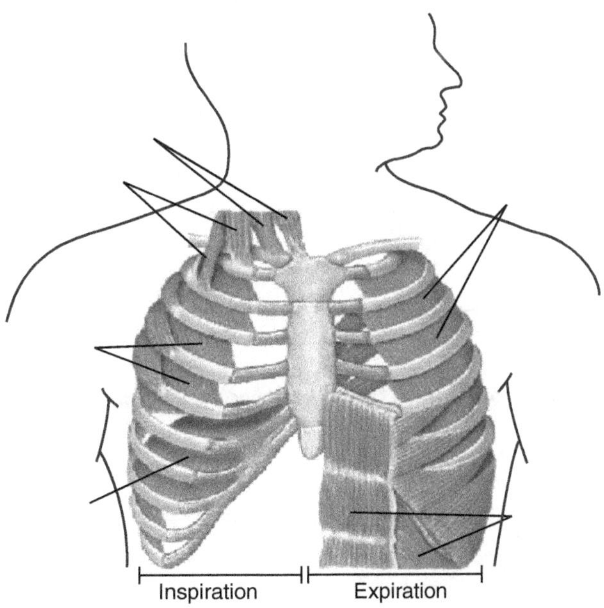

Source: Peate (2015) / Reproduced with permission of John Wiley & Sons.

(c) Label the following diagram showing the brain centres involved in the control of breathing:

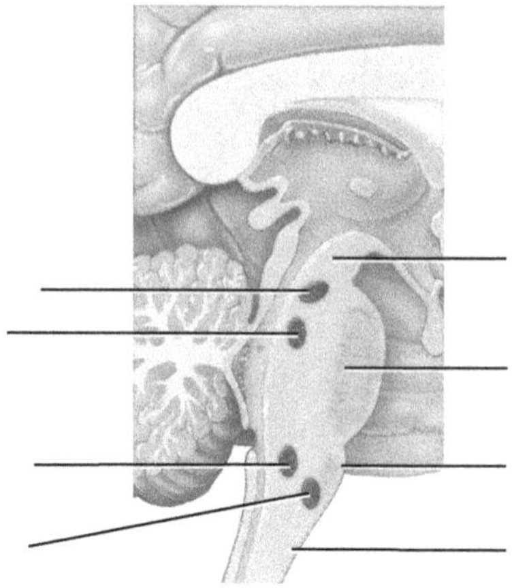

Source: Peate and Nair (2014) / Reproduced with permission of John Wiley & Sons.

(d) Complete the following diagram by naming the various lung volumes and capacities:

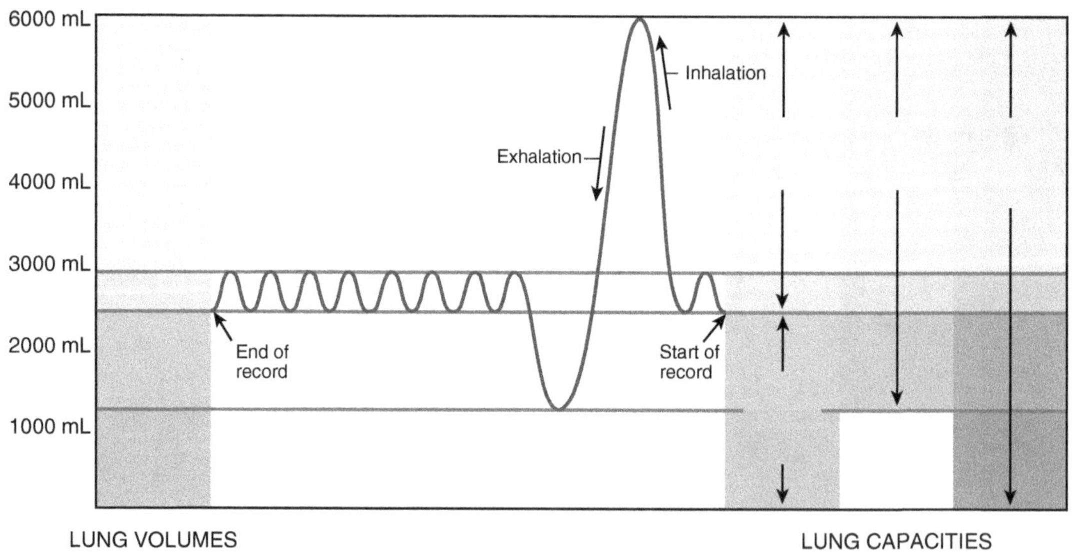

Source: Tortora and Derrickson (2017) / Reproduced with permission of John Wiley & Sons.

10 Gas exchange

(a) Label the following diagram showing an alveolus and its blood supply, and colour the blood vessels to show oxygenated vs deoxygenated blood.

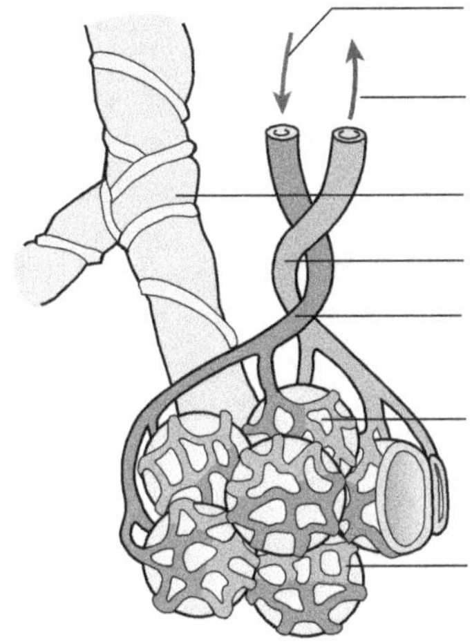

Source: Peate and Nair (2015) / Reproduced with permission of John Wiley & Sons.

(b) Label each of the arrows in the following diagram, to indicate the substances moving, and colour the blood in the capillary to show oxygenated and deoxygenated portions of the blood flowing along the alveolar wall.

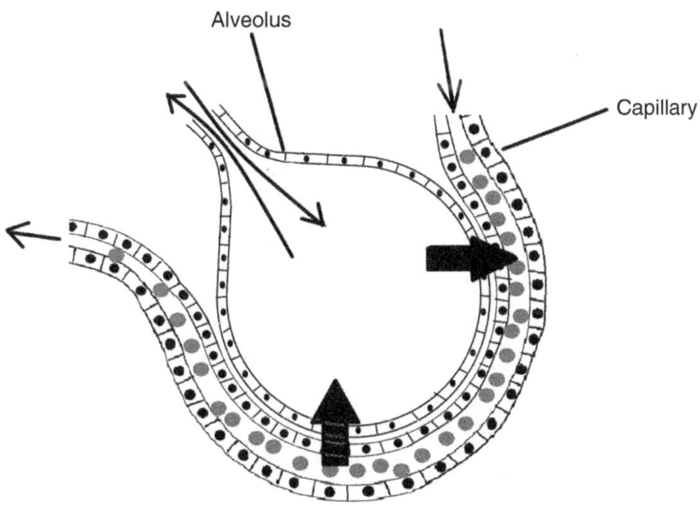

Source: Suzanne Evans (2025).

11 Match the pairs

Pulmonary ventilation concerns	air will naturally enter the lungs until the pressure difference no longer exists
External respiration concerns	the thorax expands and intrapulmonary pressure falls below atmospheric pressure
During inspiration	the respiratory centres
When intrapulmonary pressure is less than atmospheric pressure	how oxygen diffuses from the lungs to the blood and how carbon dioxide diffuses from blood to the lungs
The rate and depth of breathing are controlled by	takes place between alveolar air and the blood flowing through the lung capillaries
Exchange of gases in the lungs	how air gets in and out of the lungs

12 Gas transport

(a) Complete the following diagrams to identify the respiratory gases and to indicate the percentage of each gas transported in the forms shown:

Transport of ______________________ in the blood

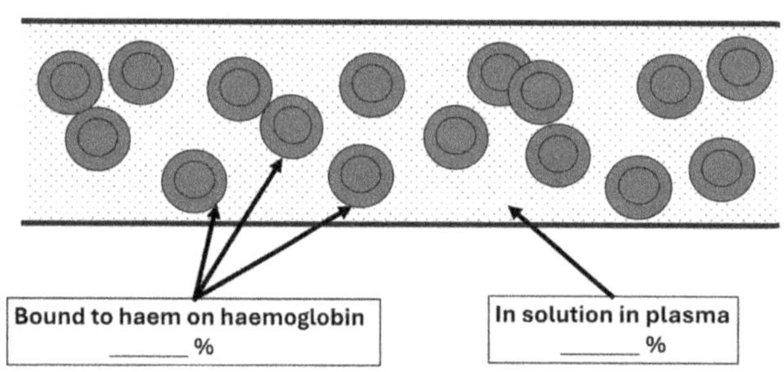

Transport of ______________________ in the blood

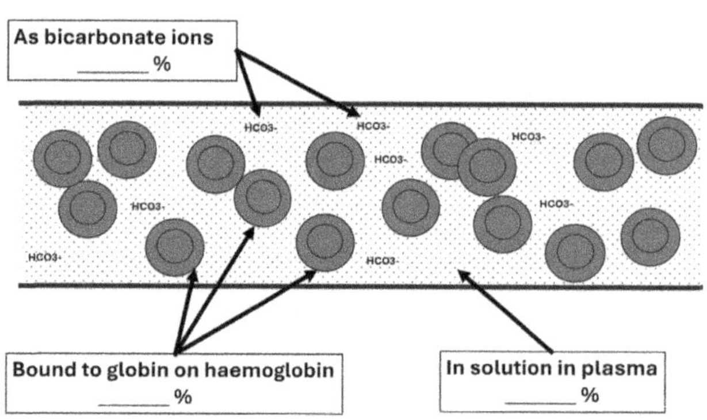

Source: Suzanne Evans (2025).

(b) Complete the following table, showing the measurement of gases transported in the blood.

Term	Abbreviation	Definition
Oxygen Saturation	SaO_2	
Partial pressure of oxygen in arteries	PaO_2	
Partial pressure of carbon dioxide in arteries	$PaCO_2$	
Arterial oxygen content	CaO_2	

13 Snap shot

Peak expiratory flow

The assessment of respiratory status is important in understanding the severity of the respiratory problem a person may have, with the intention of prioritising care, ensuring safety, providing comfort and offering support.

When a person is in the acute state of a respiratory illness, for example, if they have an infection or exacerbation of chronic obstructive pulmonary disease, the emphasis is placed on physiological assessment in order to detect life-threatening situations that require immediate interventions. Respiratory assessment requires observation, communication, measurement and clinical skills, and should include assessment of physiological factors, cognitive state, causative factors, symptoms, the impact on the person's ability to perform the activities of living and psychosocial factors. The health care provider must aim to provide care that is effective, kind, caring, with the patient at the centre of all that is done.

A series of physiological measures that are central to assessing the needs of the person with a respiratory problem fall under an umbrella term known as lung function tests. What do you understand by peak expiratory flow (PEF) and how should this important test be carried out?

14 Terminology

Hyperventilate	
Hyper- =	-ventilate =
Meaning:	

Dyspnoea	
Dys- =	-pnoea =
Meaning:	

Inspire	
In- =	-spire =
Meaning:	

Rhinitis	
Rhin- =	-itis =
Meaning:	

Pneumothorax	
Pneumo- =	-thorax =
Meaning:	

Hypercapnia (hypercarbia)	
Hyper- =	-capnia = -carbia =
Meaning:	

15 Crossword

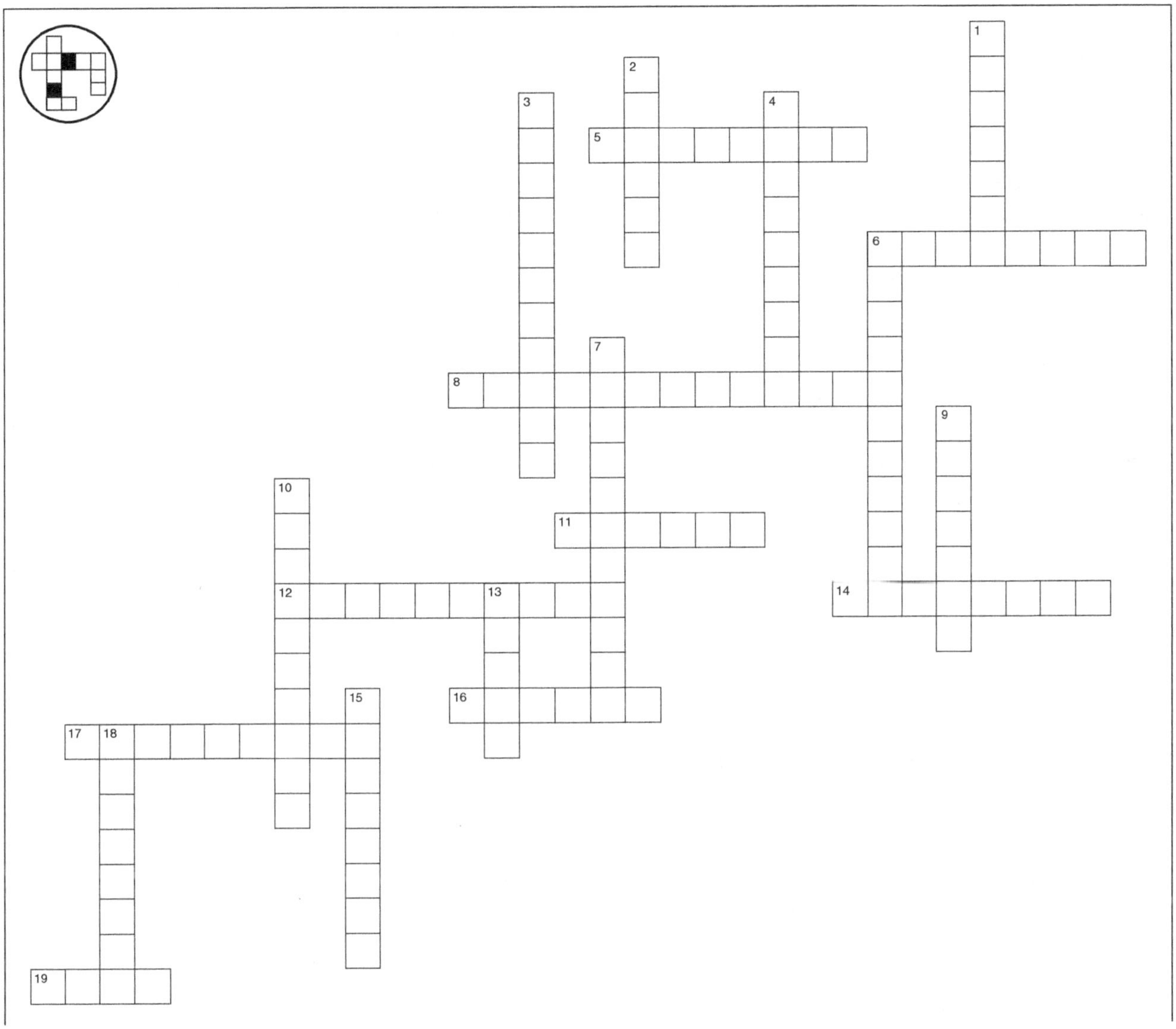

Across

5. During inspiration, the diaphragm contracts to flatten itself and moves ___________
6. The respiratory centres involved in the control of breathing are located in this part of the brain
8. Instrument for measuring the oxygen saturation of the blood
11. If a person has haemothorax, there will be blood between the ___________
12. This substance reduces the work of inspiration considerably
14. The volume of air that cannot be expired from the lungs
16. The border between the upper and lower respiratory tract
17. The process by which gas is exchanged at the lungs and at the tissues
19. Oxygen attaches to this component of haemoglobin

Down

1. Gas exchange between the lungs and the blood occurs here
2. Carbon dioxide attaches to this component of haemoglobin
3. Small airways with smooth muscle in their walls allowing them to dilate or constrict
4. The trachea is braced open by rings of ___________
6. The form in which most of the carbon dioxide in blood is carried
7. The movement of air in and out of the lungs, brought about by the muscles of respiration
9. Abnormally low oxygen level in the tissues
10. This characteristic of lungs means that expiration during quiet breathing is passive
13. The volume of air that is moved in and out of the lungs during normal quiet breathing
15. If gases are in a closed container, and the volume of the container is decreased, the pressure in the container will ___________
18. A decrease in blood pH will cause the respiratory rate to ___________

Multiple-choice questions

16. Inhalation and exhalation are:

A. caused by contraction and relaxation of the bronchiolar smooth muscle
B. caused by the relaxation of the diaphragm and intercostal muscles
C. referred to as ventilation
D. none of the above

17. The bronchi, bronchioles and alveoli are:

A. concerned with the exchange of respiratory gases
B. classed as part of the immune system
C. referred to as the bronchial tree
D. all surrounded by rings of cartilage

18. What does the diameter of the bronchioles determine?

A. Amount of mucus secreted by the lungs
B. Amount of surfactant absorbed
C. Air flow to the alveoli
D. Rate of ventilation

19. Which of the following best describes the visceral and parietal pleura?

A. They line the diaphragm
B. They line the pharynx
C. They are serous membranes
D. They are surfactant-secreting membranes

20. What happens if intrapleural pressure equals or exceeds intrapulmonic pressure?

A. Death occurs
B. The lung collapses
C. The larynx can no longer generate sound
D. Pulmonary oedema develops

21. Which of the following does NOT occur on inhalation?

A. Air is moved into the lungs
B. Thoracic volume increases
C. The diaphragm contracts
D. Pressure within the intrapleural space becomes positive

22. Boyle's law states that:

A. when the temperature of a gas is constant, the volume is inversely proportional to its pressure
B. when the temperature of a gas is constant, its volume is directly proportional to its temperature
C. there is no relationship between intrapulmonic pressure and volume
D. an increase in thoracic volume causes an increase in intrapleural pressure

23. How many pieces of cartilage are there in the larynx?

A. 3
B. 6
C. 9
D. 12

24. During an asthma attack there is often intense constriction of the:

A. bronchi
B. larynx
C. bronchioles
D. trachea

25. What are the sensory cells that detect the level of carbon dioxide and oxygen in the blood?

A. Chemoreceptors
B. Pacini corpuscles
C. Baroreceptors
D. All of the above

CHAPTER 14

The reproductive systems

1 Male reproductive system

(a) Label the following diagram of the male reproductive system and colour in the urinary bladder, the prostate and urethra:

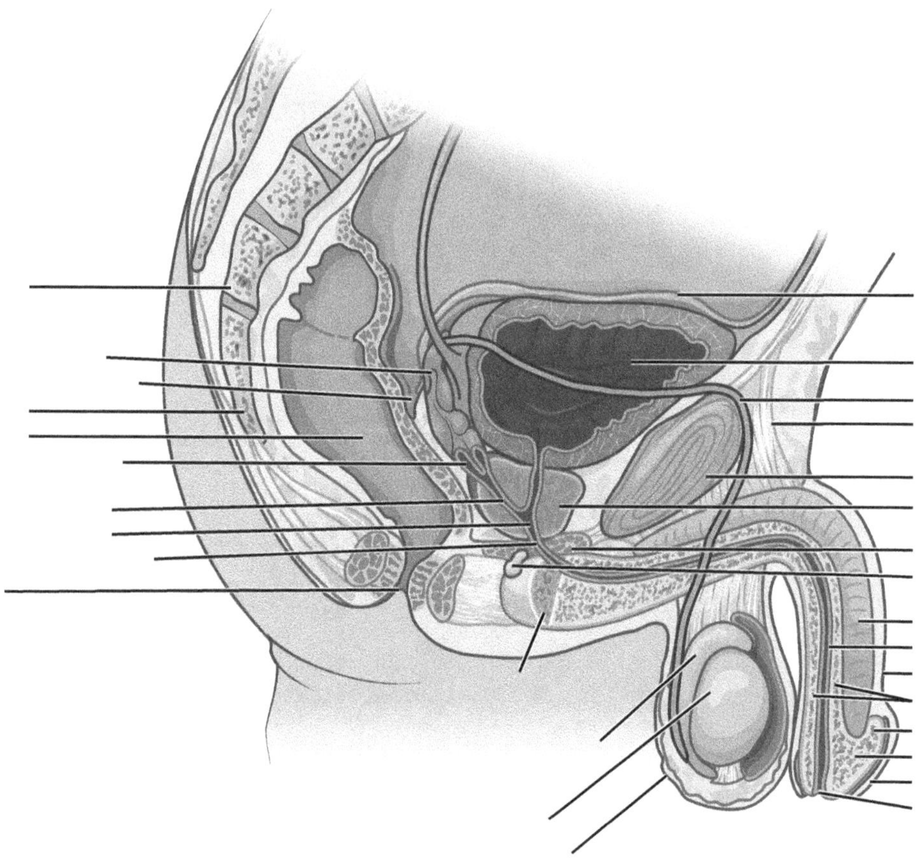

Source: Peate and Nair (2015) / Reproduced with permission of John Wiley & Sons.

(b) Label the following diagram of the testicle:

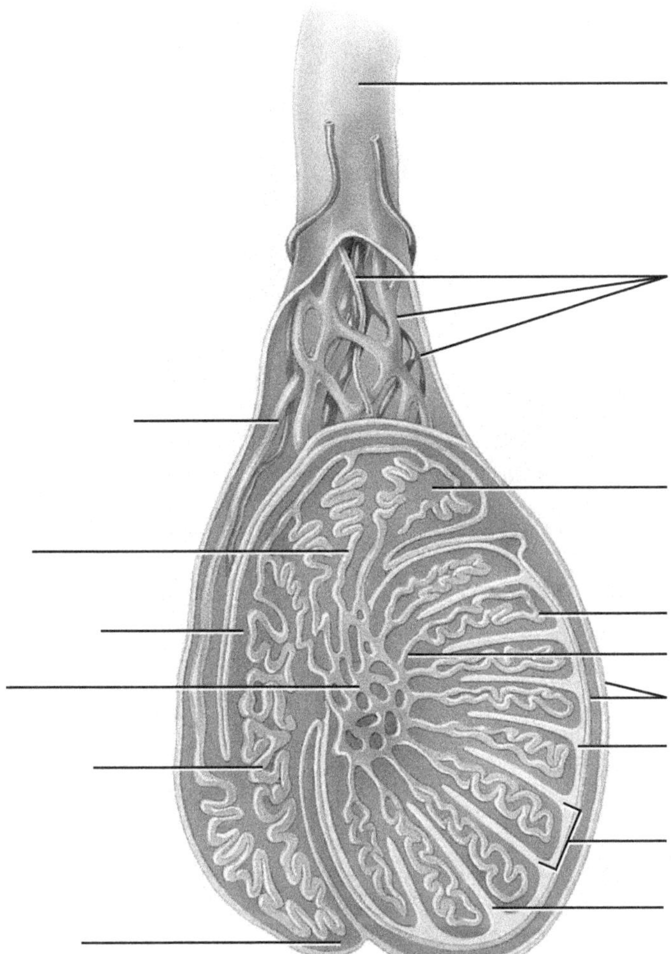

Source: Tortora and Derrickson (2009) / Reproduced with permission of John Wiley & Sons.

2 Sperm

(a) On the following diagram, write the names of the cells at each stage of spermatogenesis:

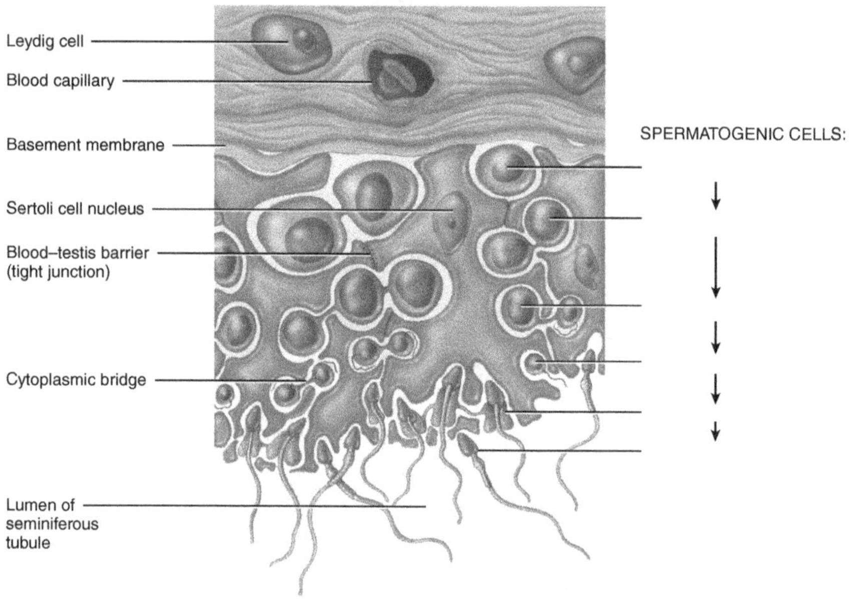

(b) Label the diagram of a sperm cell here, and colour in the nucleus and mitochondria:

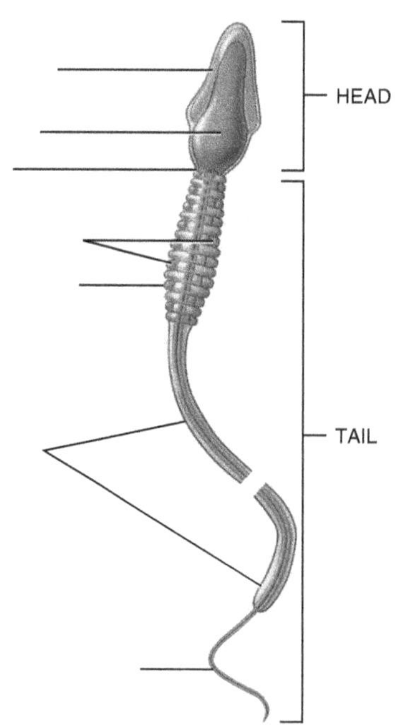

Source: Tortora and Derrickson (2009) / Reproduced with permission of John Wiley & Sons.

3 Testosterone

On the following diagram, fill in the effects of the hormone testosterone on the organs and tissues shown:

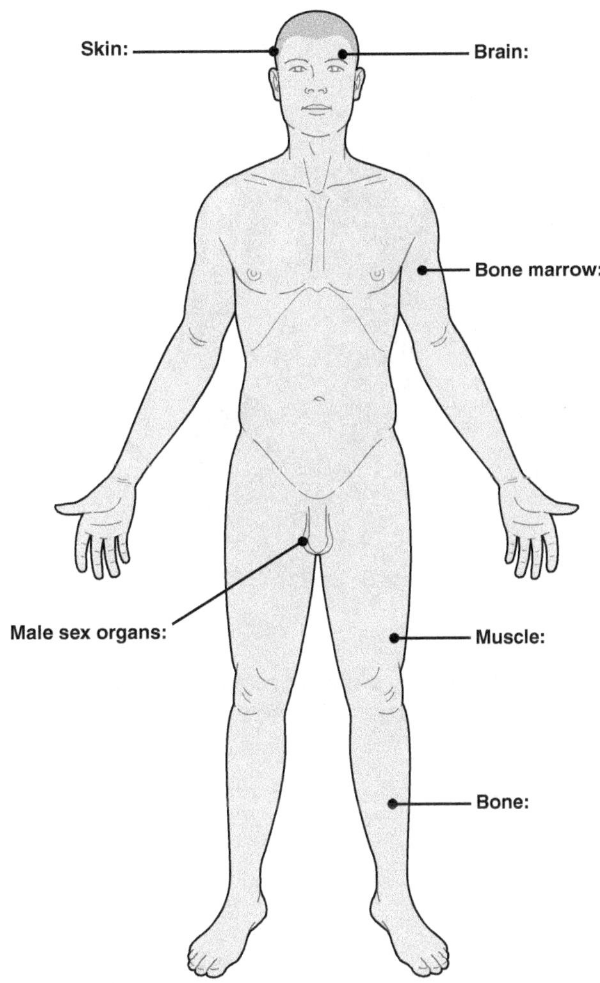

Source: Peate and Nair (2015) / Reproduced with permission of John Wiley & Sons.

4 Male external genitalia

Label the following diagram and colour in the corpus cavernosa, the corpus spongiosum and the vas deferens:

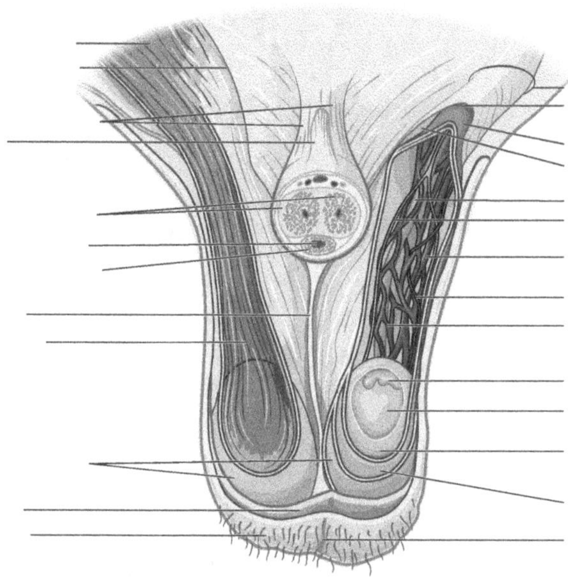

Source: Tortora and Derrickson (2009) / Reproduced with permission of John Wiley & Sons.

5 Match the pairs

The reproductive glands of the male are the testes	near the base of the bladder, they provide sperm with a source of energy and assist with motility
Leydig cells, between the seminiferous tubules,	as sperm leaving the testes are immature, and are unable to fertilise the egg
Spermatogenesis turns each diploid spermatogonium into	which transports sperm from the epididymis to the urethra
The epididymis brings sperm to maturity	these are the male equivalent of the ovaries
The vas deferens is a long, muscular tube	manufacture and secrete testosterone and other androgens
The seminal vesicles are sac-like pouches attached to the vas deferens	four haploid sperm cells, quadrupling is accomplished through meiotic cell division

6 The prostate gland

(a) Label the following diagram of the prostate and colour in the three zones:

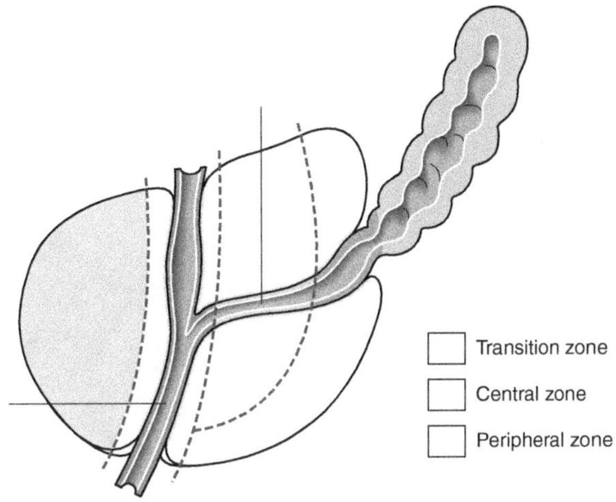

Source: Peate and Nair (2015) / Reproduced with permission of John Wiley & Sons.

(b) Complete the following table with brief descriptions of each of the zones of the prostate gland:

Zone	Description
Peripheral	
Transition	
Central	

(c) Match the pairs.

The peripheral zone of the prostate gland	check for growths in or enlargement of the prostate gland
As the transition zone enlarges, it then pushes	and is farthest from the rectum
The central zone is in front of the transition zone	is the area of the prostate that is closest to the rectum
The gland cells within the prostate produce a	the peripheral zone of the prostate toward the rectum
Prostate specific antigen counteracts the clotting enzyme in the seminal vesicle fluid	thin fluid that is rich in proteins and minerals that maintain and nourish the sperm
Digital rectal examination is usually performed to	which principally glues the semen to the cervix, located next to the uterine entrance inside the vagina.

7 Female reproductive system

(a) Label the following diagram of the internal female reproductive organs:

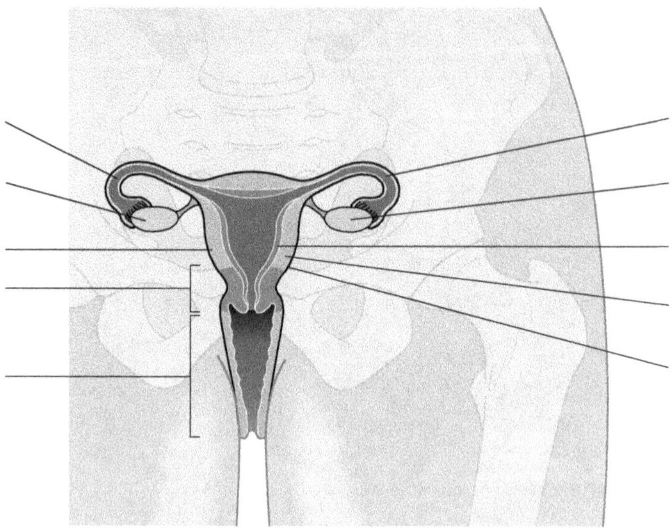

Source: Peate and Nair (2015) / Reproduced with permission of John Wiley & Sons.

(b) Label the following diagram of the uterus and associated structures and colour in the various structures:

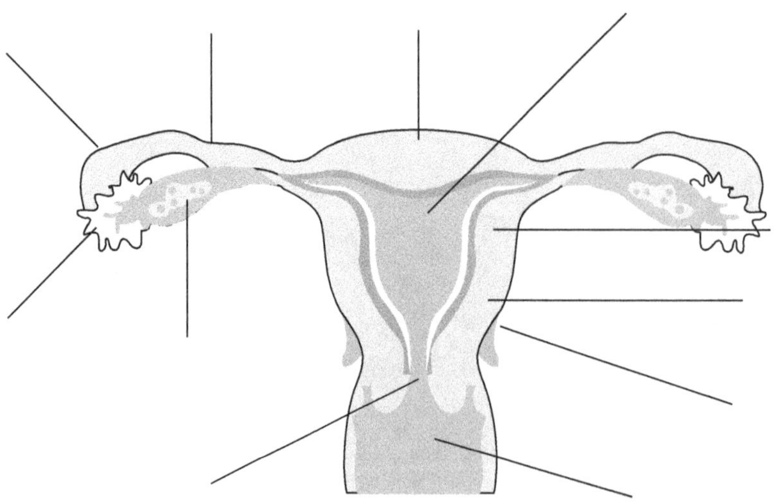

Source: Nair and Peate (2009) / Reproduced with permission of John Wiley & Sons.

(c) Complete the following table with brief descriptions of the function and location of each of the uterine layers:

Layers	Description/Role
Perimetrium	
Myometrium	
Endometrium	

8 Eggs

Fill the boxes on the diagram below with each of the stages of oogenesis:

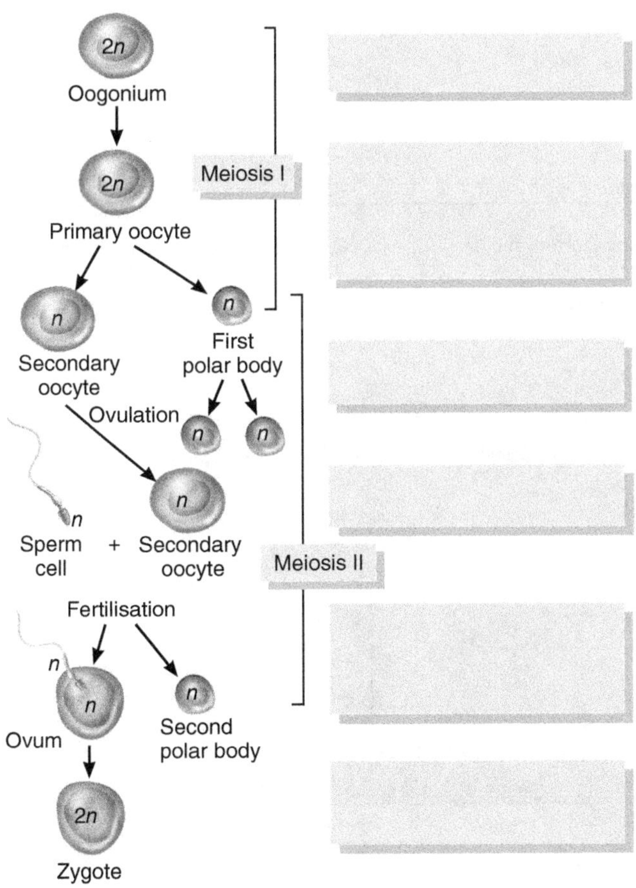

Source: Tortora and Derrickson (2009) / Reproduced with permission of John Wiley & Sons.

9 The female reproductive cycle

(a) Fill in the boxes on the diagram below to show the roles of the hormones listed:

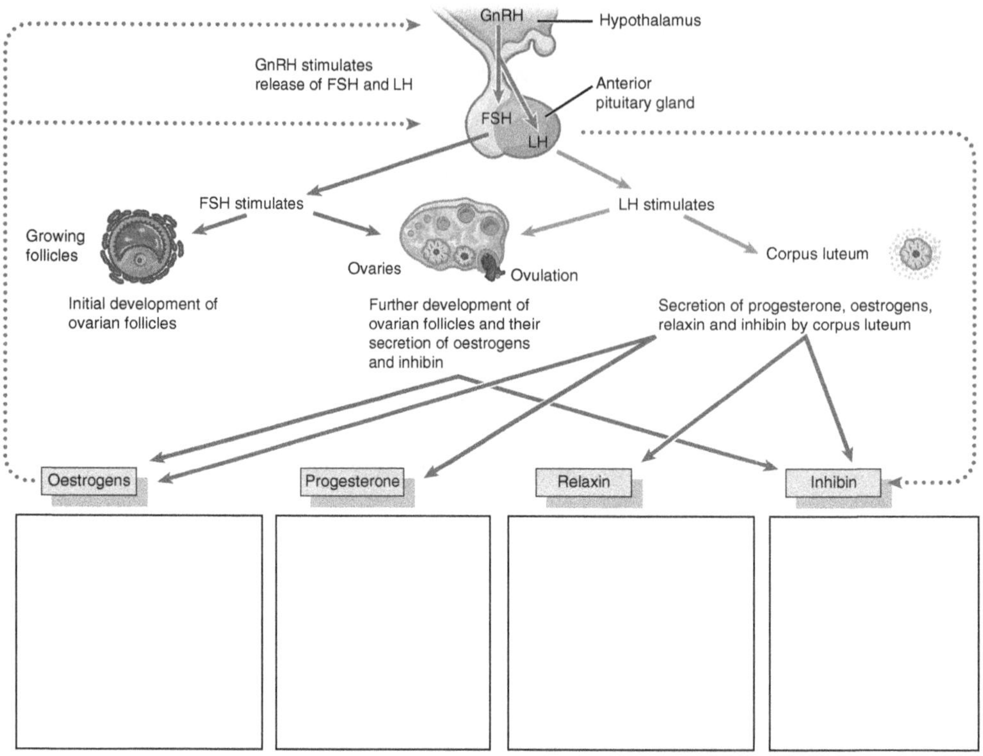

Source: Tortora and Derrickson (2009) / Reproduced with permission of John Wiley & Sons.

(b) Fill in the boxes on the diagram below with the relevant events or locations:

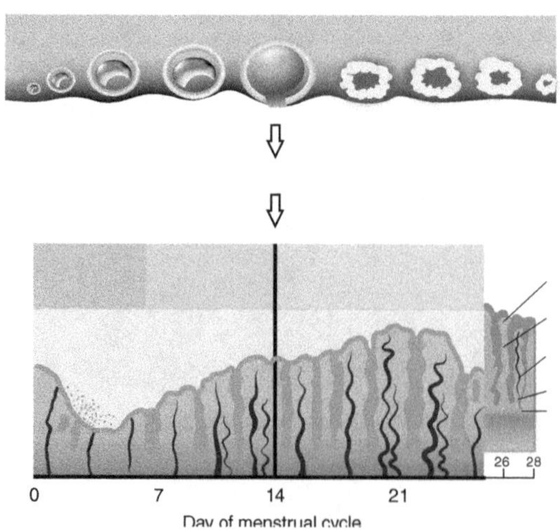

Source: Rice University (2013) / Reproduced with permission of Rice University.

10 Match the pairs

The female reproductive system produces the ova	attached to the upper part of the uterus and serve to transport the ova from the ovaries to the uterus
The vagina is a canal that joins the	located on either side of the uterus; they produce eggs and hormones
The uterus is a hollow, pear-shaped organ divided into two parts	occurs in the fallopian tubes. The fertilised egg moves to the uterus and implants into the lining of the uterine wall
The ovaries are small, oval-shaped glands	cervix to the outside of the body; it is also known as the birth canal
Fallopian tubes are narrow tubes	and transports the ova to the site of fertilisation
Conception is the fertilisation of an egg by a sperm; it normally	the cervix, which is the lower part that opens into the vagina, and the main body of the uterus, called the corpus

11 Female external genitalia

Label the following diagram of the female external genitalia:

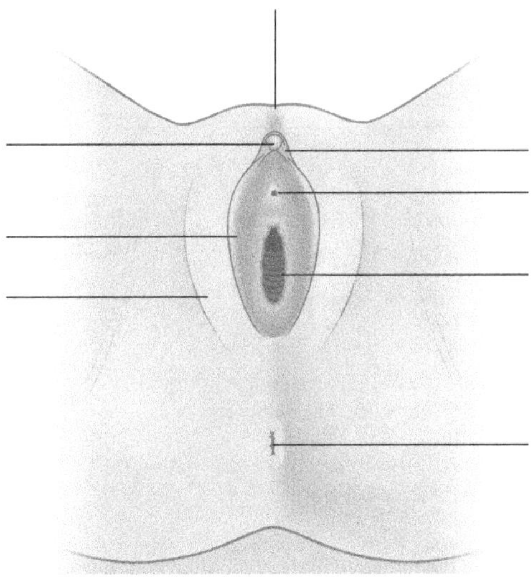

Source: Peate and Nair (2015) / Reproduced with permission of John Wiley & Sons.

12 The breast

Label the diagram of the breast here and colour in the various elements:

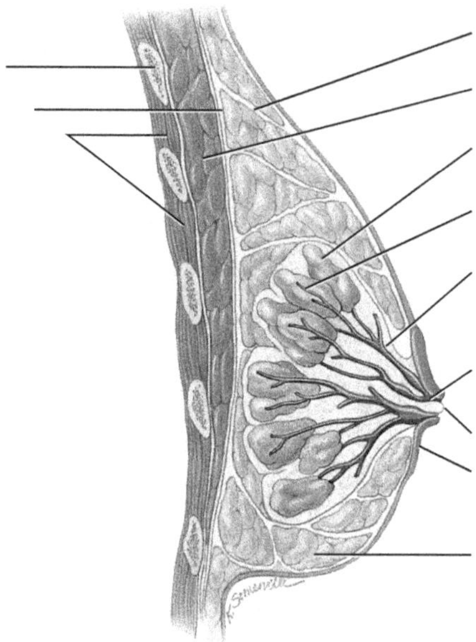

Source: Peate and Nair (2015) / Reproduced with permission of John Wiley & Sons.

13 Match the pairs

The labia majora are the outer lips of the vulva made of two symmetrical pads of fatty tissue	including nerves in the chest and arm, branches from the 4th, 5th and 6th thoracic nerves supply the breasts
Labia minora are thin folds of tissue within the labia majora	throughout the breast following stimulation by hormones produced after the woman has given birth
The clitoris is a small white body of oval tissue located at the top of the labia minora and the clitoral hood	providing protection for the urethral and vaginal openings
The key function of the breast is to produce, store and release milk produced in lobules located	it is composed of spongy tissue and is highly sexually sensitive
There are a number of major nerves in the breast area,	each month breast tissues are exposed to cycles of oestrogen and progesterone throughout a woman's childbearing years
Progesterone prepares the uterus for pregnancy and the breasts for lactation,	functioning as protective structures that surround the clitoris, urinary orifice and vaginal orifice

14 Time yourself to unscramble these words

SCRAMBLE

Scrambled	Unscrambled
YIDDIMSEPI	
IANPOLLAF	
YAROV	
LICELLOF	
GRONERESTPO	
ANIVAG	
SONETTESTROE	

15 Terminology

Progesterone		
Pro- =	- gest =	-erone =
Meaning:		

Corpus luteum	
Corpus =	luteum =
Meaning:	

Androgens	
Andro- =	-gens =
Meaning:	

Cryptorchidism		
Crypt- =	-orchid =	-ism=
Meaning:		

Endometriosis		
Endo- =	-metri =	-osis=
Meaning:		

16 Snap shot

Erectile dysfunction

Deniz Yayincilik is a 45-year-old gentleman with diabetes mellitus and has experienced erectile dysfunction for 2 years. The erectile dysfunction was causing disharmony with his wife. Treatment is with self-injection therapy; the injectable form of MUSE alprostadil is injected into the side of the penis.

How should Mr Yayincili use the medication?

17 Crossword

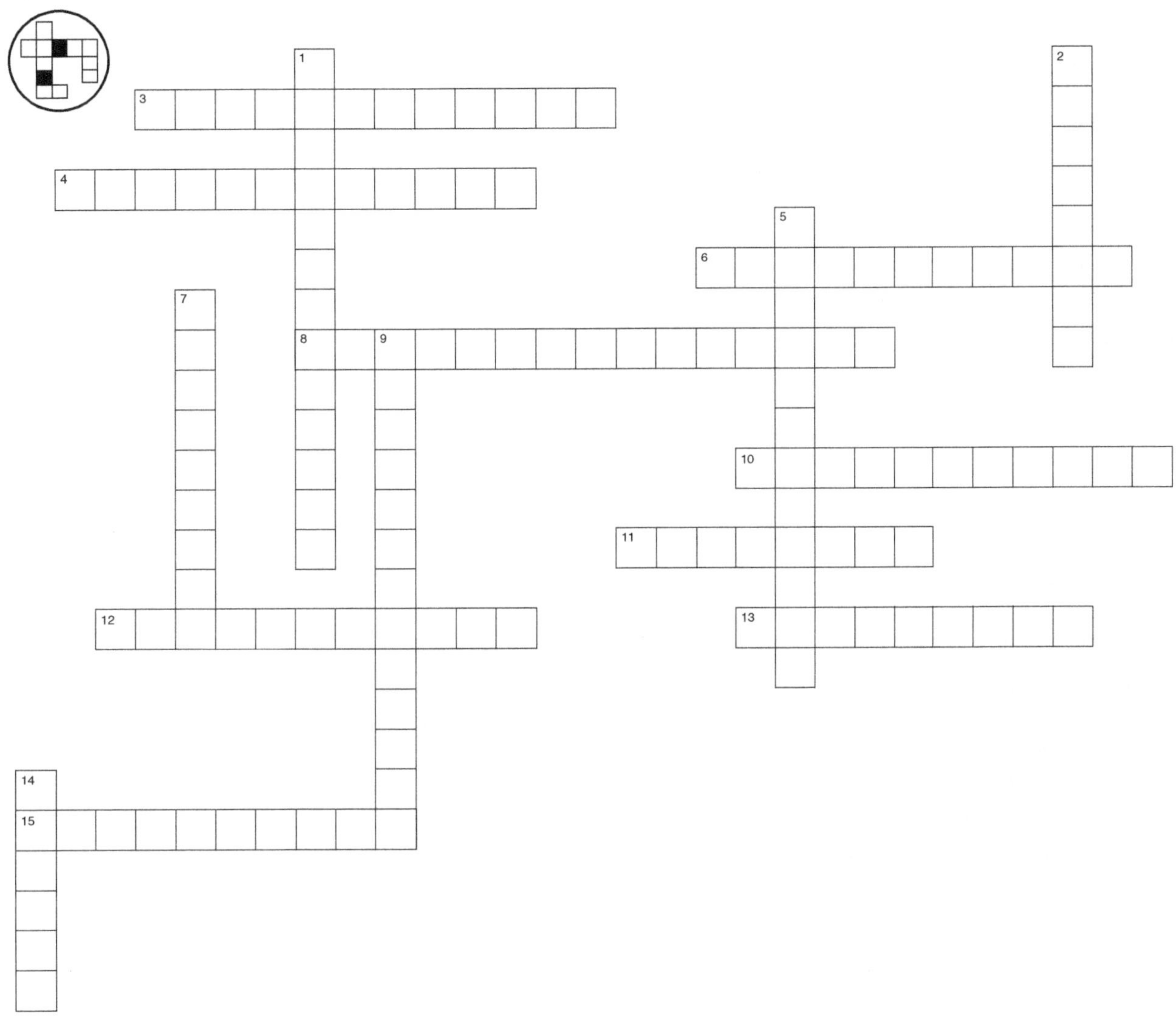

Across

3. Hormone that maintains pregnancy
4. Hormone responsible for deeper voice and male baldness
6. Reflex which elevates the testes
8. The conversion of spermatids into sperm cells
10. Hormone that stimulates ovulation
11. Gland encircling the male urethra
12. The structures cut during a vasectomy
13. The development of mature ova from oogonia
15. Sperm gain their motility here

Down

1. The point at which the ovum completes meiosis II
2. Fingerlike projections at the end of the Fallopian tubes
5. When the endometrium is shed
7. Male sex hormones
9. The growth of uterine lining tissue outside the uterus
14. Neck of the uterus

Multiple-choice questions

18. Oestrogen and progesterone:
A. are gonadotropins
B. are secreted by the liver
C. are secreted by the ovaries
D. exert their effects only on reproductive structures

19. Human chorionic gonadotropin (hCG):
A. promotes the maturation of the egg
B. is responsible for male characteristics
C. maintains the corpus luteum
D. transforms the corpus luteum into the corpus albicans

20. The luteal phase of the ovarian cycle:
A. is essential for menstruation
B. is responsible for the uterine secretory phase
C. excessively elevates plasma levels of oestrogen, progesterone and hCG
D. leads the LH surge

21. Menstruation occurs in response to:
A. sexual activity
B. diminished plasma levels of oestrogen and progesterone
C. elevated plasma levels of hCG
D. elevated plasma levels of FSH and LH

22. Which of the following is not true of testosterone?
A. Classified as androgen
B. Secreted by the anterior pituitary gland
C. Is required for the maturation of sperm
D. Is responsible for most of the male secondary sex characteristics

23. Which structure ejects both semen and urine?
A. Prostate
B. Epididymis
C. Urethra
D. Vas deferens

24. What are seminiferous tubules responsible for?
A. Producing semen
B. Producing the sperm cells
C. The sex of the child
D. All of the above

25. What is the ridge that separates the two sides of the scrotum?
A. Septum
B. Turbinate
C. Rugae
D. Raphe

26. What is the production of sperm called?

A. Semenogenesis
B. Spermatogenesis
C. Spermatogonia
D. Spermocyte

27. Testosterone:

A. level increases as a man ages
B. is absent during puberty
C. level stay the same throughout a man's life
D. None of the above is true

CHAPTER 15

The nervous system

1 Divisions of the nervous system

The following diagram shows the divisions of the nervous system arranged in a hierarchical structure. Complete the boxes in a way that reflects how the divisions relate to each other:

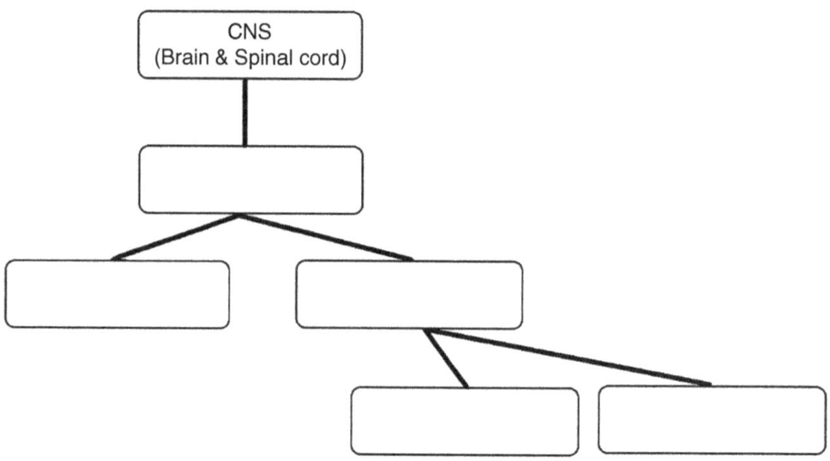

Source: Suzanne Evans (2025).

2 Cells of the nervous system

(a) Label the diagram of a neurone here and colour the myelin sheath:

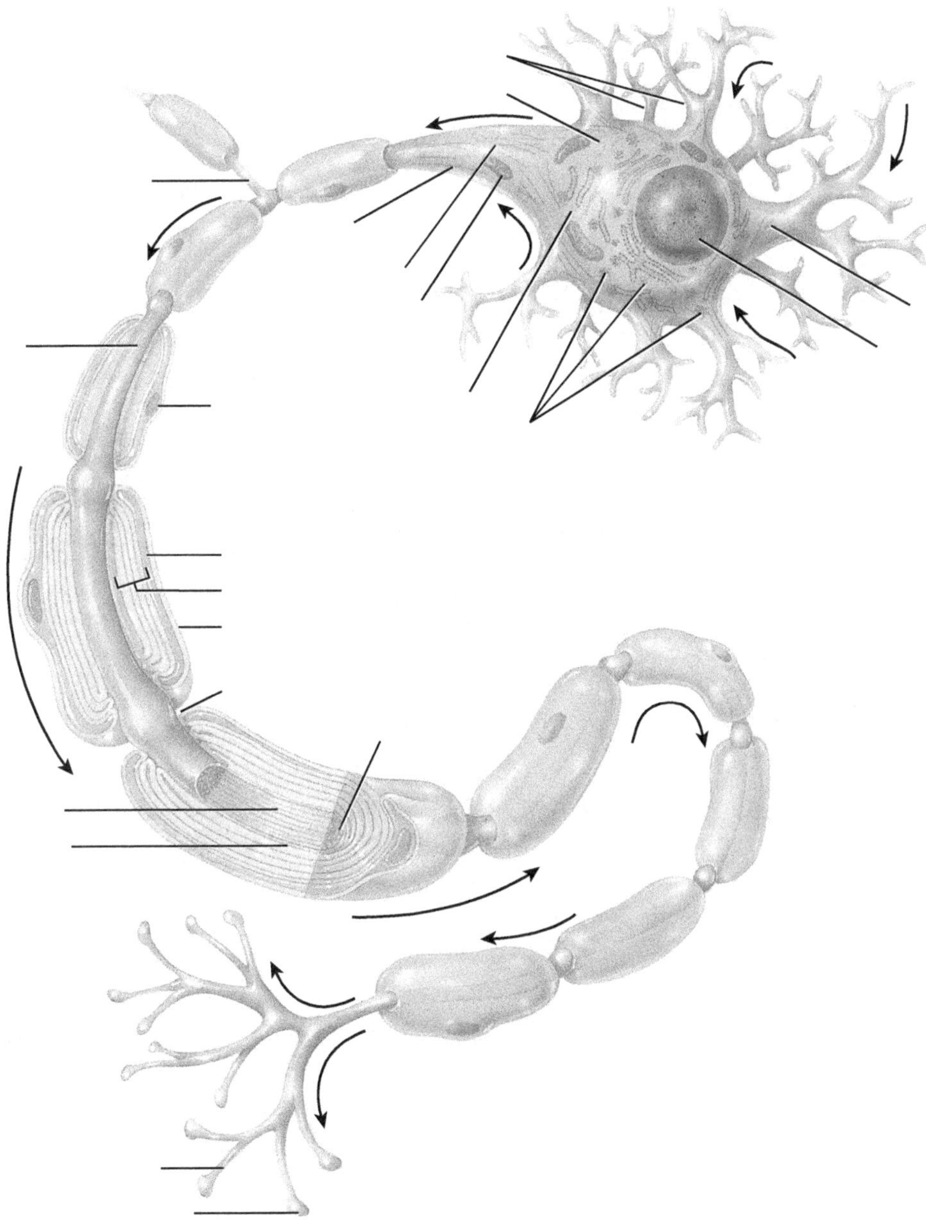

Source: Tortora and Derrickson (2009) / Reproduced with permission of John Wiley & Sons.

(b) Label the following diagram of neurones and neuroglia, and colour all the glial cells:

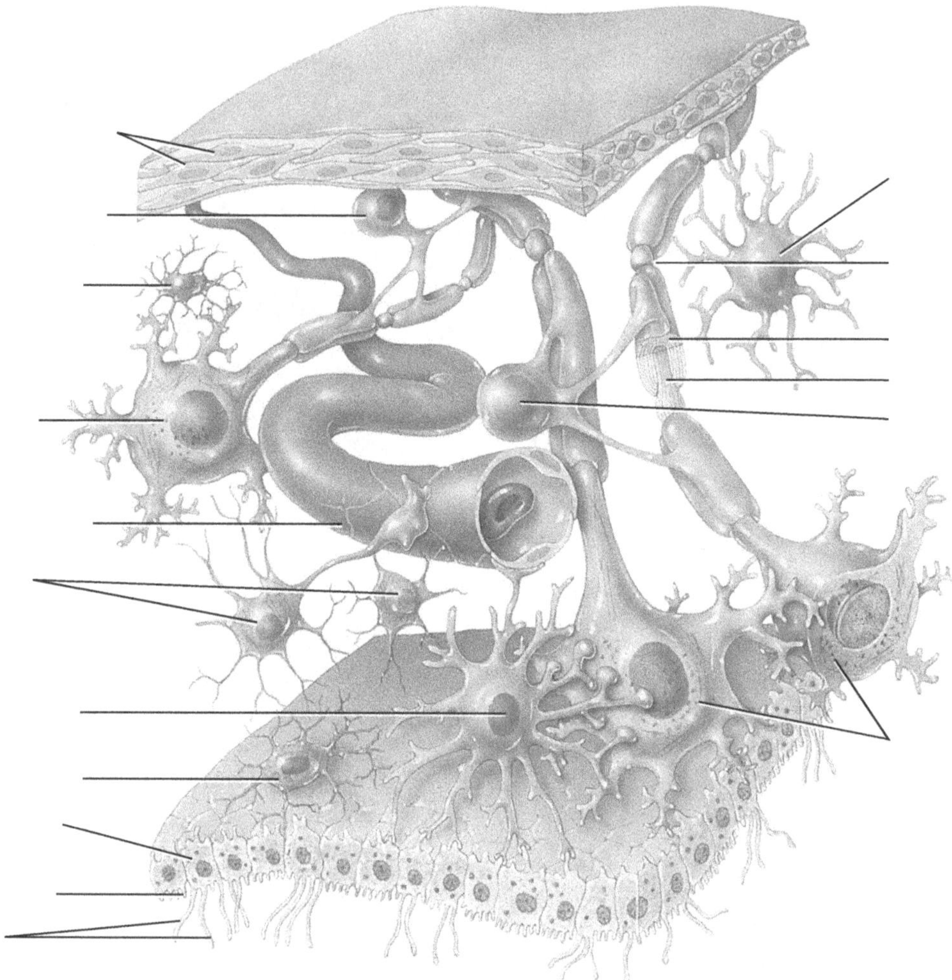

Source: Tortora and Derrickson (2009) / Reproduced with permission of John Wiley & Sons.

3 Structures of the brain

(a) Label the following diagram of a midsagittal section of the brain:

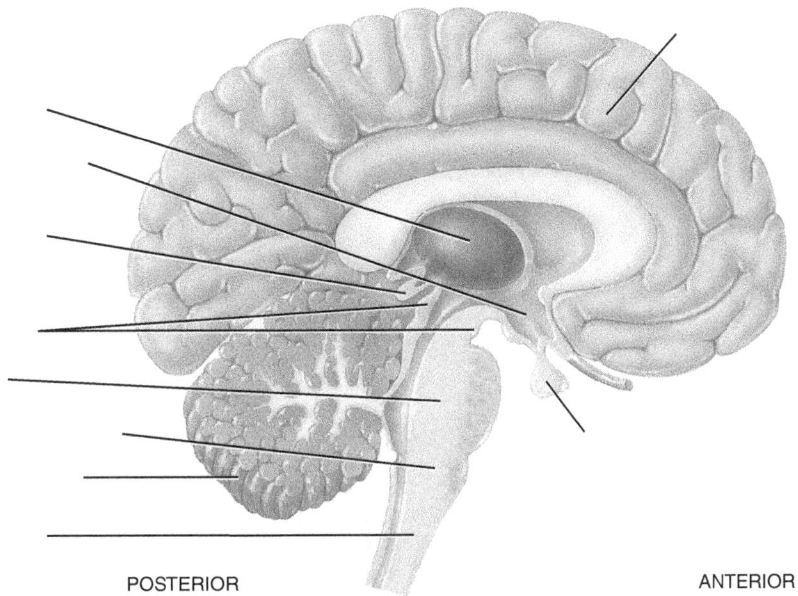

Source: Peate et al. (2014) / Reproduced with permission of John Wiley & Sons.

(b) Label the ventricles and other features of the brain in the following diagram below, and colour in the ventricles and associated ducts:

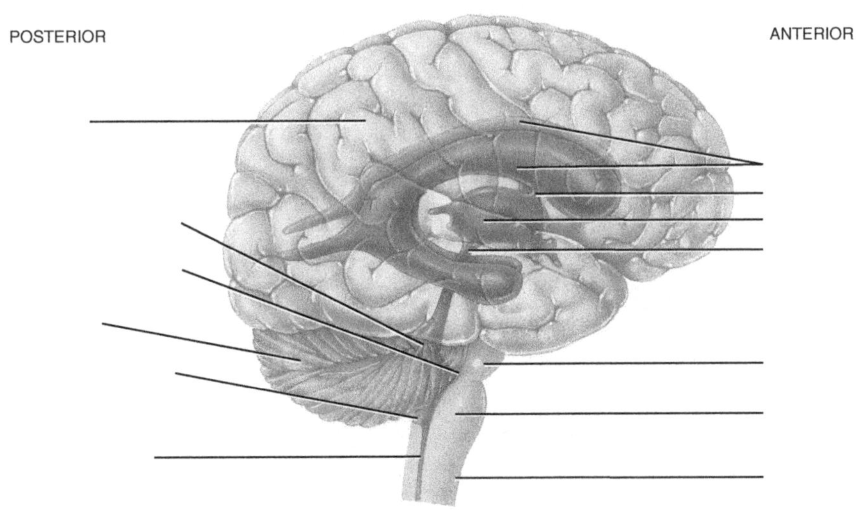

Source: Tortora and Derrickson (2009) / Reproduced with permission of John Wiley & Sons.

4 The meninges

Label the following diagram showing the meninges and the superior sagittal sinus:

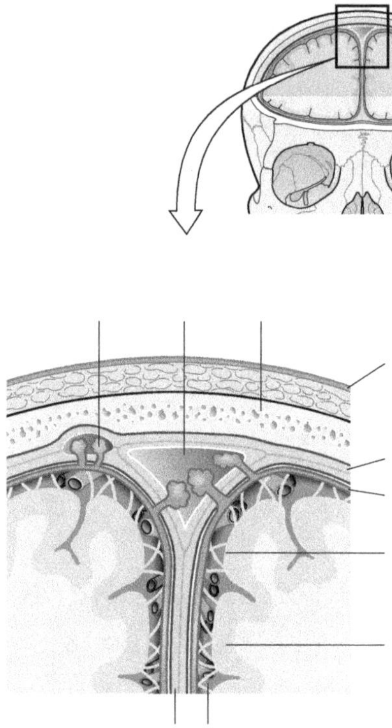

Source: Peate et al. (2014) / Reproduced with permission of John Wiley & Sons.

5 Blood supply to the brain

(a) Label the vessels in the circle of Willis in the following diagram:

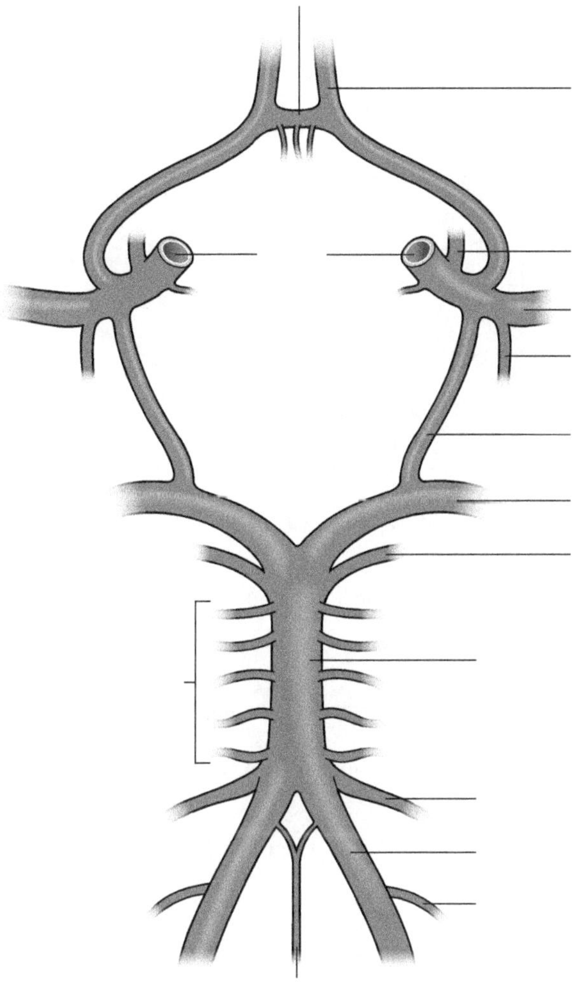

Source: Peate and Nair (2015) / Reproduced with permission of John Wiley & Sons.

(b) How does the circle of Willis protect the brain?

____

____

____

____

6 Functional areas of the forebrain

(a) Label and colour the lobes of the brain on the diagram below:

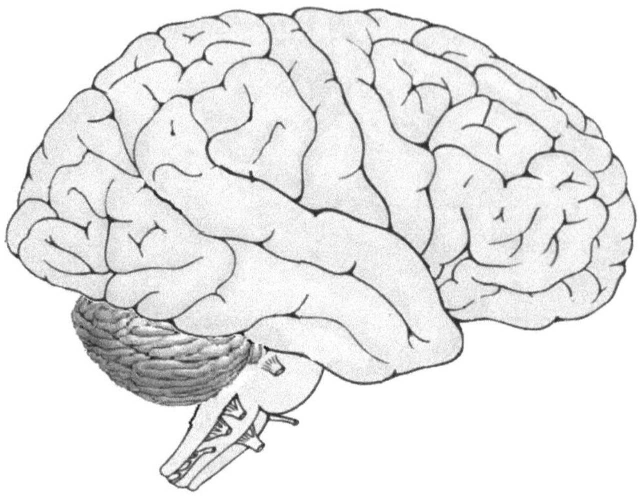

(b) On the following diagram of the brain, colour and label the:

- Primary motor area
- Primary somatosensory area
- Primary visual area
- Primary auditory area

- Premotor area
- Wernicke's area
- Broca's area

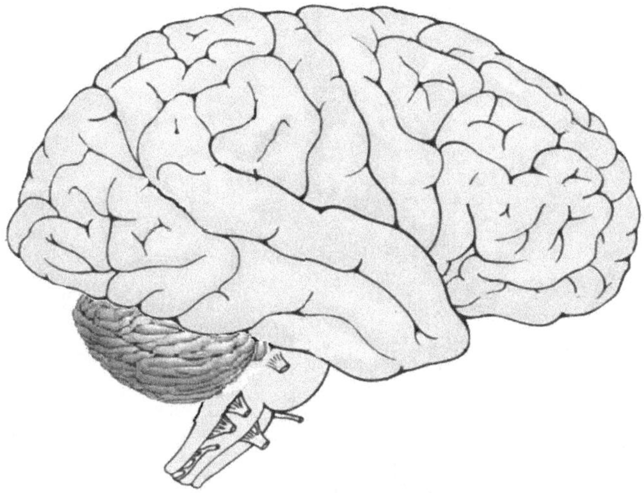

7 The diencephalon

On the diagram of the brain shown here, colour and label the structures of the diencephalon:

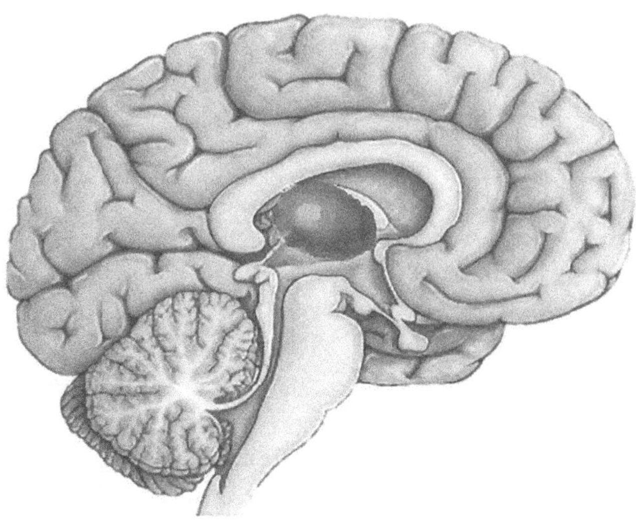

8 The brainstem

On the diagram of the brain shown here, colour and label the structures of the brainstem:

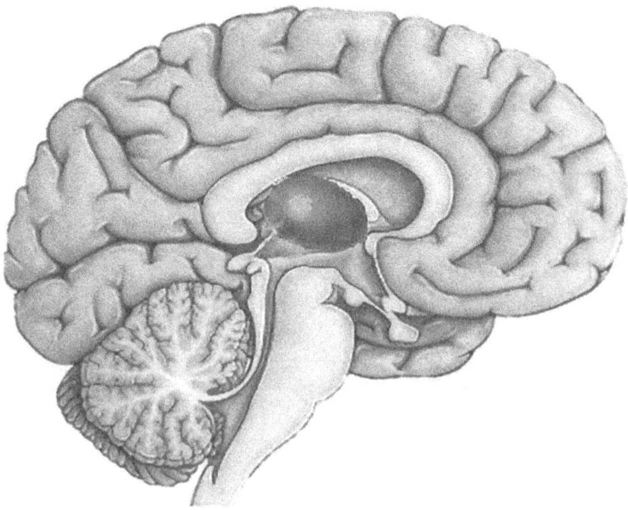

9 The spinal nerves

(a) Label the diagram of the spinal cord in the following diagram and colour in the spinal nerves and their anterior and posterior roots:

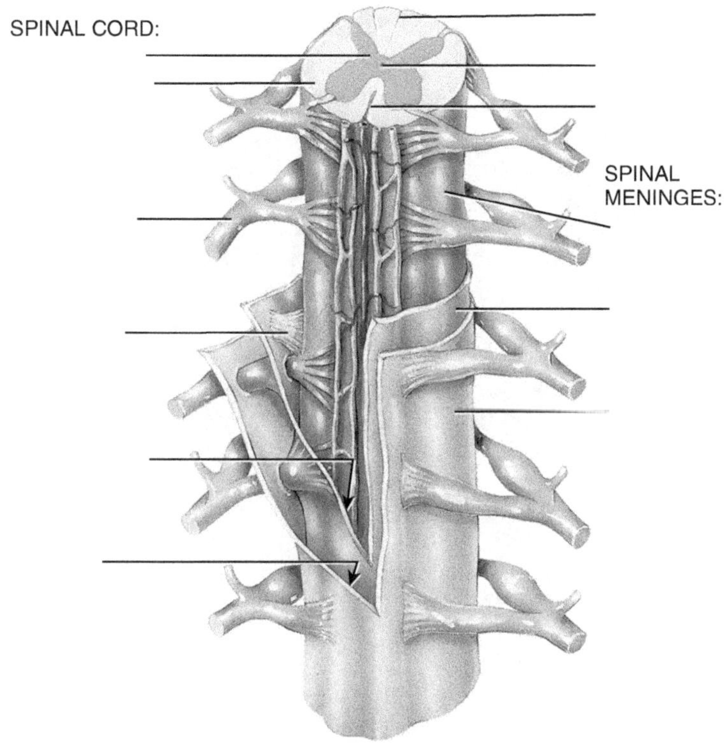

Source: Tortora and Derrickson (2009) / Reproduced with permission of John Wiley & Sons.

(b) Number the vertebrae shown in the following diagram, and colour in the spinal nerves. Note that the vertebrae are only visible as sectioned bone, as the vertebral arches have been removed to show the spinal cord.

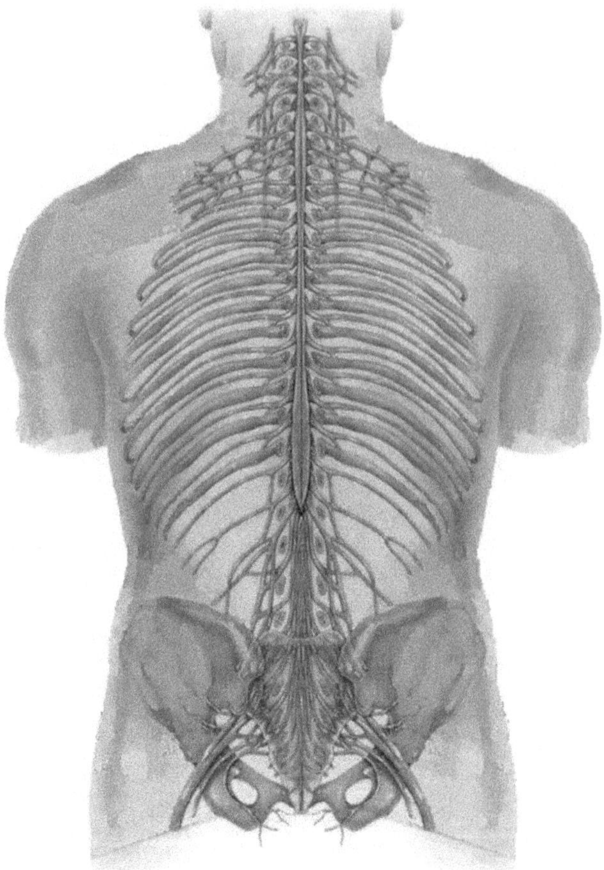

Source: Adapted from Tortora and Derrickson (2009).

(c) On the following diagram of the vertebral column, add the areas of the body supplied by the spinal nerves at each of the levels marked:

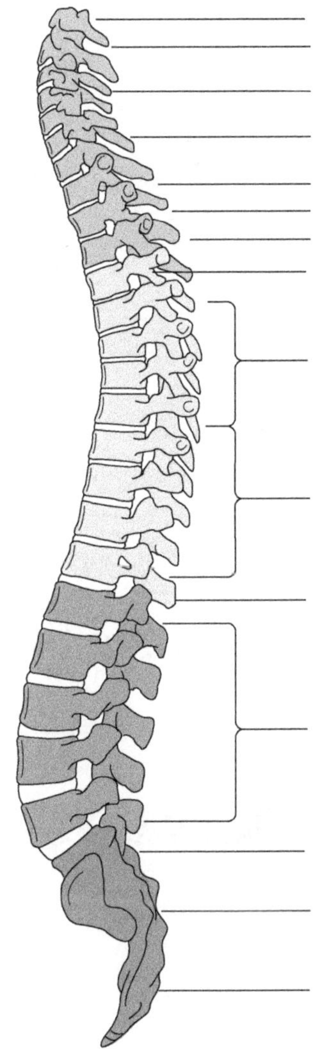

Source: Peate and Nair (2011) / Reproduced with permission of John Wiley & Sons.

10 Match the pairs

The nervous system can be divided into two parts:	the effector may be smooth or cardiac muscle (both involuntary muscles) or a gland
The somatic nervous system is under voluntary control	the central nervous system and the peripheral nervous system
The autonomic nervous system is responsible for involuntary motor responses	and the effector, the tissue or organ responding to instruction from the central nervous system, is skeletal muscle
The functional unit of the nervous system is	produces cerebrospinal fluid
The meninges protect the blood vessels that serve nervous tissue	the neurone or nerve cell
The choroid plexus in the ventricles of the brain	there is a layer of cerebrospinal fluid between the meninges

11 Time yourself to unscramble these words

Scrambled	Answer
SNIGEMEN	
LIVETRENC	
SEXPLU	
BEERSLAPCROIN	
UREOSENN	
MISTRUTTEREROSNAN	
COMSATI	
MOOTNUICA	

12 Reflexes

Annotate the following diagram with a brief description of each of the steps in the spinal reflex pathway. Using arrows, show the direction of impulse flow through the reflex arc and label the neurones.

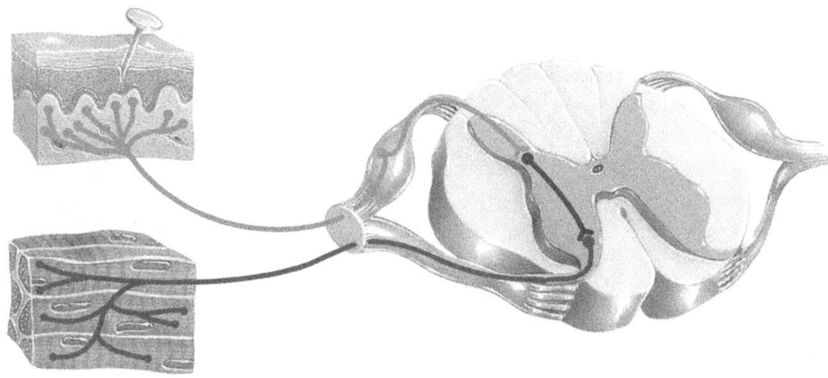

Source: Peate and Nair (2015) / Reproduced with permission of John Wiley & Sons.

13 Cranial nerves

(a) On the following diagram, label each of the cranial nerves shown with their number and name:

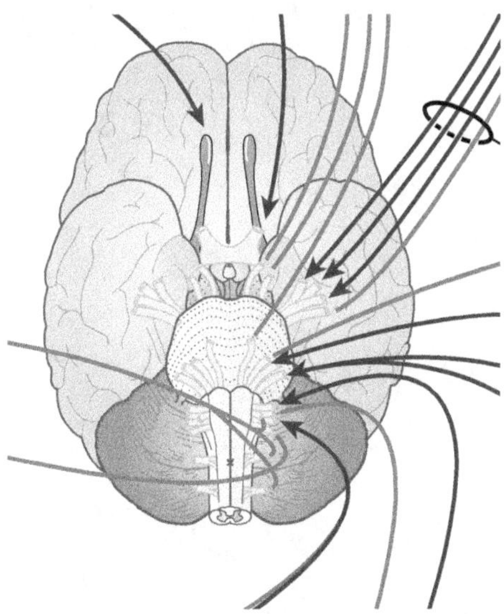

Source: Peate and Nair (2015) / Reproduced with permission of John Wiley & Sons.

(b) Fill in the following table with the functions of the cranial nerves:

	Name	Sensory/motor	Function
I			
II			
III			
IV			
V			
VI			
VII			
VIII			
IX			
X			
XI			
XII			

14 The autonomic nervous system

Complete the following table with the effects of activation of the sympathetic and parasympathetic systems on the organs listed:

Organ/system	Sympathetic effects	Parasympathetic effects
Blood vessels		
Eye		
Heart		
Lungs		
Kidneys		
Liver		
Digestive system		
Adrenal medulla		
Lacrimal glands		
Salivary glands		
Sweat glands		

15 Match the pairs

The 12 pairs of cranial nerves differ in their functions	voluntary muscle movement, balance and posture
The cerebrum is	enclosed within the vertebral canal, protected by the vertebrae
The cerebellum coordinates	the cerebrum and containing three paired structures
Diencephalon is the part of the brain surrounded by	the largest brain structure, divided into the left and right hemispheres
The spinal cord is	some are sensory nerves, some are motor nerves and some are mixed nerves

16 Terminology

Neuroglia	
Neuro- =	- glia =
Meaning:	

Meningitis	
Mening- =	- itis =
Meaning:	

Trigeminal	
Tri- =	- geminal =
Meaning:	

Vagus
Meaning:

Subarachnoid	
Sub- =	- arachnoid=
Meaning:	

17 Snap shot

Ageing and the nervous system

As we age, there are a number of changes that occur throughout our body. With regards to the nervous system, these can be grouped as:

- structural changes with ageing
- cellular changes associated with ageing
- cerebrovascular changes related to ageing
- changes that have an impact on a person's function

It must be remembered that all of the areas of change will impact on each other.
Make notes on the changes related to these aforementioned points.

18 Crossword

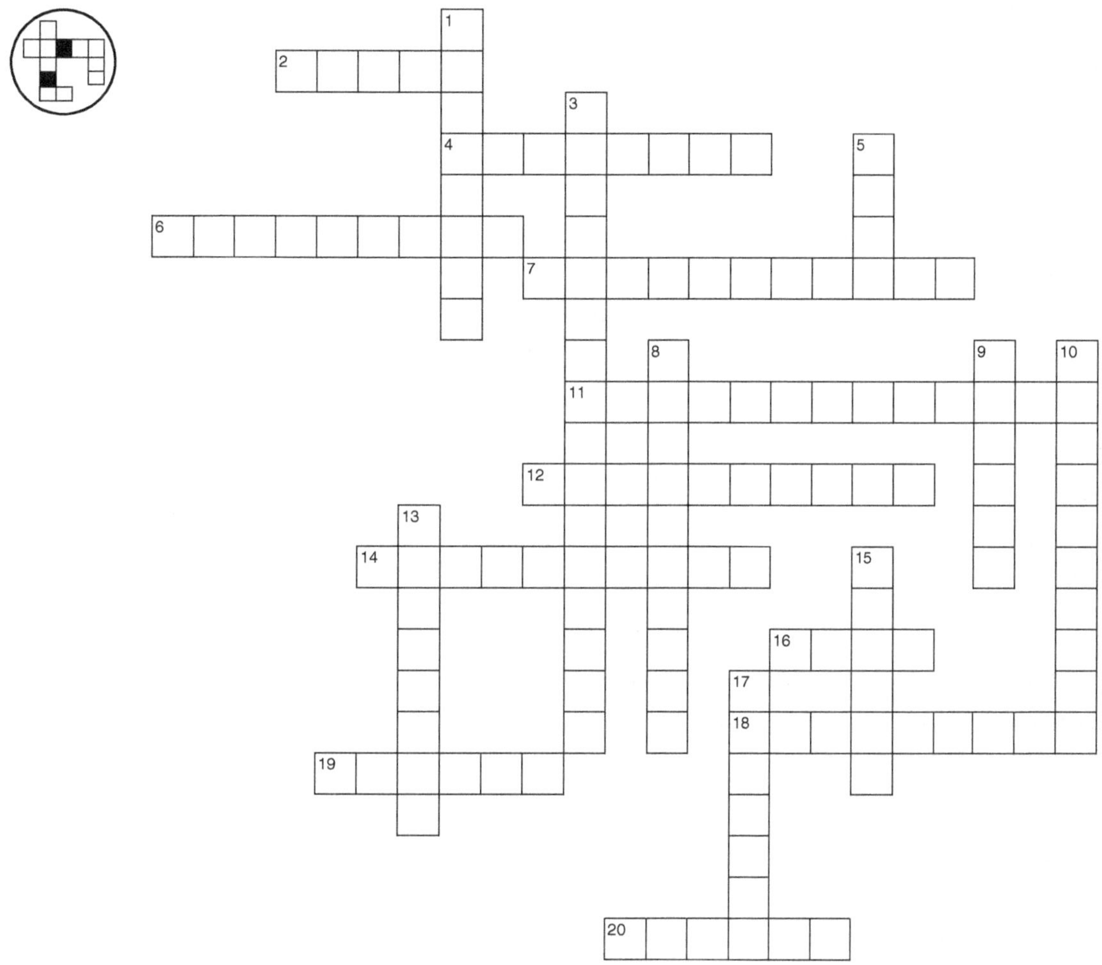

Across

2. Sense associated with the gustatory area of the brain
4. Any part of the body that produces a response to stimuli
6. Cranial nerve which has a role in the sense of smell
7. The parasympathetic nervous system attempts to maintain ___________
11. Neurotransmitter which acts at the neuromuscular junction
12. Star-shaped glial cells
14. Number of ventricles in the brain
16. The meningeal layer which lies closest to the bone of the skull
18. Specialised sensory cells
19. Fatty insulator of axons
20. Clusters of cell bodies grouped together in the central nervous system

Down

1. The largest brain structure
3. Chemical that signals between two neurones, or between a neurone and a muscle cell
5. Brainstem structure with a role in regulating breathing
8. The outermost part of the Schwann cell
9. The circle of __________ forms part of the blood supply to the brain
10. Photophobia and a stiff, sore neck are symptoms associated with _________
13. Membranes that cover the central nervous system
15. Axons bundled together
17. Collective term for the nerves that emerge from the base of the brain

Multiple-choice questions

19. The precentral gyrus is:
- A. situated in the parietal lobe
- B. the primary motor cortex
- C. the primary visual cortex
- D. a part of the brainstem

20. Which of the following is true?
- A. The medulla oblongata is a cerebral structure
- B. The hypothalamus is a brainstem structure
- C. The medulla oblongata is continuous with the spinal cord
- D. The midbrain, pons and medulla oblongata are supratentorial structures

21. The postcentral gyrus:
- A. is found in the parietal lobe
- B. regulates all voluntary motor activity
- C. is where Broca's area can be found
- D. contains the primary visual cortex

22. Cerebrospinal fluid:
- A. drains out of the subarachnoid space into the choroid plexus
- B. circulates within the subarachnoid space
- C. is also known as mucus
- D. flows up the central canal into the fourth, third and lateral ventricles

23. Which of the following pairs is a correct match?
- A. Temporal lobe: motor planning
- B. Frontal lobe: somatosensory (touch, pressure, pain)
- C. Occipital lobe: vision
- D. Parietal lobe: hearing

24. Neuroglia:
- A. are categorised as sensory and motor
- B. include astrocytes and oligodendrocytes
- C. fire action potentials when stimulated
- D. contain cerebrospinal fluid (CSF), dendrites and axons

25. Activation of the emetic centre:
- A. decreases blood pressure
- B. increases body temperature
- C. stops diaphoresis
- D. causes vomiting

26. The hypothalamus:
- A. is within the diencephalon
- B. synthesises antidiuretic hormone and oxytocin
- C. regulates pituitary gland activity
- D. All of the above are true

27. The meninges consist of how many connective tissue layers?

A. 1

B. 2

C. 3

D. 4

28. What is the name of cranial nerve IV?

A. Trochlear

B. Optic

C. Trigeminal

D. Vagus

CHAPTER 16

The senses

1 Receptors

Complete the following table by filling in examples of where the sensory receptors listed can be found:

Receptor	Stimulus	Example
Chemoreceptors	Alterations in concentrations of chemical substances	
Nociceptors (pain receptors)	Damage to tissues	
Thermoreceptors	Temperature changes	
Sensory receptor (mechanoreceptors)	Changes in pressures (can also include change in the movement of fluids)	
Photoreceptors	Light energy	

2 The chemical senses

Label the following diagram and colour in the olfactory bulbs:

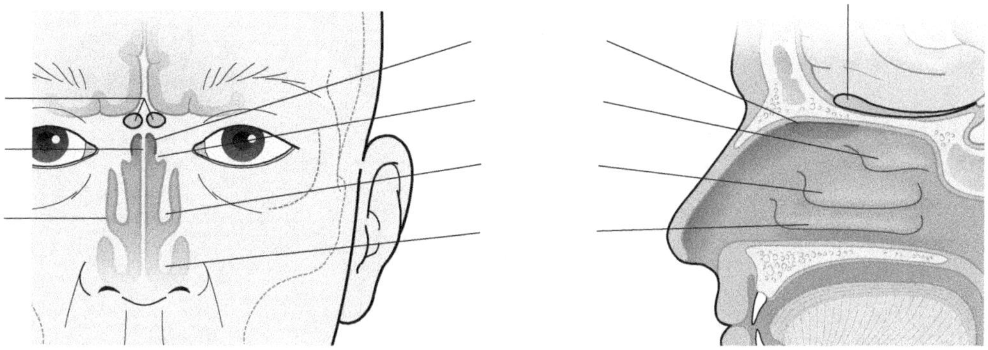

Source: Peate and Nair (2015) / Reproduced with permission of John Wiley & Sons.

3 Olfaction

Label the following diagram of the olfactory pathway:

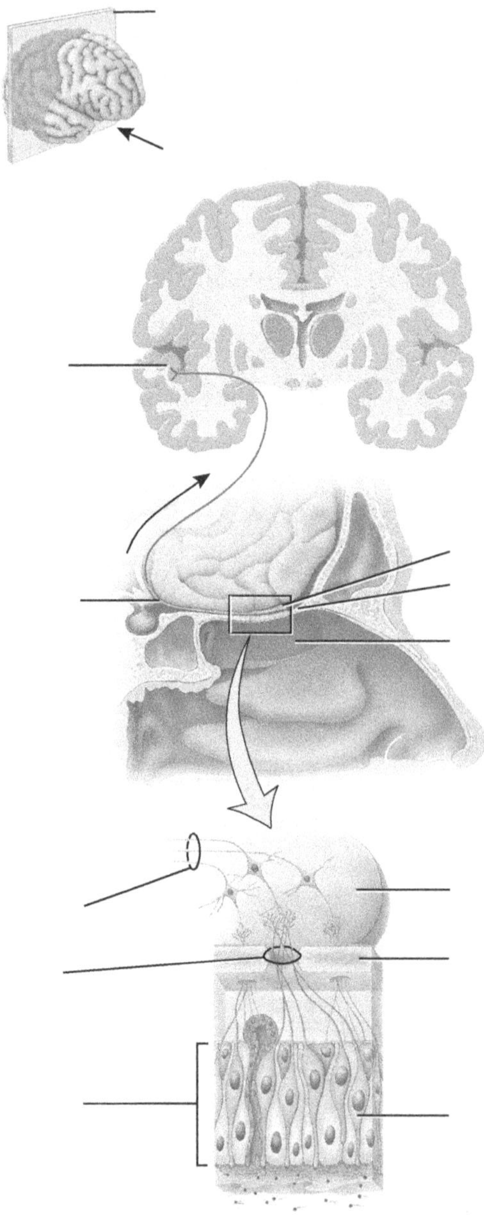

Source: Tortora and Derrickson (2009) / Reproduced with permission of John Wiley & Sons.

4 Match the pairs

The sense of smell aids survival by	in the nasal cavity there are paired olfactory organs made up of two layers
Olfaction is dependent on	the identification of food that is safe to eat and that which has gone rotten
On either side of the nasal septum	receptors that respond to airborne particles
When air is inhaled through the nasal cavity	highly modified neurones contained within the olfactory epithelium
The olfactory receptors are	that respond to certain irritants such as ammonia, chilies and menthol
The nasal cavity contains pain receptors	it is subject to turbulent flow ensuring that airborne smell particles are brought to the olfactory organs

5 Time yourself to unscramble these words

SCRA-MBLE

Scrambled	Unscrambled
TAYFORCLO	
CREEPROST	
LUBB	
BLICIM	
IMCHELAC	
LLEMS	
IRCIMBFORR	
DRATOON	

6 Tongue and taste buds

(a) Label the following diagram of the tongue and colour in the papillae:

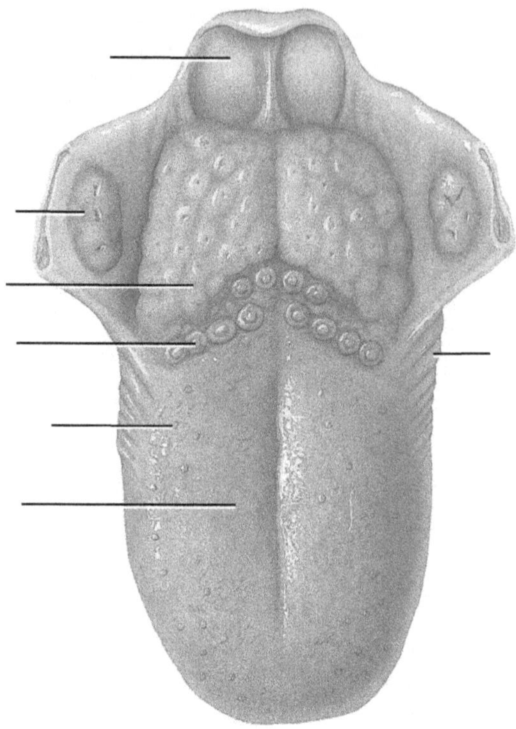

Source: Tortora and Derrickson (2009) / Reproduced with permission of John Wiley & Sons.

(b) Label the following diagram of the taste bud and colour the gustatory receptor cell:

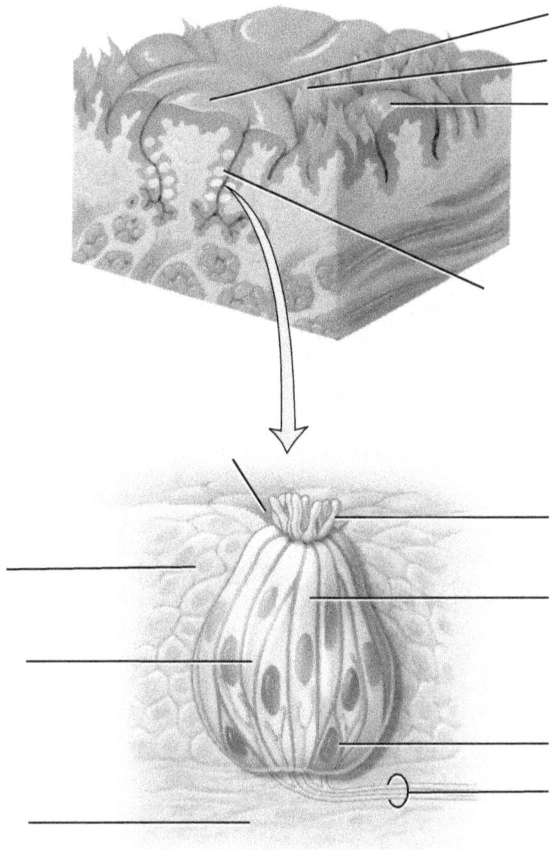

Source: Tortora and Derrickson (2009) / Reproduced with permission of John Wiley & Sons.

7 Match the pairs

Bitter or sour flavours usually taste unpleasant because	in conjunction with the needs of the body
The tongue is a muscular structure	a number of efferent neural pathways important to digestive function are activated
The papillae are projections of a connective tissue core covered	through which microvilli from the taste cells extend
The taste cells within a bud are arranged so that their tips form a small taste pore	poisons are bitter, while foods that have gone off taste acidic
When the taste signals are transmitted to the brain	with squamous epithelium
Taste preferences often change	with a rough surface created by papillae with thousands of taste buds on them

8 Hearing and equilibrium

(a) Label the following diagram of the ear and colour in the cochlea, semicircular canals and ossicles:

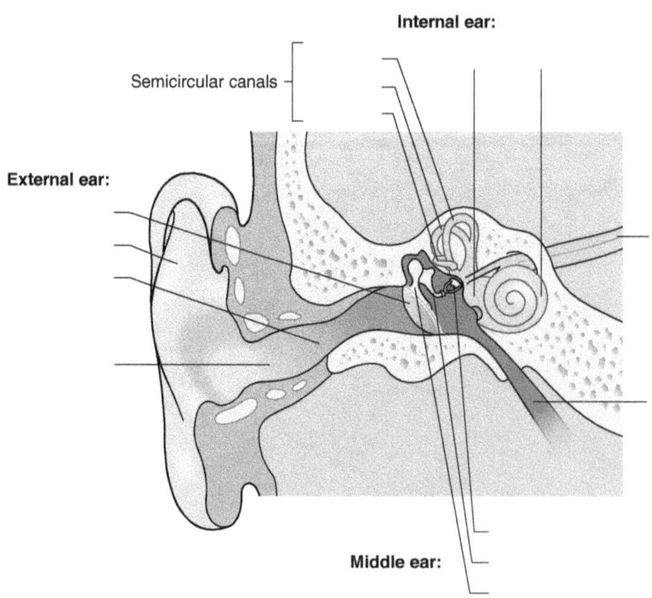

Source: Peate et al. (2014) / Reproduced with permission of John Wiley & Sons.

(b) Label the following diagram of the middle ear and colour in the malleus and incus:

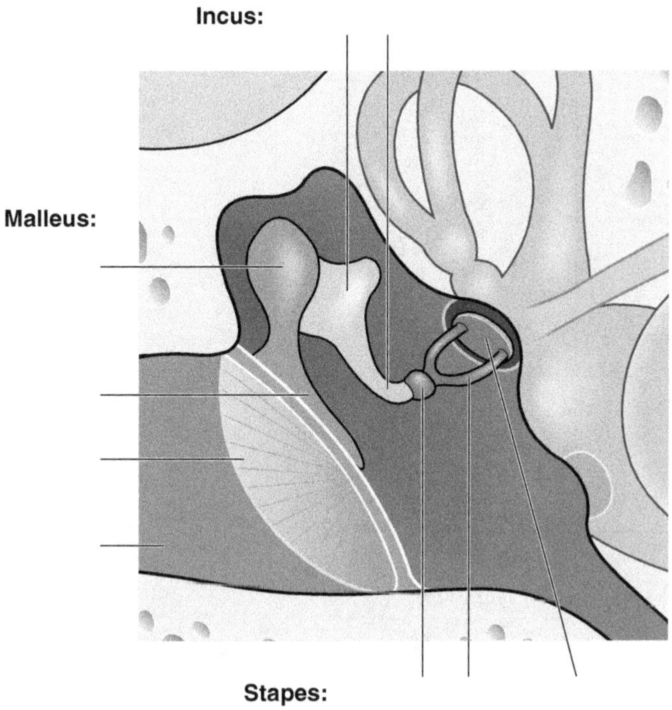

Source: Peate et al. (2014) / Reproduced with permission of John Wiley & Sons.

(c) Label the following diagram of the inner ear and colour the semicircular canals:

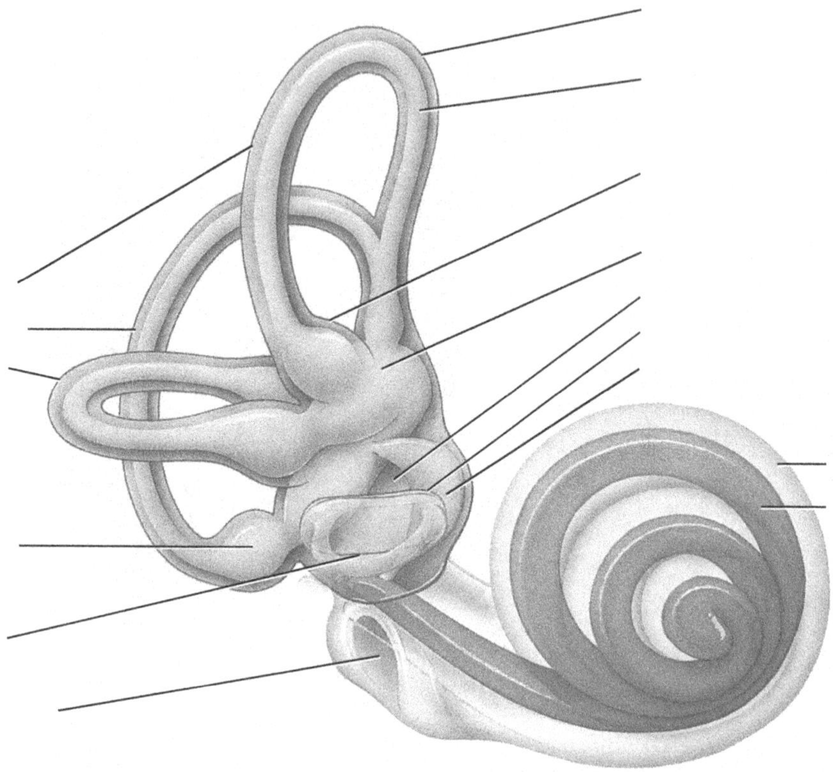

(d) Label the following diagram of the unfolded cochlea and colour the perilymph in the scala vestibuli and scala tympani:

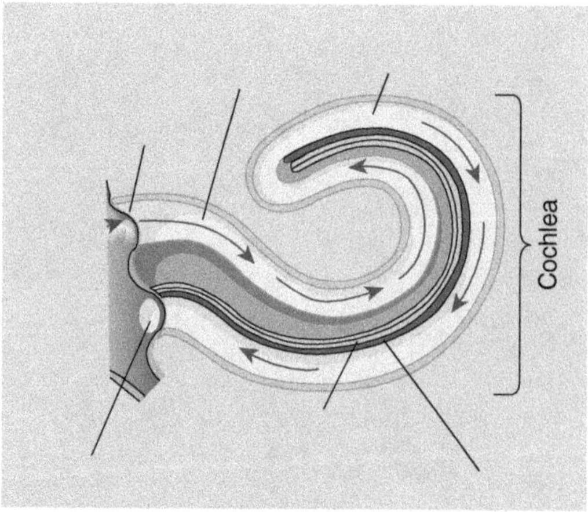

Source: Tortora and Derrickson (2009) / Reproduced with permission of John Wiley & Sons.

9 Match the pairs

The cochlea is a bony, spiral chamber	kill bacteria and, in conjunction with the hairs, keep the canal free of debris
The purpose of the oils and the cerumen is to lubricate the ear canal	containing the cochlear duct of the membranous labyrinth
The tympanic cavity is a small, air-filled cavity	and is controlled by receptors in the semicircular ducts, the utricle and the saccule of the inner ear
The inner ear is also known as the labyrinth due to its complicated series of canals	lined with mucosa and contained within the temporal bone
The sense of equilibrium is part of the sense of balance	they are hair cells similar to those of the semicircular canals and vestibule
The sense of hearing is provided by receptors in the cochlear duct,	composed of two main fluid-filled parts

10 The eye

(a) Fill the functions of the accessory structure of the eye listed in the following table:

Structure	Function
Eyelids (palpebrae)	
Eyelashes	
Commissure	
Conjunctiva	
Eyebrows	

(b) Label the structures of the eye shown in the following photograph:

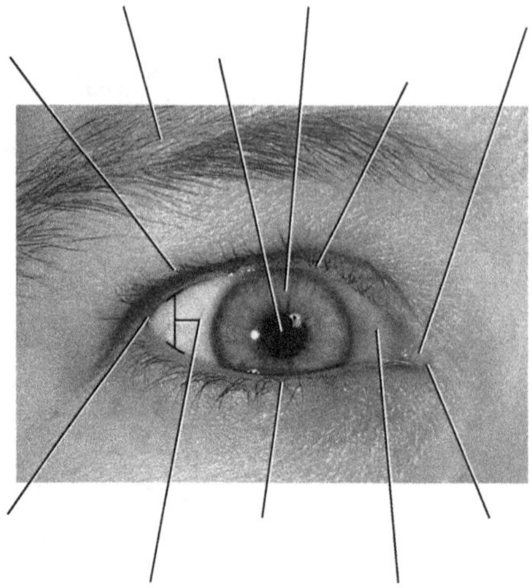

Source: Tortora and Derrickson (2009) / Reproduced with permission of John Wiley & Sons.

(c) Label the following diagram of the lacrimal apparatus:

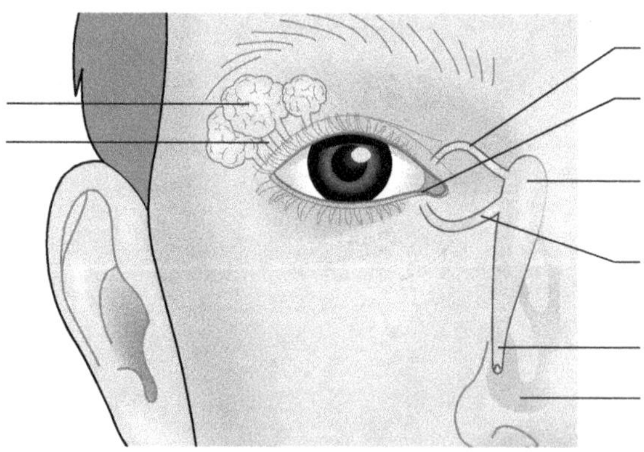

Source: Peate et al. (2014) / Reproduced with permission of John Wiley & Sons.

11 Match the pairs

Continual blinking keeps the surface of the eye	the tarsal glands which produce a lipid-rich secretion that helps to prevent the eyelids from sticking together
Eyelashes are robust hairs that help to keep foreign matter out of the eyes associated with	occupied by adipose tissue
The conjunctiva is	arched protecting the eyeball from foreign bodies, dust and sweat
The eyebrows are	the optic nerve (cranial nerve II)
The eye is innervated by	the epithelial cell layer that lines the inside of the eyelids and the outer surface of the eye
The space between the eye and the orbital cavity is	lubricated and removes dirt. The gap between the eyelids is known as the palpebral fissure

12 Photoreceptors

(a) Label the following diagram of the eye and colour in the lens and the photoreceptors:

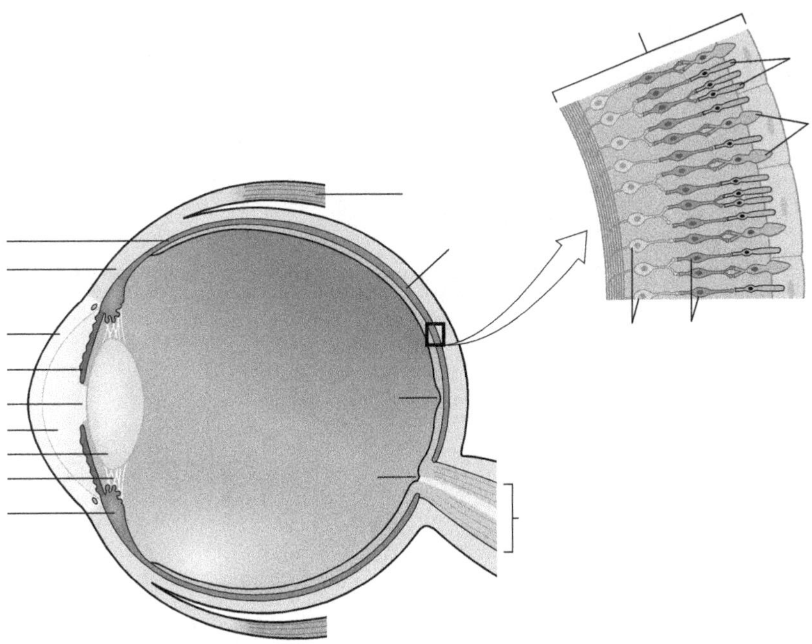

Source: Peate and Nair (2015) / Reproduced with permission of John Wiley & Sons.

(b) Label the following diagram of the retina:

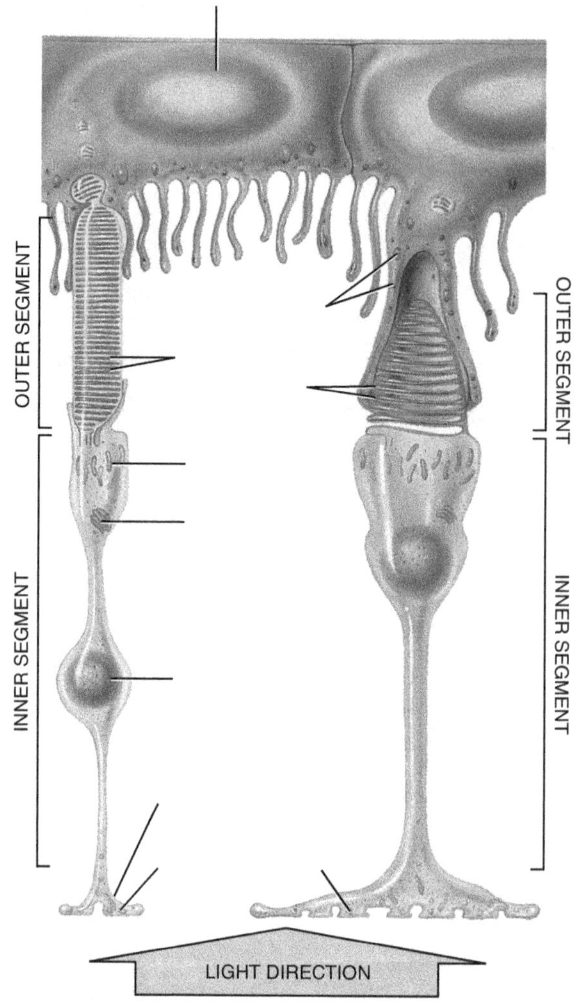

Source: Tortora and Derrickson (2009) / Reproduced with permission of John Wiley & Sons.

13 Muscles moving the eye

Identify the six extrinsic muscles of the eye shown in the following diagram:

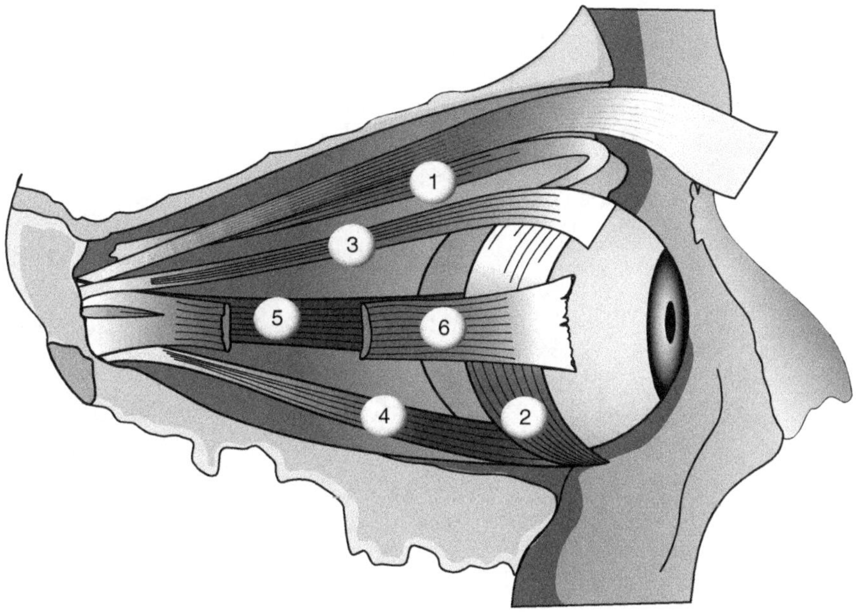

1 ______________ 2 ______________

3 ______________ 4 ______________

5 ______________ 6 ______________

Source: Adapted from Edelhart Kempeneers. Gray's Anatomy, 1918.

14 The visual pathway

Label the following diagram of the visual pathway and colour in the two sides of the visual image in contrasting colours.

Visual pathways

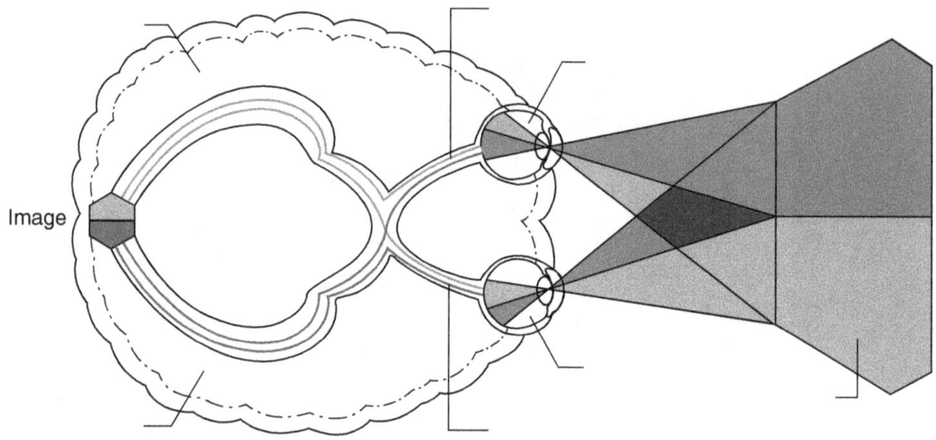

15 Match the pairs

The retina is a thin transparent tissue	for peripheral vision and vision under low light conditions
In the retina there are two types of receptors	to discern colour and fine detail
Cones provide the ability	rods and cones
Rods are mainly responsible	designed to capture photons of light
The extrinsic eye muscles move	structures within the eyeball
The intrinsic muscles move	the eyeball in the bony orbit

16 Terminology

Presbyopia	
Presby- =	-opia =
Meaning:	

Otolith	
Oto- =	-lith =
Meaning:	

Ossicles
Meaning:

Cochlea
Meaning:

Perilymph	
Peri- =	-lymph =
Meaning:	

17 Snap shot

Visual acuity

The term 20/20 vision is used to express normal visual acuity; this is the clarity or sharpness of vision. 20/20 vision is cited when the imperial system is used, with the metric system normal visual acuity quoted as being 6/6.
What does 6/6 vision mean?

____

____

____

____

18 Crossword

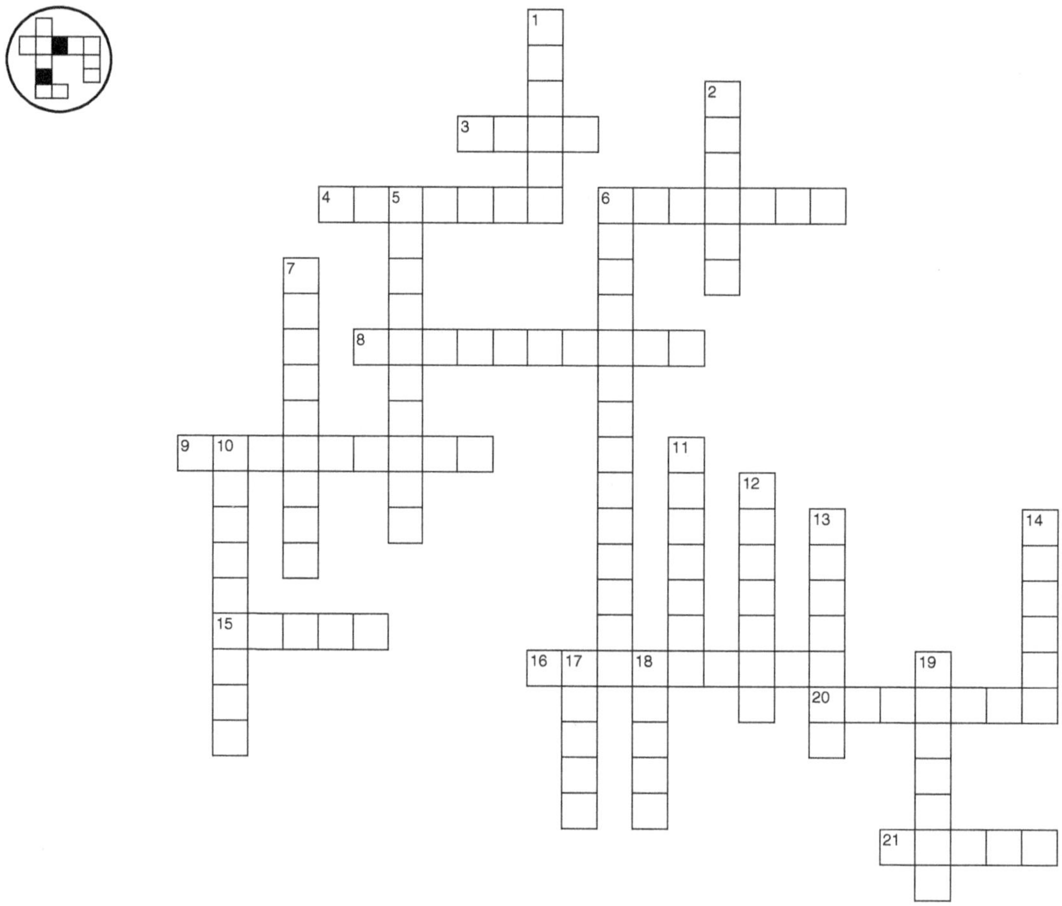

Across

3. The central, coloured portion of the eye
4. Complete loss of sense of taste
6. Ear wax
8. Anosmia can be an early indicator of this degenerative neurological condition
9. The sense of smell
15. Bone which contacts the malleus and the stapes
16. Taste
20. Bony spiral
21. Dissolved chemicals interact with odorant-binding proteins on the cell's ________

Down

1. The innermost layer of the eye
2. The area of the retina with the highest concentration of cones
5. Tube which connects the middle ear to the nasopharynx
6. Sensors for the chemical senses
7. Pain receptors in the nasal cavity respond strongly to ________
10. The inner ear
11. Singular of papillae
12. Loss of the sense of smell
13. Equilibrium
14. Tissue that covers most of theouter surface of the eye
17. Basic taste associated with the proteins found in meat and fish
18. Number of bones in the middle ear
19. The vascular layer between the retina and sclera

Multiple-choice questions

19. The retina:
  A. is avascular
  B. contains rods and cones
  C. covers the eyelid
  D. secretes vitreous humour

20. Diminished blood flow to the choroid can result in:
  A. an increase in intraocular pressure
  B. pupillary constriction
  C. death of retinal cells
  D. none of the above

21. A drug that is described as mydriatic:
  A. increases intraocular pressure
  B. dilates the pupil
  C. decreases the secretion of aqueous humour
  D. increases the number of rods

22. Which of the following is not true of the middle ear?
  A. It contains the malleus, incus and stapes
  B. It connects with the pharynx via the eustachian tube
  C. It is the location of the organ of Corti
  D. It is concerned with bony conduction of sound

23. The organ of Corti:
  A. is the receptor for hearing
  B. refers to the bones within the middle ear
  C. is easily identified with an ophthalmoscope
  D. deactivates CN II

24. Touch, pressure, pain and temperature are:
  A. mediated through mechanoreceptors
  B. classified as general senses
  C. processed in the precentral gyrus
  D. processed in the occipital lobe

25. Cranial nerves III, IV and VI:
  A. carry sensory information from the iris to the occipital lobe
  B. carry sensory information from the organ of Corti to the primary auditory cortex
  C. innervate the extrinsic eye muscles
  D. are the motor nerves involved in tear production

26. Which of the following is not a sense?
  A. Gustation
  B. Lacrimation
  C. Olfaction
  D. Proprioception

27. What are these structures: superior oblique, inferior oblique, superior rectus, inferior rectus, medial rectus and lateral rectus?

A. Cranial nerves that stimulate the extrinsic eye muscles

B. Muscles that form the iris

C. Structures of the middle ear

D. Extrinsic eye muscles

28. What is ptosis?

A. Drooping of the upper eyelid

B. Constricted pupils

C. An intense earache

D. None of the above

CHAPTER 17

The endocrine system

1 Endocrine vs nervous control

Complete the following table showing comparisons between the endocrine and nervous systems:

	Nervous system	Endocrine system
Speed of action		
Duration of action		
Commands are in the form of		
Commands distributed by		

2 Major endocrine glands

Label the major endocrine glands on the following diagram:

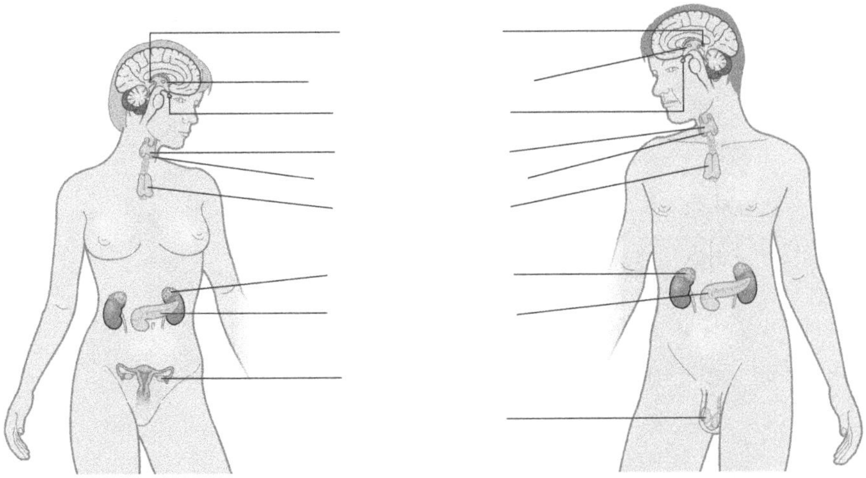

Source: Peate and Nair (2015) / Reproduced with permission of John Wiley & Sons.

3 Definition of terms

Define the terms in the following table:

	Definition
Endocrine	
Paracrine	
Autocrine	
Exocrine	

4 Endocrine responses

Fill in the missing components of the endocrine feedback loops shown in (a) to (d):

(a)

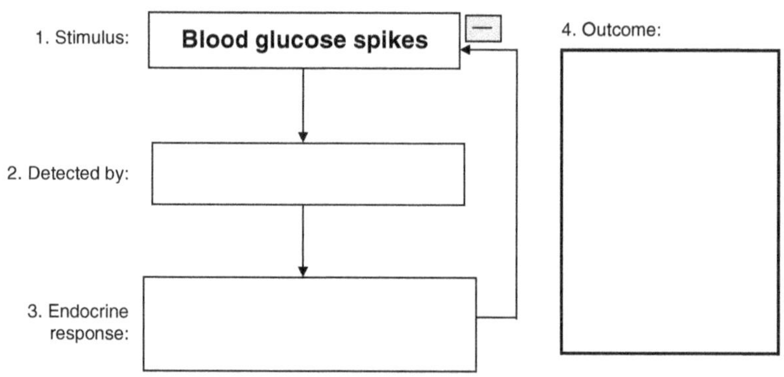

(b)

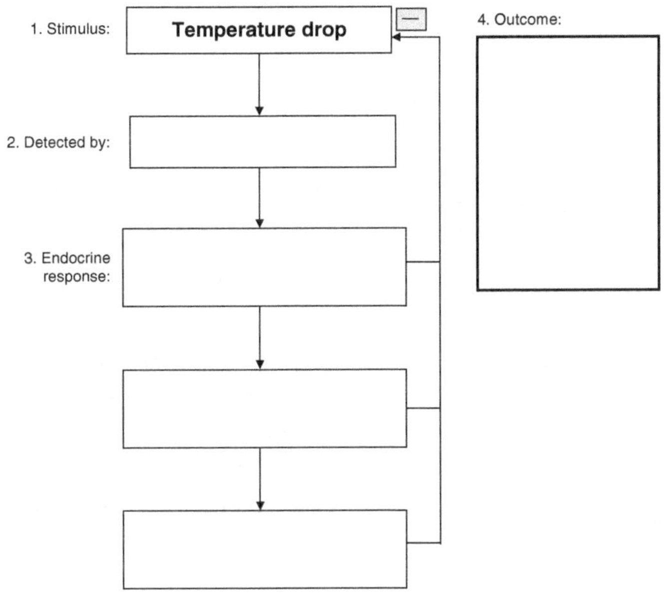
1. Stimulus:
Temperature drop
–
2. Detected by:
3. Endocrine response:
4. Outcome:

(c)

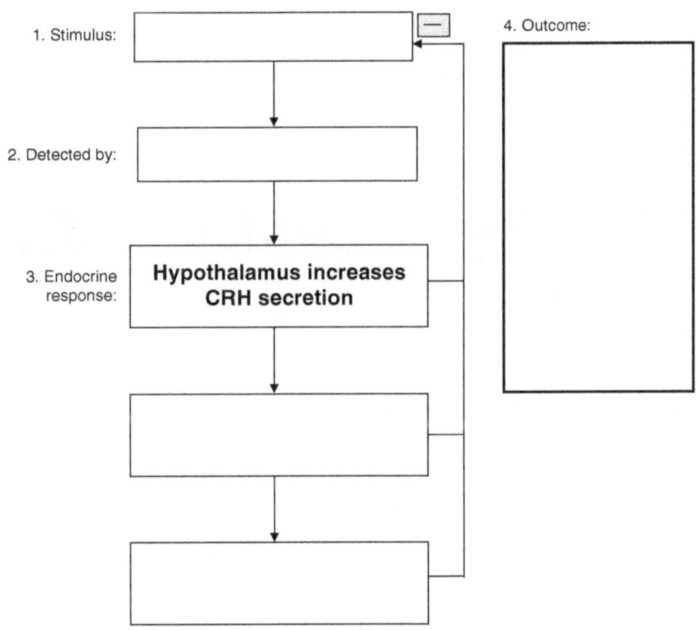
1. Stimulus:
–
2. Detected by:
3. Endocrine response:
Hypothalamus increases CRH secretion
4. Outcome:

(d)

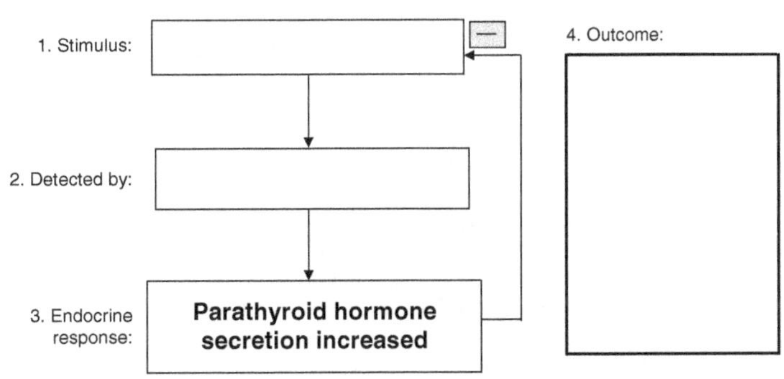
1. Stimulus:
–
2. Detected by:
3. Endocrine response:
Parathyroid hormone secretion increased
4. Outcome:

5 Match the pairs

A change in the numbers of a particular receptor is known as	and excreted mostly in the urine
The endocrine system is made up of	hormones that act locally and diffuse to the cells in the immediate neighbourhood to produce their action
Paracrine refers to	chemical messengers that are secreted into the blood or the extracellular fluid by one cell and influence the functioning of other cells
Hormones are	up-regulation and down-regulation
Most hormones are inactivated by enzyme systems in the liver and kidneys	organs scattered throughout the body which release hormones into the blood

6 Time yourself to unscramble these words

Scrambled	Unscrambled
SHOREMON	
CREEDINON	
CROXEINE	
RATGET	
BEEFCAKD	
USMUTLIS	
PORCESTER	
RINCETOAU	

7 Control of the endocrine system by the brain

(a) Label the following diagram of the pituitary gland, and colour the anterior and posterior pituitary in contrasting colours:

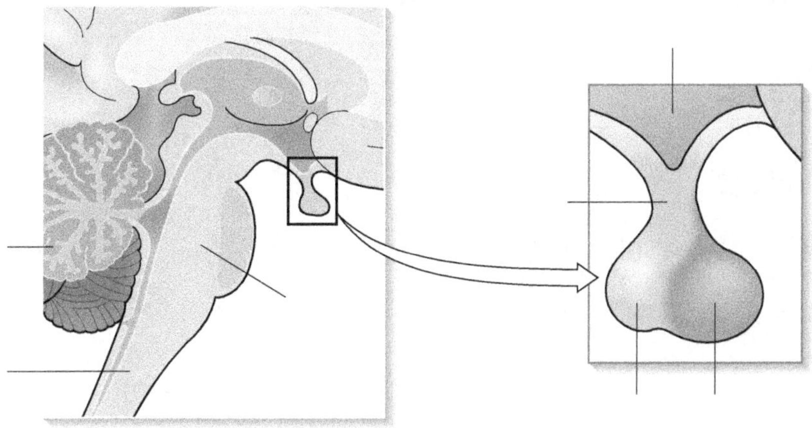

Source: Peate and Nair (2015) / Reproduced with permission of John Wiley & Sons.

(b) Add the names of the pituitary hormones corresponding to the target tissues shown in the following diagram:

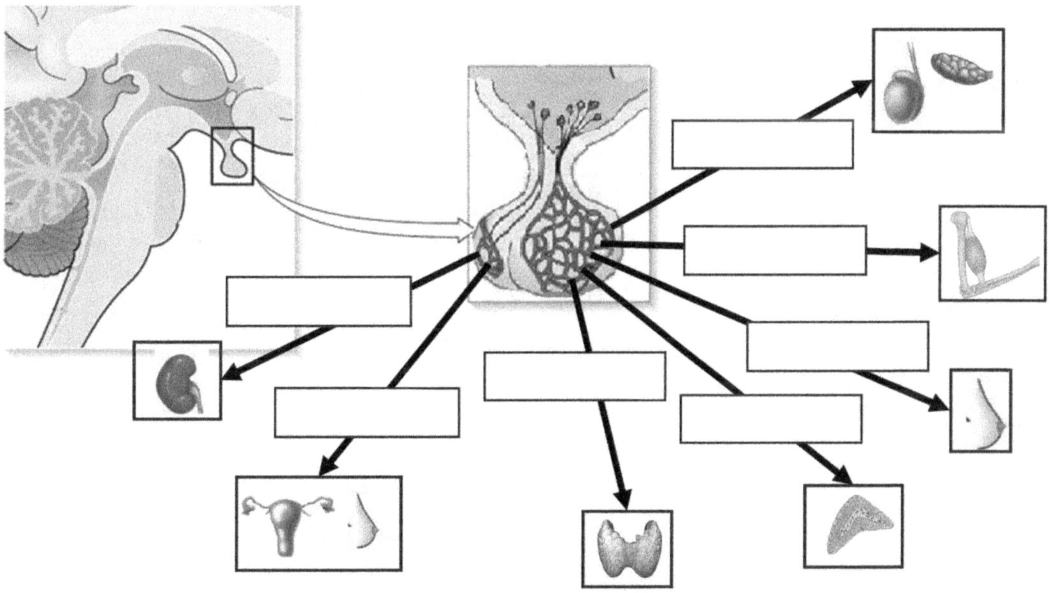

Source: Adapted from Peate and Nair (2015) / Reproduced with permission of John Wiley & Sons.

(c) Complete the following table by filling in the names of the hypothalamic and pituitary hormones and their target tissues:

Hypothalamic hormone	Anterior pituitary hormone	Target tissue	Action
Growth-hormone-releasing hormone (GHRH)			
Thyroid-releasing hormone (TRH)			
Corticotropin-releasing hormone (CRH)			
Prolactin-inhibiting hormone (dopamine)			
Gonadotropin-releasing hormone (GRH)			

8 Thyroid and parathyroid

(a) Label the following diagram and colour the two endocrine organs in contrasting colours:

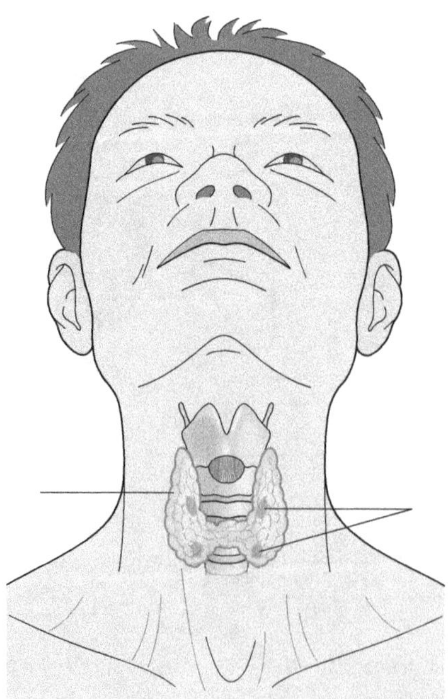

Source: Peate (2015) / Reproduced with permission of John Wiley & Sons.

(b) Complete the following table with the effects of hyperthyroidism and hypothyroidism:

Hyperthyroidism (excessive secretion of T_3 and T_4)	Hypothyroidism (inadequate secretion of T_3 and T_4)
Increased basal metabolic rate	

9 Adrenal gland

(a) Label the following diagram, and colour in the adrenal glands:

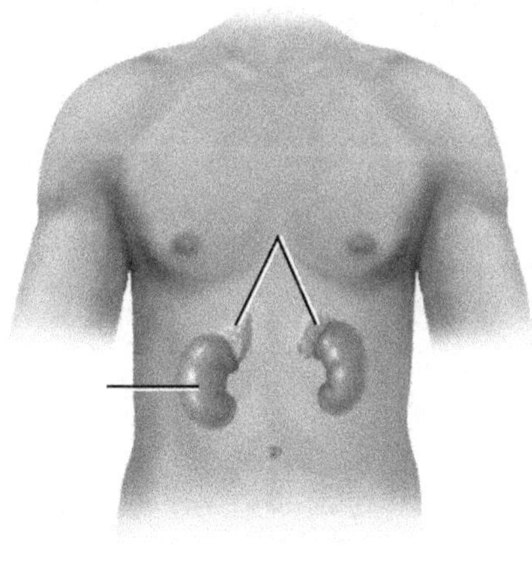

Source: Tortora and Derrickson (2009) / Reproduced with permission of John Wiley & Sons.

(b) Label the following diagram of the adrenal gland, and colour the various parts:

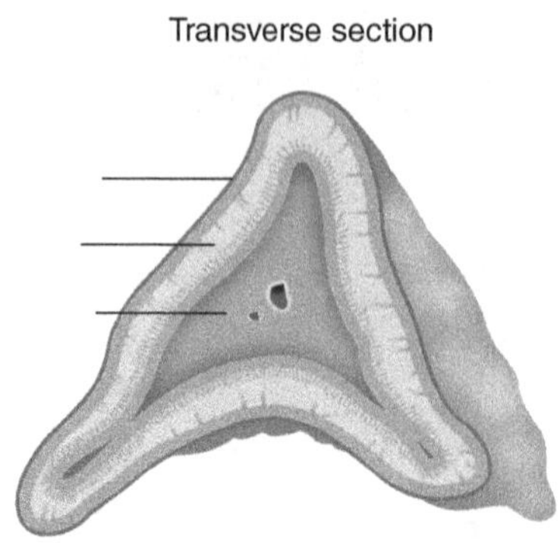

Source: Nair and Peate (2009) / Reproduced with permission of John Wiley & Sons.

10 Match the pairs

The thyroid is made up of two lobes	made up of three distinct functional layers
One unique feature of the thyroid gland is	the top of each of the two kidneys
The parathyroid glands are located on	its ability to create and store large amounts of hormone
The two adrenal glands are found on	the posterior of the thyroid gland
The outer part of each adrenal gland is	the regulation of the concentration of electrolytes in the blood
Mineralocorticoids are the group of hormones whose main function is	joined by an isthmus

11 The pancreas

Label the following diagram of the pancreas, and colour the component parts:

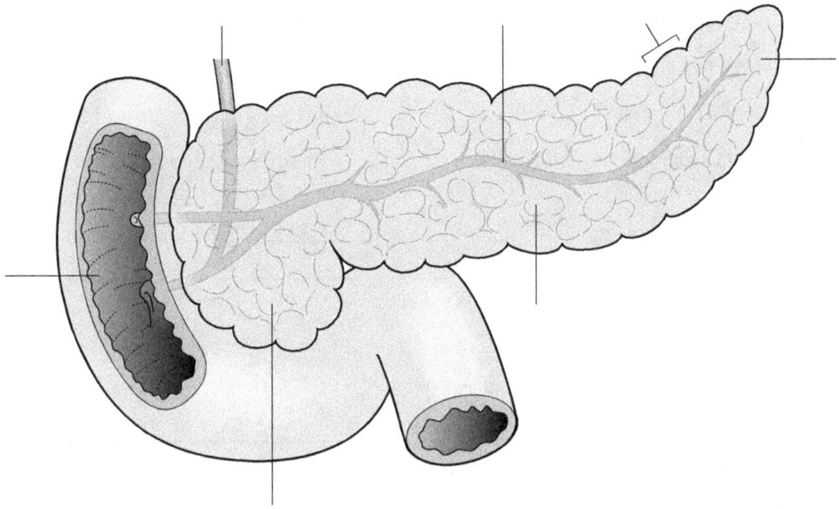

Source: Peate and Nair (2015) / Reproduced with permission of John Wiley & Sons.

12 Other organs with endocrine functions

Complete the following table with the endocrine functions of the organs listed:

Organ	Description
Thymus gland	
Stomach	
Small intestine	
Heart	
Placenta	

13 Match the pairs

The gonads are the primary reproductive organs:	the gastric mucosa produces gastrin
The pancreas is an elongated organ and	exocrine tissue and its associated ducts
The pancreas is innervated	is located next to the duodenum
Special cells in the wall of the atria produce	the testes in the male and the ovaries in the female
The majority of the pancreas is made up of	by the parasympathetic and sympathetic nervous systems
When food is present in the stomach	atrial natriuretic hormone

14 Terminology

Look up the meanings of the prefixes and suffixes in the following terms, write them into the table and then give the meaning of the complete terms.

Corticotropin	
Cortico- =	- tropin =
Meaning:	

Hyperglycaemia	
Hyper- =	- glycaemia=
Meaning:	

Hypothalamus	
Hypo- =	- thalamus =
Meaning:	

Adenohypophysis		
Adeno- =	- hypo =	-physis =
Meaning:		

Neurohypophysis		
Neuro- =	- hypo =	-physis =
Meaning:		

15 Snap shot

Polydipsia and polyuria

John James, a 46-year-old, has been referred to and admitted to a specialist centre by his general practitioner. He has been complaining of intense thirst that is not relieved by drinking copious amounts of fluid (he has a preference for ice-cold water). John is passing large amounts of very pale diluted urine. Today, he has passed over 7 L, has been experiencing nocturia and has wet his bed on two occasions.

What might the diagnosis and treatment be?

____

____

____

What is the term for drinking copious amounts of fluid?

____

What is the term for producing large volumes of dilute urine?

____

16 Crossword

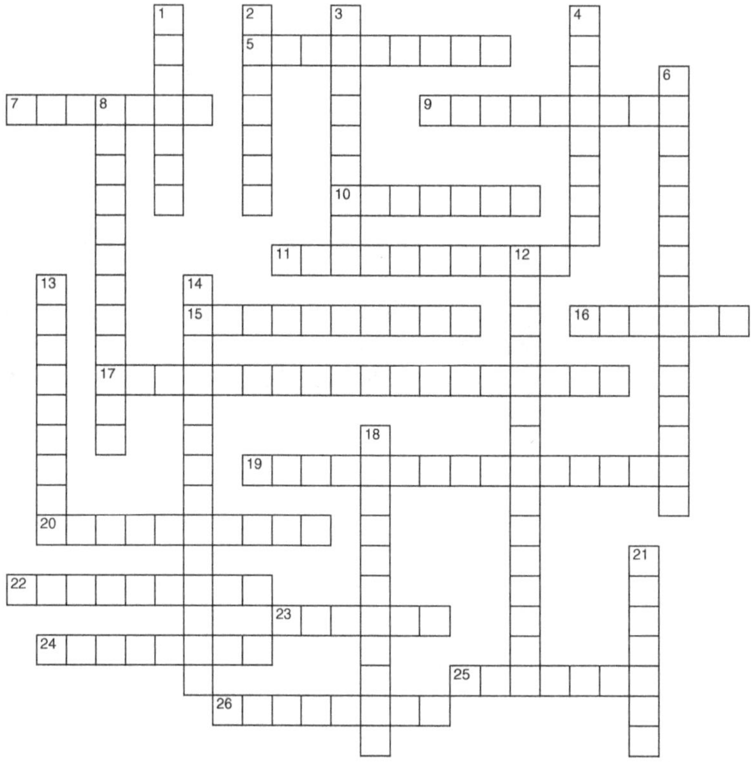

Across

5. T4
7. A narrow strip
9. The" master gland" of the endocrine system
10. Gland which allows adaptation to changes in temperature
11. Islets of endocrine tissue in the pancreas
15. Fight-or-flight hormone
16. Effect produced by the nervous system
17. Hormones which regulate the concentration of the electrolytes in the blood
19. The anterior lobe of the pituitary gland
20. A normal blood volume
22. Hormones which produce their action in the immediate area
23. The outer part of the adrenal gland
24. Organ with endocrine and exocrine tissue
25. Hormone which reduces blood glucose levels
26. Glands/organs that secrete substances into ducts that eventually lead outside the body

Down

1. The inner part of the adrenal gland
2. Chemical class of hormone that includes mineralo-corticoids, glucocorticoids and sex hormones
3. Hormone that stimulates the secretion of milk
4. Hormone that produces powerful contractions in the pregnant uterus
6. An overactive thyroid gland
8. Part of the diencephalon in which the nervous and endocrine systems interact
12. The posterior lobe of the pituitary gland
13. Hormones that are secreted into the blood and influence distant cells
14. The class of hormones secreted by the adrenal medulla
18. The process of maintaining a stable internal environment
21. Glands found on the top of the kidneys

Multiple-choice questions

17. Which of the following is true of cortisol?
A. It is an enzyme
B. It is secreted by the adrenal cortex in response to ACTH
C. It stimulates the secretion of ATP
D. It is released by the adrenal medulla in response to CRH

18. Cortisol is:
A. a mineralocorticoid
B. a glucocorticoid
C. an enzyme
D. a carbohydrate

19. The pancreas:
A. secretes hormones that regulate plasma calcium
B. is controlled by a hormone secreted by the ovaries
C. secretes both insulin and glucagon
D. secretes hormones that only lower blood glucose levels

20. What is the best way to describe the function of insulin?
A. Regulates blood viscosity
B. It is only concerned with gluconeogenesis
C. Causes ketone body formation
D. Lowers blood glucose

21. As calcium decreases in the blood:
A. insulin ceases to be secreted
B. the parathyroid glands secrete calcitonin
C. the kidneys excrete more calcium and phosphate
D. PTH is secreted

22. Hypocalcaemic tetany:
A. could be caused by a deficiency of PTH
B. could be caused by retention of carbon dioxide
C. could be a consequence of osteoclast inactivity
D. is a natural phenomenon when a person is obese

23. Autocrine:
A. refers to hormones that act on the cells they are produced by
B. refers to hormones that act locally on cells in the immediate area
C. refers to an immune disorder
D. None of the above

24. Hyperglycaemia, polyuria, polydipsia and ketoacidosis may indicate a deficiency of:
A. thyroxine
B. insulin
C. epinephrine
D. oestrogen

25. Which of the following is not a steroid?
A. Adrenocortical hormones
B. ACTH
C. Oestrogen
D. Androgens

26. The hormone that stimulates production of milk by the breast is:
A. prolactin
B. oxytocin
C. dopamine
D. follicle-stimulating hormone

CHAPTER 18

The immune system

1 Cells of the immune system

Complete the labelling of the following diagram showing the cells of the immune system, and colour in the nuclei of the cells:

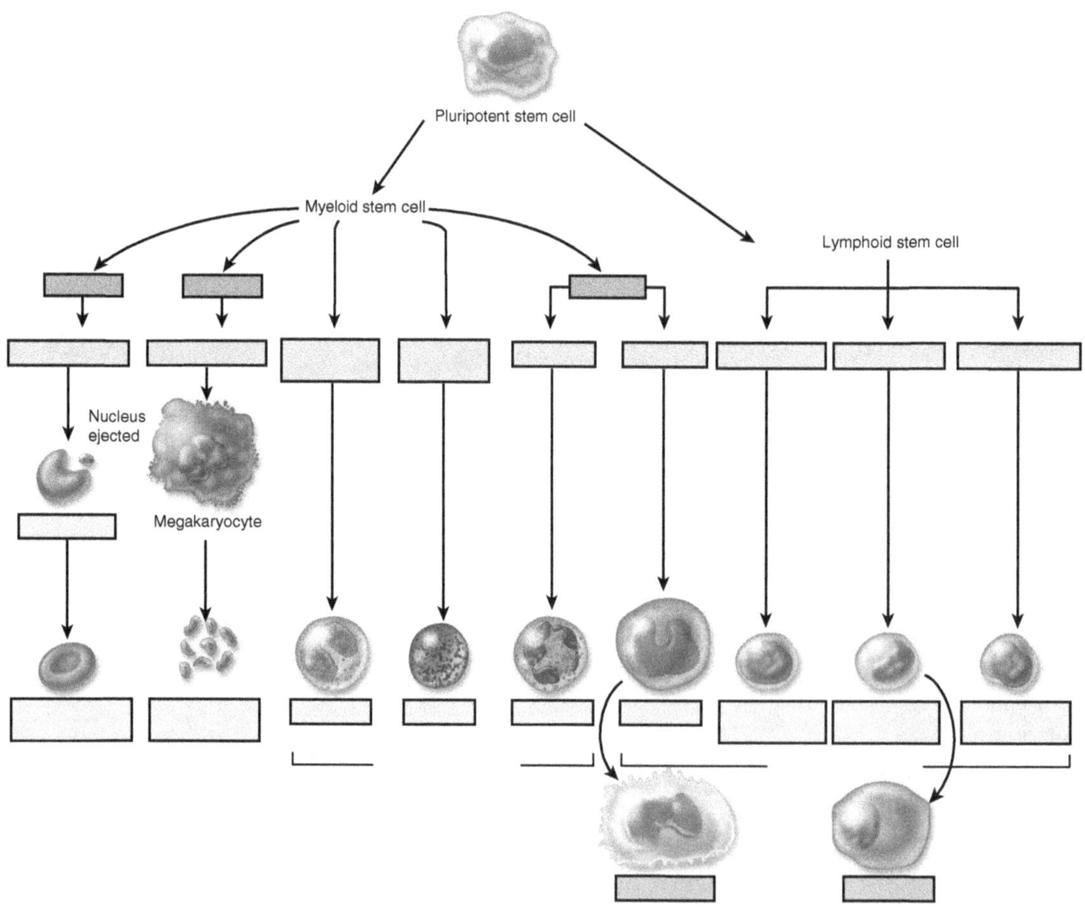

Source: Peate and Nair (2015) / Reproduced with permission of John Wiley & Sons.

2 Lymphatic system and lymphoid organs

(a) Label the following diagram showing the components of the lymphatic system, and colour the lymphatic ducts and nodes:

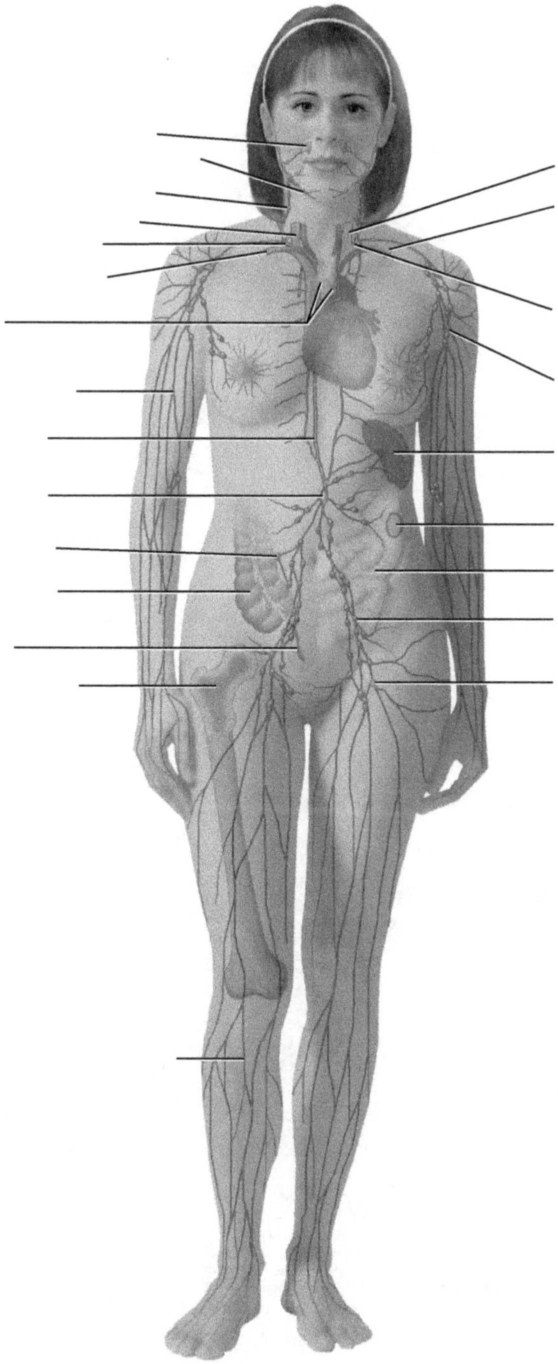

Source: Tortora and Derrickson (2020) / Reproduced with permission of John Wiley & Sons.

(b) Label the following diagram of a lymph node, and colour in the inner and outer cortex:

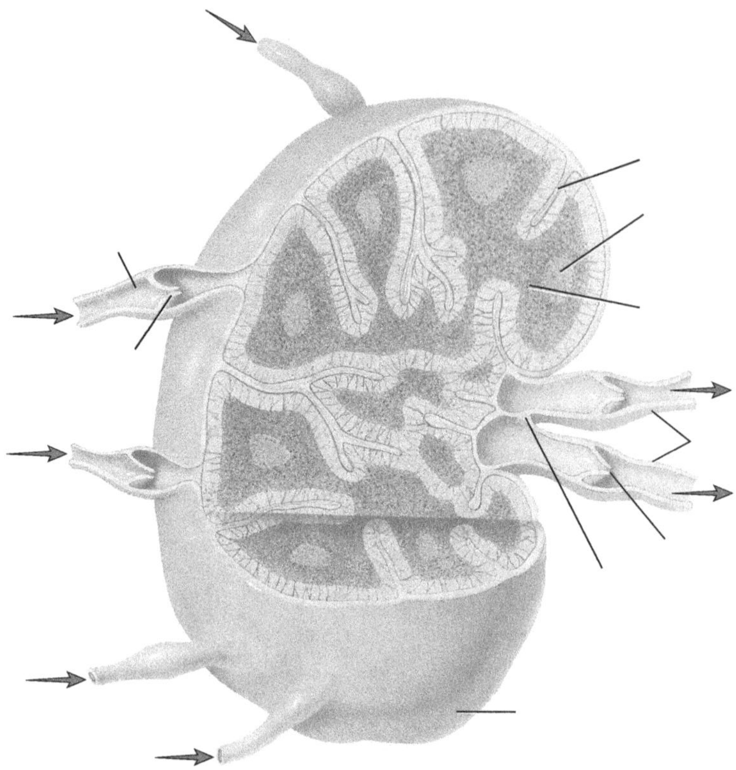

Source: Peate et al. (2014) / Reproduced with permission of John Wiley & Sons.

(c) Match the pairs.

The thymus is largest and most active during the neonatal and pre-adolescent periods of development	but it does not have a pump like the heart
Red bone marrow	the right lymphatic duct and the thoracic duct
Lymphatic capillaries are similar to blood capillaries	conduits called lymphatic vessels that carry a clear fluid called lymph towards the heart
The lymph vessels and capillaries form a network throughout the body	in that their walls consist of a layer of endothelial cells
The lymphatic vessels are drainage vessels that	collect the excess interstitial fluid and return it to the bloodstream
The lymphatic system can be thought of as a parallel system to the blood circulatory system	by the early teens it begins to atrophy
The lymphatic system is a part of the circulatory system, comprising a network of	is a key element of the lymphatic system, being one of the primary lymphoid organs that generates lymphocytes
The lymph eventually flows into two large lymph ducts,	and connect the tissues of the body to the lymphoid organs

(d) Place a mark in the appropriate column to indicate whether each of the tissues/organs listed is a primary or secondary lymphoid organ:

	Primary lymphoid organ	Secondary lymphoid organ
Spleen		
Lymph nodes		
Thymus		
Appendix		
Mucosal-associated lymphoid tissue (MALT)		
Bone marrow		

(e) Complete the following table with brief descriptions of the immune organs listed:

	Description
Thymus	
Spleen	
Lymph nodes	

(f) Label the following diagram showing the position of the thymus, and colour in the thymus:

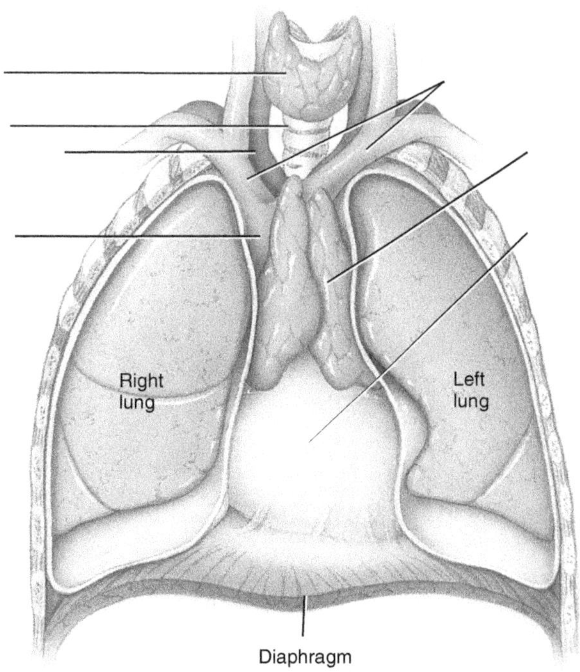

Source: Tortora and Derrickson (2009) / Reproduced with permission of John Wiley & Sons.

3 Innate and acquired immunity

Complete the following table by listing the components of innate and acquired immunity:

Innate immunity	Acquired immunity

4 Inflammation

(a) Fill in the boxes on the following diagram showing causes of an inflammatory response:

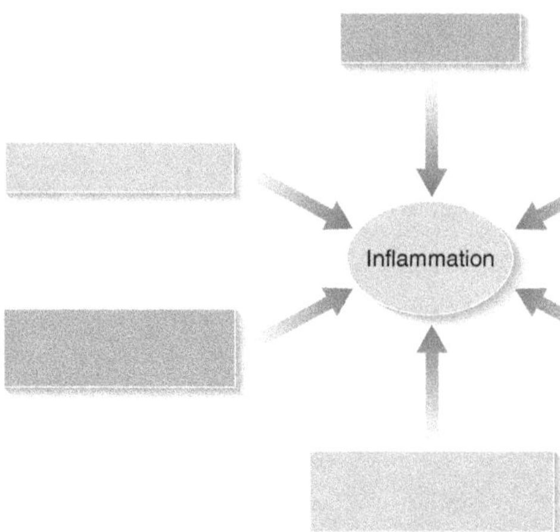

Source: Peate and Glencross (2015) / Reproduced with permission of John Wiley & Sons.

(b) Fill in the steps of the inflammatory response on the following diagram, and colour the phagocytes, platelets and bacteria in contrasting colours:

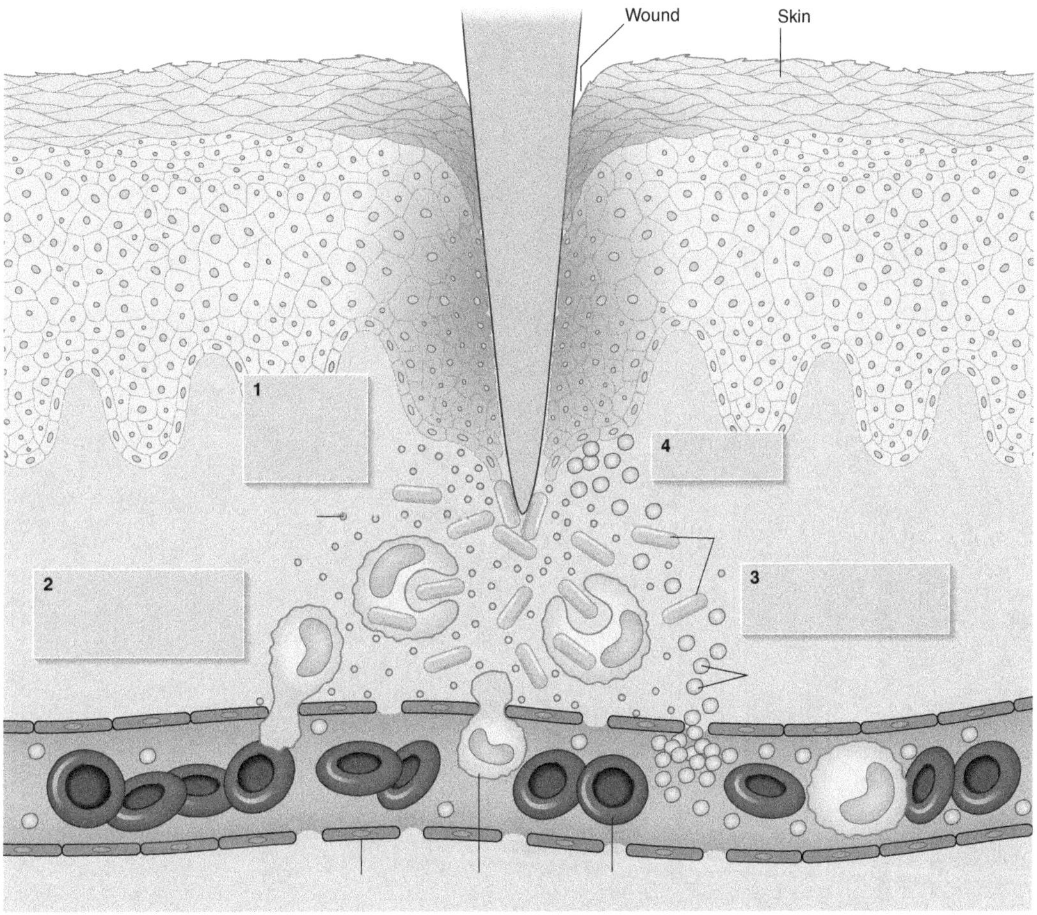

Source: Peate and Glencross (2015) / Reproduced with permission of John Wiley & Sons.

(c) Match the pairs.

Inflammation is	three processes occur at the same time
The inflammatory process involves the movement of	and immunoglobulins help in the destruction of bacteria
Following injury or other damage to the body	an immediate reaction to tissue injury or damage
The complement system activates and assists the inflammatory and immune processes	are cytokines which promote inflammation, attracting white blood cells to the affected area
The kinin system helps to control vascular permeability	playing a major role in the destruction of bacteria
Other factors involved in vascular permeability	white cells, complement and other plasma proteins

5 Specific cellular and humoral immunity

(a) Complete the labelling on the following diagram showing the cellular and humoral specific immune responses:

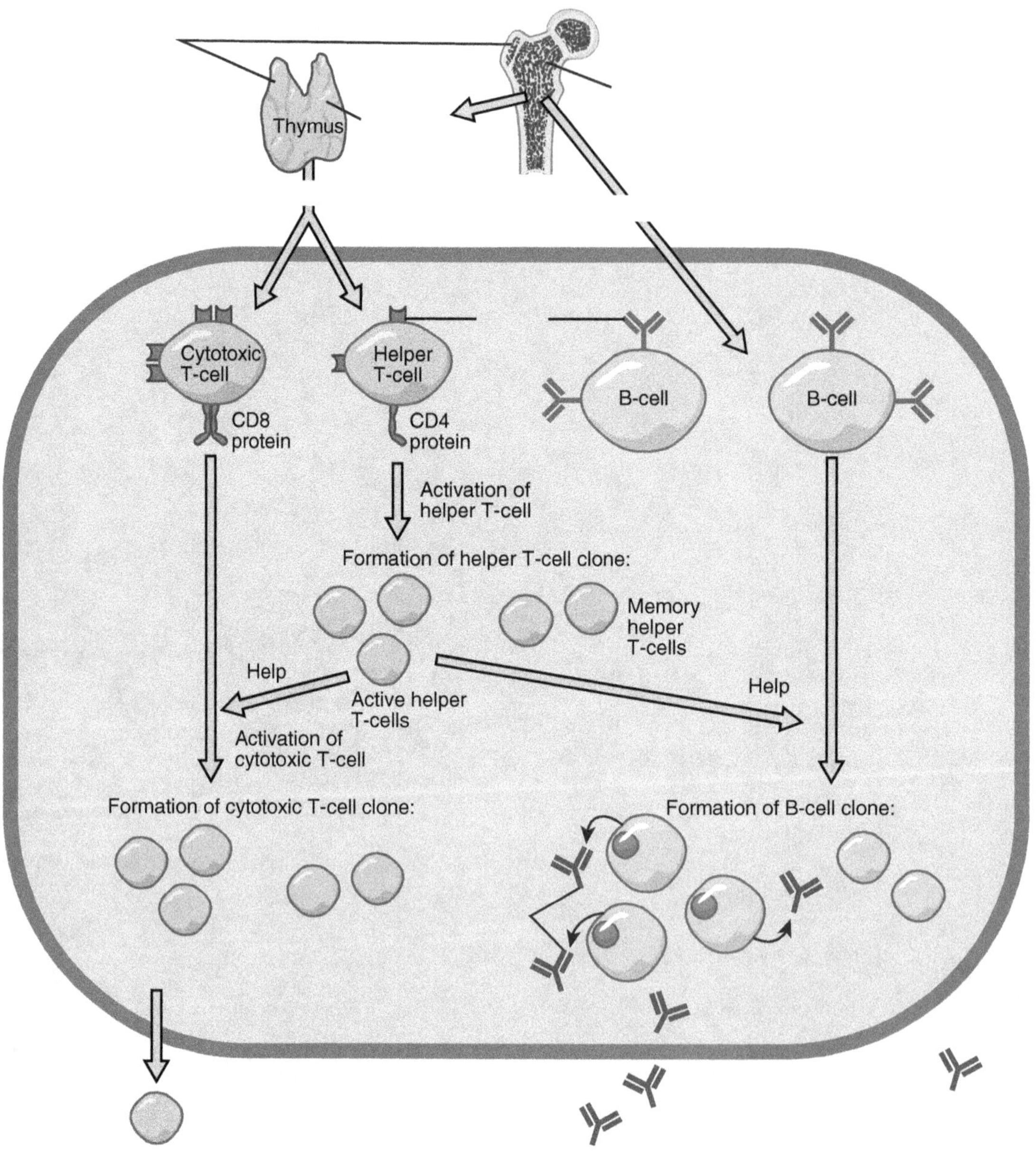

Source: Adapted from Tortora and Derrickson (2020).

(b) Complete the following table with the functions of the various immunoglobulins:

Type of antibody	Functions
IgA	
IgD	
IgE	
IgG	
IgM	

(c) Fill in the boxes in the following table, with descriptions of each type of acquired immunity and provide an example of each type of immunity:

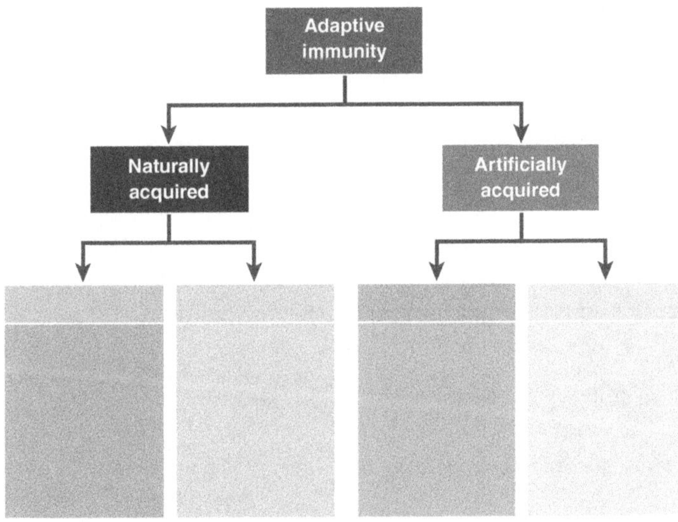

Source: Peate and Nair (2015) / Reproduced with permission of John Wiley & Sons.

Example of natural active immunity: ______________________

Example of natural passive immunity: ______________________

Example of artificial active immunity: ______________________

Example of passive artificial immunity: ______________________

(d) Label the following diagram of an antibody, and colour the light and heavy chains in contrasting colours:

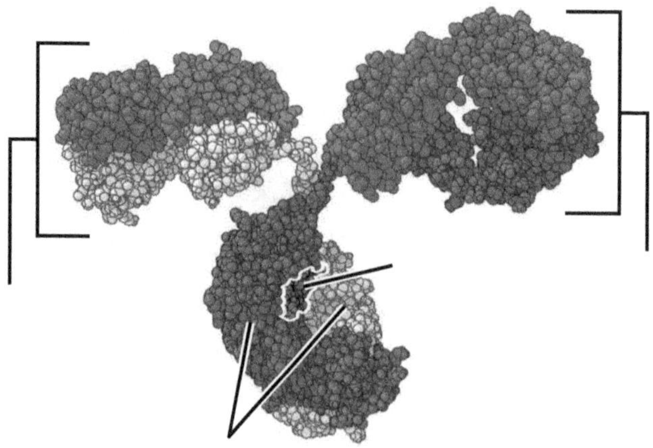

Source: Adapted from Tortora and Derrickson (2020).

6 Match the pairs

Innate immunity is acquired at birth	been met and overcome known as immunological memory
A central role of the innate immune responses is to prevent or restrict	the fetus acquires some immunity via the placenta; this is called passive immunity
Acquired immunity has the ability to remember when a particular immunological threat has	associated with activation of the T-lymphocyte system that stimulates B-lymphocyte separation
The primary response generates a slow and delayed rise in antibody levels	the entrance of microorganisms into the body, so that tissue damage is limited
The secondary response occurs on subsequent exposure to the same antigen	this is relatively short acting as the antibodies eventually break down
Passive immunity occurs when the person has been given antibodies	the response is much faster as the memory B-lymphocytes generated after the first infection divide and separate a faster rate

7 Time yourself to unscramble these words

SCRAMBLE

Scrambled	Unscrambled
VESPASI	
TABIESDINO	
TENAGIN	
QUACREDI	
TUMMYINI	
CHYMESYPOTL	
GRAPHSOMEAC	
SYMHUT	

8 Primary and secondary immune responses

Fill in the following table to show the major differences between a primary and a secondary specific immune response:

	Primary immune response	Secondary immune response
Speed of response		
Size of response		
Immunoglobulin type involved		

9 Terminology

Look up the meanings of the prefixes and suffixes in the following terms, write them into the table and then give the meaning of the complete terms.

Immunoglobulin	
Immuno- =	-globulin =
Meaning:	

Lymphoma	
Lymph- =	-oma =
Meaning:	

Cytokines	
Cyto- =	-kines =
Meaning:	

Kinins	
Kin- =	-in =
Meaning:	

Innate	
In- =	- nate =
Meaning:	

10 Snap shot

Immunisations

Immunisation protects people against harmful infections before they come into contact with them in the community. Immunisation is the most important way of protecting people from vaccine-preventable diseases.

All health professionals who become involved in immunisation in any context, administering or advising, should have an understanding of the key issues associated with immunisation.

People are advised to have a number of vaccines during their lifetimes. Outline the vaccination programme in your country.

____

____

____

____

____

____

____

____

11 Crossword

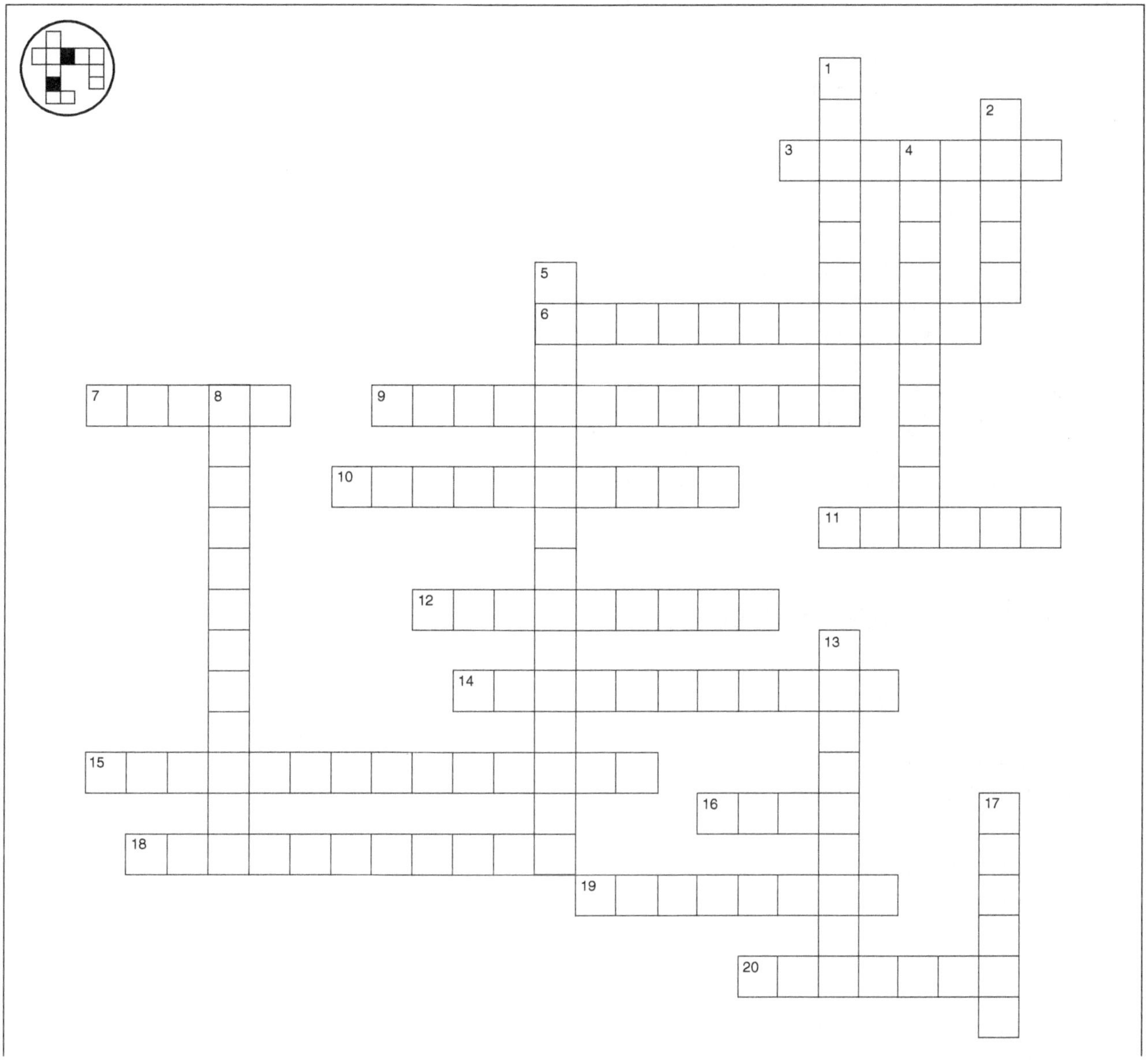

Across

3. Anything that provokes an antibody response
6. Stem cell with the ability to differentiate into many different cells
7. Fluid within lymphatic vessels
9. Neutrophils, eosinophils and basophils
10. The type of white blood cell involved in acquired immunity
11. Primary lymphoid organ that shrinks with age
12. Poisonous to cells
14. White blood cells specialised to kill bacteria
15. Range of lipid molecules involved in pain, inflammation and other physiological processes, whose synthesis is inhibited by NSAIDs
16. Number of classes of immunoglobulin
18. Cells that makes up 1% of white blood cells
19. A form of immunity that requires exposure to a pathogen to be activated
20. Immunisation in which the individual is injected with antibodies

Down

1. Large white blood cells that can differentiate into macrophages
2. Fluids from the eyes that act as a mechanical barrier
4. The study of the immune system
5. Antibodies
8. Destruction of infectious organisms by a cell engulfing and digesting the organism
13. Thrombocytes
17. A secondary lymphoid organ that destroys erythrocytes

Multiple-choice questions

12. What are complement and interferons?
A. Protective proteins in specific immunity
B. Protective proteins in non-specific immunity
C. Secreted by B-cells and T-cells
D. None of the above

13. What are T- and B-cells?
A. Types of red blood cells
B. Platelets
C. Viruses
D. Lymphocytes

14. Active immunity is protection that is:
A. produced by the person's own immune system
B. only activated when the person becomes seriously ill
C. only activated during times of stress
D. None of the above

15. B-cells:
A. can only connect to virus antigens on the outside of infected cells
B. are types of red blood cells
C. All of the above are true
D. None of the above are true

16. Pyrexia, pyrogens and febrile seizures are most related to which component of the non-specific immune response?

A. Hypotension
B. Fever
C. Anaphylaxis
D. Hypertension

17. Plasma cells:

A. are also called T-cells
B. are known as NK cells
C. secrete antibodies
D. secrete viruses

18. With which of the following is anaphylaxis most associated?

A. Interferons
B. IgA
C. IgE
D. IgG

19. What is the primary concern in the care of a patient experiencing anaphylaxis?

A. Development of rash
B. Inability to breathe
C. Development of seizure
D. Inability to communicate

20. Where is the thymus located?

A. Abdomen
B. Brain
C. Thorax
D. Small intestine

21. Inflammation is:

A. related to anxiety
B. characterised by redness, heat, swelling and pain
C. known as cell-mediated immunity
D. the same as infection

CHAPTER 19

The skin

1 Skin structure

(a) Label the following diagram of a cross section through the skin, and colour the three layers:

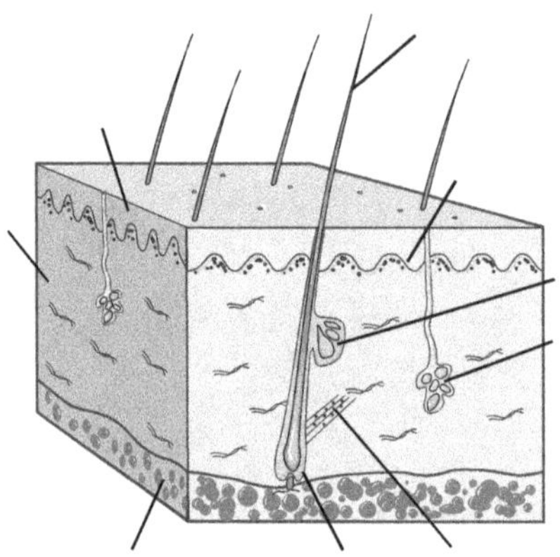

Source: Nair and Peate (2009) / Reproduced with permission of John Wiley & Sons.

(b) Match the pairs.

The skin is sometimes referred to as	nearly one third of all blood that flows thorough the body
The thinnest part of the skin is	the brain
The skin is composed of two distinct regions	modifications of the skin
The skin is twice as heavy as	the epidermis
The appendages are	the dermis and epidermis
The skin receives	the integumentary system

2 Time yourself to unscramble these words

SC R A-MBLE

Scrambled	Unscrambled
DRMIES	
ENCOUTASSUBU	
SNLAGD	
OSCUMU	
SPIDEREMI	
PAILLEAP	
SIREGD	
ROPE	

3 The epidermis

(a) Label the diagram of the epidermis shown here, and colour the five strata:

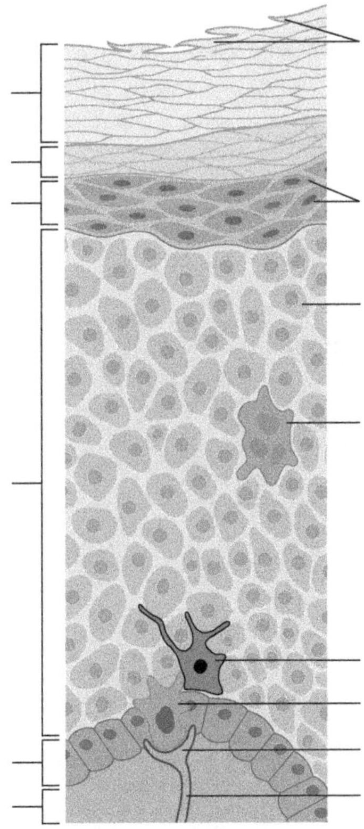

Source: Peate and Nair (2015) / Reproduced with permission of John Wiley & Sons.

(b) Label the following diagram showing the cell types in the epidermis:

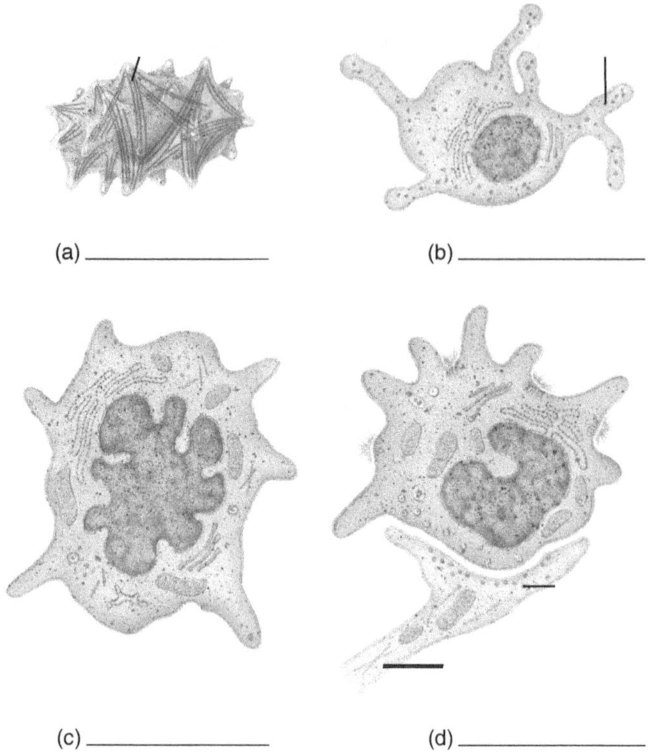

Source: Tortora and Derrickson (2009) / Reproduced with permission of John Wiley & Sons.

(c) Match the pairs.

Also known as a tactile cell	Keratinocytes
The most numerous cell in the skin	Merkel cell
Associated with immunity	Melanocyte
Located in the stratum basale	Langerhans cells

4 Hair follicles and glands of the skin

(a) Label the following diagram of a pilosebaceous unit, and colour the sebaceous glands:

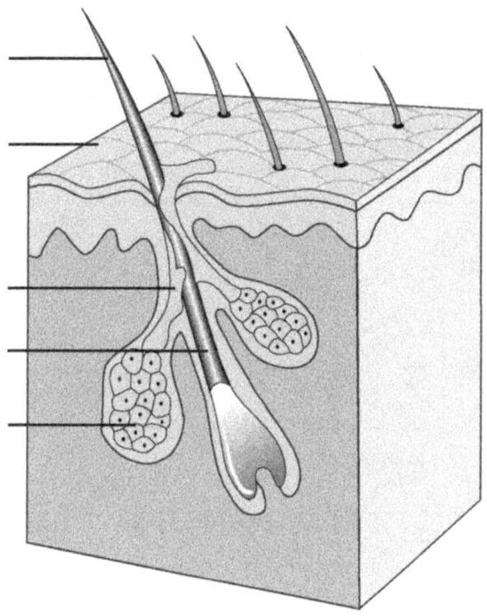

(b) Match the pairs.

Found on most surfaces of the body	Follicles
Accompanies hair follicles	Sebum
Hair follicles are found here	Sebaceous gland
Secretion of the sebaceous glands	Hair
Most of the skin has these	Skin surface

(c) Label the following diagram of a sweat gland, and colour in the sweat gland and duct:

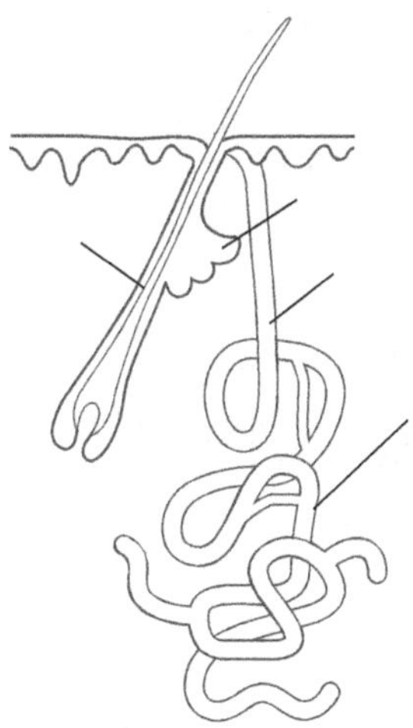

Source: Nair and Peate (2009) / Reproduced with permission of John Wiley & Sons.

(d) Match the pairs.

Supply lubrication to the skin	Apocrine glands
Coiled glands, more prominent in some sites, such as axillae, activated during stress	Eccrine glands
Every pore is an opening for one of these	Sebaceous glands
Mainly thermoregulatory and located all over the body	Hair follicle

5 Nails

(a) Label the following diagram of the nail, and colour in the phalanges and the nail bed:

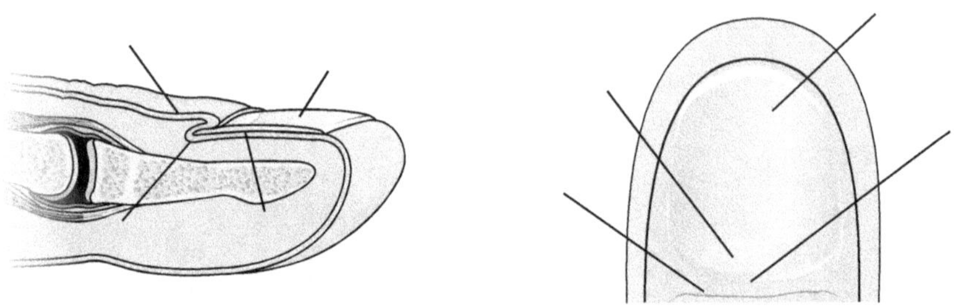

Source: Nair and Peate (2009) / Reproduced with permission of John Wiley & Sons.

(b) Match the pairs.

White crescent located at the proximal end of the nail	Nails
Mainly composed of keratin	Lunula
The formative layer of cells at the base of the fingernail or toenail	Cuticle
Also called the eponychium	Nail matrix
Tightly packed, dead, hard, keratinised epidermal cells that form a clean, solid covering over the digits	Nail plate

SCRAMBLE

(c) Time yourself to unscramble these words.

Scrambled	Unscrambled
NULALU	
ELICTUC	
TAXMIR	
LAHAPXN	

6 Skin damage and healing

(a) On the following graph showing the events of wound healing, label the proliferation phase, the remodelling/maturation phase and the inflammatory phase:

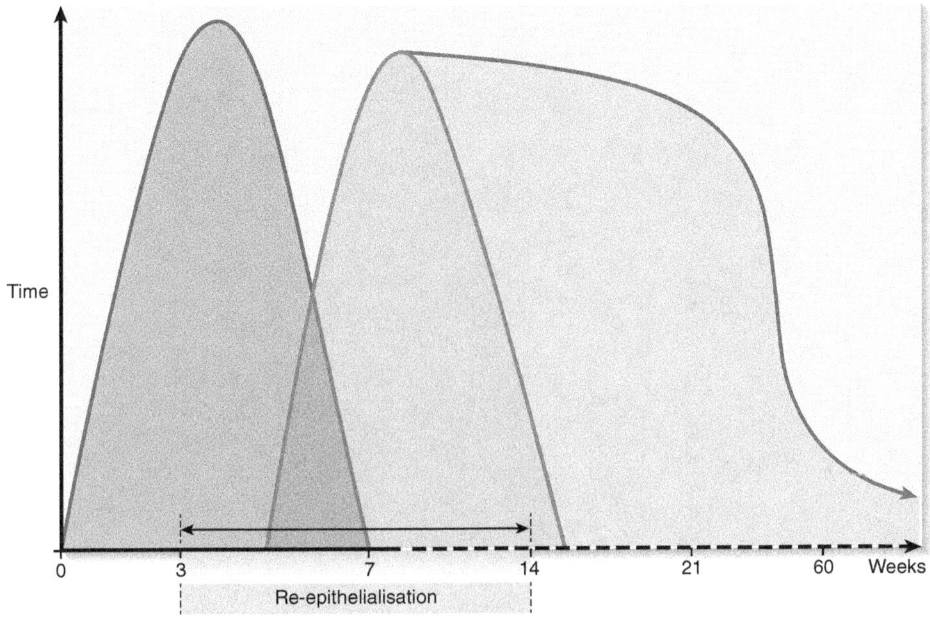

Source: Peate and Nair (2015) / Reproduced with permission of John Wiley & Sons.

(b) What is the tissue shown in the following picture? Colour it in its natural colour:

____

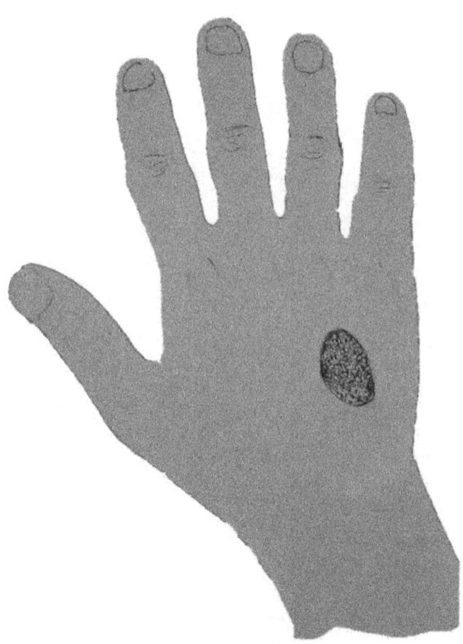

Source: Suzanne Evans (2025).

(c) Complete the following table to indicate the tendency of each of the skin tones to burn under ultraviolet (UV) light:

Natural skin colour		UV sensitivity and tendency to burn
1	Very fair, pale white, often freckled	
2	Fair, white skin	
3	Light brown	
4	Moderate brown	
5	Dark brown	
6	Deeply pigmented, dark brown to black	

Source: Peate and Nair (2015) / Reproduced with permission of John Wiley & Sons.

7 Terminology

Look up the meanings of the prefixes and suffixes in the following terms, write them into the table and give the meaning of the complete terms.

Keratin	
Kera- =	-tin =
Meaning:	

Melanin	
Mela- =	-nin =
Meaning:	

Melanocyte	
Melano- =	-cyte =
Meaning:	

Transdermal	
Trans- =	-dermal =
Meaning:	

Apocrine	
Apo- =	-crine =
Meaning:	

8 Skin sensations

Complete the following grid with all the senses that skin is equipped with:

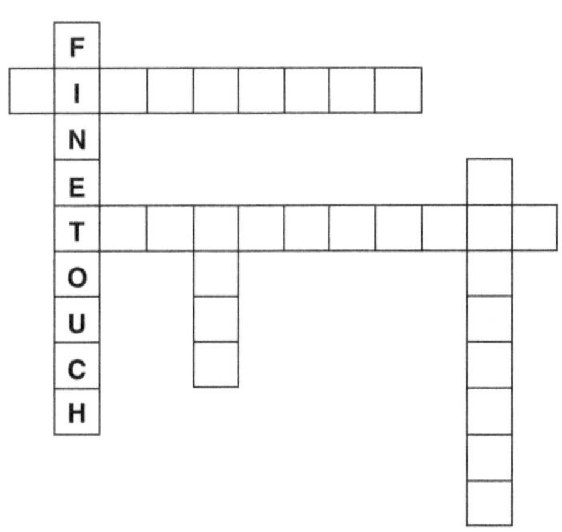

9 Snap shot

Capillary nail bed refill (also called the nail blanch test)

(a) What is the purpose of the nail blanch test?

(b) How is it performed?

(c) What are the normal parameters?

(d) What should you remove prior to performing the test?

(e) Who should abnormalities be reported to?

(f) Where should the outcome of the test be recorded?

10 Crossword

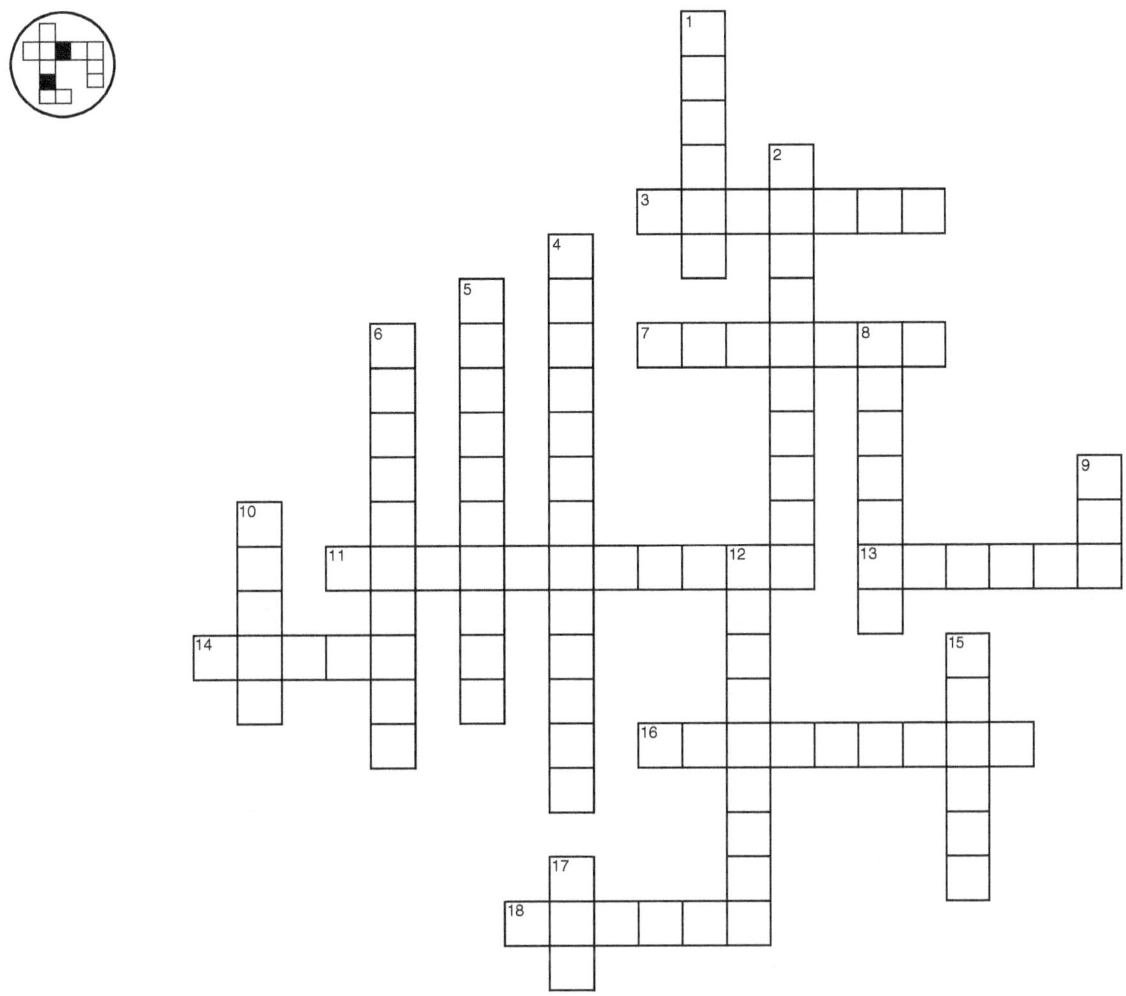

Across

3. Nails are made of this

7. Sebaceous glands are most active during __________

11. Cells that produce melanin

13. Very fine, downy, non-pigmented hair

14. Secretion of sebaceous glands

16. Chemical substance that drives behavioural responses between individuals of the same species

18. The deepest part of the skin

Down

1. Apocrine glands have a ____________ form

2. Cells that provide immune protection for the skin

4. Secrete the protein that gives skin its waterproofing

5. Accessory structures of the skin

6. The subcutaneous fascia

8. Pertains to touch

9. Number of distinct layers in the skin

10. Stratum

12. The thinnest aspect of the skin

15. The crescent shape at the base of the nail

17. The hormones that influence the manufacture of sebum

Multiple-choice questions

11. Which of the following is most likely to increase body temperature?
   A. Dilation of the blood vessels in the skin
   B. Shivering
   C. Secretion of cerumen
   D. Secretion of sebum

12. A person's unique fingerprint is derived from ridges in the:
   A. epidermis
   B. stratum corneum
   C. dermis
   D. subcutaneous layer

13. The epidermis is nourished by:
   A. inhaled air that diffuses into the pores
   B. blood vessels in the hair shafts
   C. blood vessels in the underlying dermis
   D. oxygen and glucose in the cerumen

14. Which of the following is true of the stratum corneum?
   A. It always produces epidermal cells
   B. It secretes keratin for making the skin supple
   C. It is the dead layer sloughed off
   D. It continuously secretes mucus

15. Which word best describes the function of the stratum granulosum?
   A. Meiosis
   B. Mitosis
   C. Keratinisation
   D. Thermogenesis

16. Secretion of the eccrine glands:
   A. lubricates the hair shafts
   B. produces vernix caseosa to protect the skin of the fetus
   C. lowers body temperature
   D. blocks the production of sebum

17. Cyanosis is a sign of:
   A. low levels of oxygenation in the cutaneous blood
   B. rapid flow of blood through cutaneous vessels
   C. dilation of cutaneous vessels
   D. none of the above

18. The skin's role in the synthesis of vitamin D is conversion of:
   A. pro-vitamin D3 (7dehydroxycalciferol) to vitamin D3 (cholecalciferol)
   B. vitamin D2 (ergocalciferol) to vitamin D3 (cholecalciferol)
   C. calcidiol (hydroxycholecalciferol) to calcitriol (dihydroxycholecalciferol)
   D. None of the above is true

19. Thermoregulatory cooling responses involving the skin include:
   A. dilation of skin blood vessels to allow blood to radiate heat directly through the skin
   B. activation of sweat glands to cool the skin by evaporation of sweat
   C. stretching out to increase the surface area of exposed skin
   D. all of the above

20. Where are the receptors that provide skin sensation located?
   A. Epidermis
   B. Dermis
   C. Subcutaneous layer
   D. Through all the skin layers